HANDBOOK OF ESSENTIAL PSYCHOPHARMACOLOGY

SECOND EDITION

By

Ronald W. Pies, M.D.

Clinical Professor of Psychiatry
Tufts University School of Medicine
Formerly Lecturer on Psychiatry, Harvard Medical School
Boston, Massachusetts

With editorial contributions by

Donald P. Rogers, Pharm.D., B.C.P.S.

Assistant Professor of Pharmacy
Massachusetts College of Pharmacy and Health Sciences
Manchester, New Hampshire

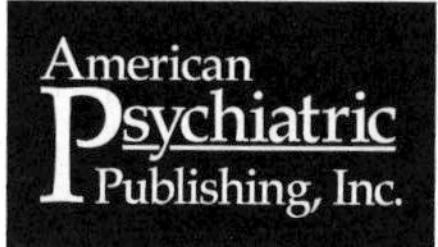

Washington, DC
London, England

Note: The authors have worked to ensure that all information in this book is accurate at the time of publication and consistent with general psychiatric and medical standards, and that information concerning drug dosages, schedules, and routes of administration is accurate at the time of publication and consistent with standards set by the U.S. Food and Drug Administration and the general medical community. As medical research and practice continue to advance, however, therapeutic standards may change. Moreover, specific situations may require a specific therapeutic response not included in this book. For these reasons and because human and mechanical errors sometimes occur, we recommend that readers follow the advice of physicians directly involved in their care or the care of a member of their family.

Books published by American Psychiatric Publishing, Inc., represent the views and opinions of the individual authors and do not necessarily represent the policies and opinions of APPI or the American Psychiatric Association.

Copyright © 2005 American Psychiatric Publishing, Inc.
ALL RIGHTS RESERVED

Manufactured in the United States of America on acid-free paper
09 08 07 06 05 5 4 3 2 1
First Edition

Typeset in Adobe's AGaramond and Frutiger

American Psychiatric Publishing, Inc.
1000 Wilson Boulevard
Arlington, VA 22209-3901
www.appi.org

Library of Congress Cataloging-in-Publication Data
Pies, Ronald W., 1952–
Handbook of essential psychopharmacology / by Ronald W. Pies ; with editorial contributions by Donald P. Rogers.—2nd ed.
p. ; cm.
Includes bibliographical references and index.
ISBN 1-58562-168-4 (pbk. : alk. paper)
1. Psychopharmacology—Handbooks, manuals, etc.
[DNLM: 1. Psychotropic Drugs—pharmacology—Examination Questions.
2. Psychotropic Drugs—pharmacology—Handbooks. QV 39 P624h 2005] I. Rogers, Donald P. (Donald Patrick), 1969– II. Title.
RM315.P495 2005
615′.78–dc22

2004021390

British Library Cataloguing in Publication Data
A CIP record is available from the British Library.

HANDBOOK OF ESSENTIAL PSYCHOPHARMACOLOGY

SECOND EDITION

West Sussex Health Libraries
COPY NUMBER 2050107

CONTENTS

Preface to the Second Edition. xvii

CHAPTER 1

Introduction to Pharmacodynamics and Pharmacokinetics 1

Pharmacodynamics 2

Ligands and Receptors 2

Neurotransmitters and Signal Transduction 3

Figure 1–1 Drug mechanism of action (pharmacodynamics) 5

Pharmacokinetics 6

Absorption 6

Distribution 7

Elimination. 8

Drug Metabolism 9

General Issues 9

Cytochrome Families 10

Table 1–1 Selected substrates, inhibitors, and inducers of major cytochrome P450 enzymes 11

Glucuronidation 15

Drug–Drug Interactions 15
Conclusion 16
References 17

CHAPTER 2

Antidepressants. 19

Overview. 19

Drug Class 19
Indications 20
Mechanisms of Action 20
Pharmacokinetics 21
Main Side Effects 22
Drug–Drug Interactions 23
Potentiating Maneuvers 24
Use in Special Populations 25

Tables 27

Drug Class 27

Table 2–1 Classification of antidepressants by putative neurotransmitter effects 27
Table 2–2 Non-MAOI antidepressants: formulations, strengths, and usual maintenance dosage 28
Table 2–3 Monoamine oxidase inhibitors (MAOIs): tablet strengths and usual adult dosage. 30
Table 2–4 Relative monthly cost of selected antidepressants (low/middle therapeutic dosage range) 31

Indications 32

Table 2–5 "Off-label" and non–mood disorder indications for antidepressants 32

Mechanisms of Action 36

Table 2–6 Neurotransmitter effects of selected antidepressants. 36

Table 2–7 Effects of reuptake blockade and receptor antagonism. 37

Table 2–8 Effects of serotonin (5-HT) receptor stimulation . . . 38

Pharmacokinetics 39

Table 2–9 Pharmacokinetics of selected antidepressants 39

Table 2–10 Pharmacodynamic and pharmacokinetic profiles of newer antidepressants 42

Table 2–11 Putative optimal plasma levels for tricyclic antidepressants. 48

Main Side Effects 49

Table 2–12 Side-effect profiles of commonly used antidepressants. 49

Table 2–13 Side effects of tricyclic vs. selected nontricyclic antidepressants (% of patients reporting, placebo adjusted) 51

Figure 2–1 Cardiac and autonomic side effects of selected antidepressants. 52

Figure 2–2 Gastrointestinal and sexual side effects of selected antidepressants. 53

Figure 2–3 Neurobehavioral side effects of selected antidepressants. 54

Table 2–14 Some comparative side effects of selective serotonin reuptake inhibitors (placebo-adjusted %) 55

Table 2–15 Basic management of antidepressant side effects . . . 56

Table 2–16 Selected co-prescribed agents for antidepressant-induced sexual dysfunction 59

Drug–Drug Interactions 60

Table 2–17 Drug–drug interactions with tricyclic antidepressants (TCAs) 60

Table 2–18 Some drugs used in clinical practice that may interact with selective serotonin reuptake inhibitors (SSRIs) and related antidepressants 61

Table 2–19 Drug–drug interactions with monoamine oxidase inhibitors (MAOIs) 65

Table 2–20 Food restrictions for patients taking conventional monoamine oxidase inhibitors (MAOIs) 66

Table 2–21 The serotonin syndrome: differential diagnosis 67

Table 2–22 Serotonin syndrome 70

Potentiating Maneuvers 71

Table 2–23 Agents used to potentiate or augment antidepressants 71

Table 2–24 Psychostimulants and related agents: main features. 73

Use in Special Populations 75

Table 2–25 Selection of nontricyclic antidepressants for patients with special needs or comorbid conditions 75

Table 2–26 Antidepressant dosing in children and adolescents 78

Questions and Answers 79

Drug Class 79

Indications 79

Mechanisms of Action 85

Pharmacokinetics 90

Main Side Effects 94

Drug–Drug Interactions 101

Potentiating Maneuvers 103

Use in Special Populations 111

Vignettes/Puzzlers 117

References 123

CHAPTER 3

Antipsychotics . . . 139

Overview . . . 139

Drug Class . . . 139

Indications . . . 140

Mechanisms of Action . . . 140

Pharmacokinetics . . . 142

Main Side Effects . . . 143

Drug–Drug Interactions . . . 144

Potentiating Maneuvers . . . 145

Use in Special Populations . . . 145

Tables . . . 148

Drug Class . . . 148

Table 3–1 Dosages and putative therapeutic levels of currently available antipsychotics . . . 148

Table 3–2 First-generation ("typical" or "neuroleptic") antipsychotic dosage equivalents of 10 mg of haloperidol . . . 150

Table 3–3 Second-generation ("atypical") antipsychotic dosage equivalents of 10 mg of haloperidol . . . 151

Table 3–4 Comparative costs of some atypical antipsychotics . . . 152

Indications . . . 153

Table 3–5 Indications for use of antipsychotics . . . 153

Mechanisms of Action . . . 159

Table 3–6 Relative receptor affinities of haloperidol versus available atypical agents . . . 159

Pharmacokinetics . . . 160

Table 3–7 Pharmacokinetic profiles of first-generation (neuroleptic) antipsychotics . . . 160

Table 3–8 Pharmacokinetic profiles of second-generation (atypical) antipsychotics 161

Main Side Effects 162

Table 3–9 Comparative side effects among available first-generation (typical) antipsychotics 162

Table 3–10 Comparative side effects among selected second-generation (atypical) antipsychotics 163

Table 3–11 Motor and mental symptoms of neuroleptic-induced extrapyramidal side effects 164

Table 3–12 Selected agents for treatment of extrapyramidal side effects (EPS) of first-generation (neuroleptic) antipsychotics. 165

Table 3–13 Neuroleptic malignant syndrome (NMS): differential diagnosis 166

Table 3–14 Management of antipsychotic (AP) side effects . . . 171

Table 3–15 Clozapine and white blood cell count (WBC): managing abnormalities 173

Drug–Drug Interactions 175

Table 3–16 Antipsychotic (AP) drug interactions 175

Table 3–17 Second-generation (atypical) antipsychotics (APs): potential drug–drug interactions 177

Potentiating Maneuvers 178

Table 3–18 Potentiation of antipsychotics (APs) 178

Use in Special Populations 182

Table 3–19 Antipsychotics (APs) in special populations 182

Questions and Answers. 186

Drug Class 186

Indications 188

Mechanisms of Action 195

Pharmacokinetics 200

Main Side Effects 201

Drug–Drug Interactions 212

Potentiating Maneuvers 214
Use in Special Populations 219
Vignettes/Puzzlers 227
References 236

CHAPTER 4

Anxiolytics and Sedative-Hypnotics 253
Overview. 253
Drug Class 253
Indications 254
Mechanisms of Action 255
Pharmacokinetics 256
Main Side Effects 256
Drug–Drug Interactions 257
Potentiating Maneuvers 258
Use in Special Populations 258
Tables 260
Drug Class 260
Table 4–1 Commonly used benzodiazepine anxiolytics. 260
Table 4–2 Commonly prescribed benzodiazepine and nonbenzodiazepine hypnotics. 261
Table 4–3 Nonbenzodiazepine anxiolytics and hypnotics 262
Table 4–4 Dosage and cost of selected benzodiazepines 265
Indications 266
Table 4–5 Indications for benzodiazepines (BZDs) 266
Table 4–6 Selective serotonin reuptake inhibitors (SSRIs) or related antidepressants with FDA-approved labeling for use in treating DSM-IV-TR anxiety disorders. 270

Table 4–7 Off-label uses for beta-blockers and clonidine for anxiety/agitation in selected disorders. 271

Mechanisms of Action 272

Table 4–8 Effect of various agents on $GABA_A$ receptors 272

Table 4–9 Pharmacodynamic aspects of hypnotic agents. 273

Pharmacokinetics 274

Table 4–10 Pharmacokinetics of orally administered benzodiazepine anxiolytics 274

Table 4–11 Pharmacokinetics of benzodiazepine hypnotics . . .275

Table 4–12 Pharmacokinetics of nonbenzodiazepine hypnotics 276

Figure 4–1 Simplified metabolic pathways of benzodiazepines 277

Main Side Effects 278

Table 4–13 Frequency (%) of benzodiazepine (BZD) and buspirone side effects (average for various BZDs) 278

Table 4–14 Side effects and management of benzodiazepines (BZDs) 279

Drug–Drug Interactions 282

Table 4–15 Benzodiazepine (BZD) drug interactions 282

Table 4–16 Nonbenzodiazepine (non-BZD) hypnotic drug interactions 285

Potentiating Maneuvers 286

Table 4–17 Agents used in combination with benzodiazepines (BZDs) for augmentation of effect 286

Use in Special Populations 287

Table 4–18 Potential concerns of benzodiazepine (BZD) use during pregnancy 287

Table 4–19 Risks of benzodiazepine (BZD) use in elderly and/or dementia patients. 288

Questions and Answers 289
Drug Class 289
Indications 290
Mechanisms of Action 302
Pharmacokinetics 304
Main Side Effects 306
Drug–Drug Interactions 310
Potentiating Maneuvers 313
Use in Special Populations 315
Vignettes/Puzzlers 320
References 324

CHAPTER 5

Mood Stabilizers 337
Overview 337
Drug Class 337
Indications 338
Mechanisms of Action 340
Pharmacokinetics 340
Main Side Effects 342
Drug–Drug Interactions 343
Potentiating Maneuvers 344
Use in Special Populations 344
Tables 346
Drug Class 346
Table 5–1 Selected mood stabilizers: preparations, usual daily doses, and putative therapeutic blood levels 346
Indications 349
Table 5–2 Indications for lithium 349

Table 5–3 Preferred treatments of acute manic or mixed episodes in bipolar disorder 351

Table 5–4 Preferred treatments of acute depressive episodes in bipolar disorder 353

Table 5–5 Preferred treatments of rapid cycling in bipolar disorder 355

Table 5–6 Preferred maintenance treatments in bipolar disorder 356

Mechanisms of Action 357

Table 5–7 Mood stabilizer and anticonvulsant mechanisms of action. 357

Pharmacokinetics 358

Table 5–8 Pharmacokinetics of selected mood stabilizers 358

Main Side Effects 360

Table 5–9 Lithium side effects 360

Table 5–10 Stages of lithium toxicity .361

Table 5–11 Five most common side effects of carbamazepine 362

Table 5–12 Management of common anticonvulsant mood stabilizer side effects (non-placebo-adjusted rates) 363

Table 5–13 Management of lithium side effects 366

Table 5–14 Potential risk factors for antidepressant-induced mania (AIM) or cycling .369

Drug–Drug Interactions 370

Table 5–15 Drug–drug interactions with lithium 370

Table 5–16 Drug–drug interactions with carbamazepine (CBZ) 373

Table 5–17 Drug–drug interactions with valproate 377

Table 5–18 Drug–drug interactions with lamotrigine 379

Potentiating Maneuvers 381

Table 5–19 Augmenting strategies in treating patients with bipolar disorder 381

Use in Special Populations 387

Table 5–20 Use of mood stabilizers in special populations 387

Questions and Answers. 389

Indications 389

Mechanisms of Action 403

Pharmacokinetics 407

Main Side Effects 410

Drug–Drug Interactions 416

Potentiating Maneuvers 420

Use in Special Populations 423

Vignettes/Puzzlers 428

References 434

CME Questions and Answers. 449

Index 469

PREFACE TO THE SECOND EDITION

In the course of only 6 years, since the publication of the first edition of this book, the art and science of psychopharmacology have undergone many changes. If there have been no radical cures or breakthroughs, there has at least been substantial refinement and elaboration. It is difficult, in the brief compass of a "handbook," to include all these developments in great detail. I have aimed, rather, at incorporating the most important changes and research findings into the four main groupings of psychotropic medications: *antidepressants, antipsychotics, anxiolytics,* and *mood stabilizers.* I have also added an introductory chapter, designed to equip the reader with a basic understanding of pharmacodynamics and pharmacokinetics.

A more ambitious text would have included chapters on a number of other agents used in psychiatric practice, such as cognitive enhancers, anticholinergic agents, and medications for various eating disorders. Separate chapters covering child and adolescent psychopharmacology and geriatric psychopharmacology would have been an option as well. But such a text would begin to expand well beyond the confines of the "white coat pocket" within which real handbooks ought to fit. To remedy these omissions, I have tried to include such specialized, supplementary material in the discussion of the major drug classes, whenever feasible. On the other hand, notwithstanding their infrequent use nowadays, I have included a substantial amount of material on the "old" tricyclic antidepressants and the monoamine oxidase inhibitors (MAOIs). The rationale for this will be clear to anyone who has spent time teaching residents and younger psychiatrists: with few exceptions, these clinicians have had very little experience with these agents, and I believe this represents a genuine loss to the field.

Given a handbook's limited scope, I frequently have referred the reader to this text's more substantial sibling, the excellent *The American Psychiatric Publishing Textbook of Psychopharmacology,* 3rd Edition, edited by Drs. Alan Schatzberg and Charles Nemeroff (Washington, DC, American Psychiatric Publishing, 2004). And, in the area of the infamous cytochrome P450 enzymes—the bane of many a psychiatric resident and attending—I have drawn extensively on the comprehensive text by Dr. Kelly Cozza and colleagues, *Concise Guide to Drug Interaction Principles for Medical Practice: Cytochrome P450s, UGTs, P-Glycoproteins,* 2nd Edition (Washington, DC, American Psychiatric Publishing, 2003). To the editors and authors of these texts, I wish to express my great appreciation. However, any errors that have crept into my synopsis are fully my responsibility.

One important caveat, with respect to the tables of side effects: the data on incidence of side effects in the tables are almost never based on direct, head-to-head comparisons of multiple agents. Unfortunately, such studies are all too rare. Rather, the percentages shown usually reflect published data from the pharmaceutical companies or data from several different studies, using varying methods and populations. (Precedent for this approach is set in, e.g., Sheldon Preskorn's book *Outpatient Management of Depression: A Guide for the Primary Care Practitioner,* 2nd Edition [Caddo, OK, Professional Communications, 1999]). Thus, the reader should take these figures with at least one grain of salt, since they may not always reflect actual drug–drug differences.

I have been fortunate to have had the editorial assistance of Donald Rogers, Pharm.D., B.C.P.S., in revising and updating this text. Don has been instrumental in keeping the text as up-to-date as possible—though every textbook, at publication, is already behind the times—as well as in preparing a new feature of the current edition: an appendix containing 50 CME questions and answers, designed to test the reader's knowledge and comprehension of the text.

I also wish to thank the expert readers who devoted their valuable time to commenting on individual chapters and suggesting areas for improvement: Marianne Kardos, M.D.; David Osser, M.D.; Robert Dunn, M.D., Ph.D.; James Ellison, M.D.; and Bertram G. Katzung, M.D., Ph.D. My appreciation also extends to the reviewers and editors at American Psychiatric Publishing, Inc. (APPI), and to the many clinicians, colleagues, psychiatric residents, and medical students who have helped shape my understanding of psychopharmacology. Special mention goes to Amit Rajparia, M.D., who helped inspire and edit a key table in the antidepressant chapter. In addition, I would like to thank Dr. Robert Hales and Mr. John McDuffie at APPI for their encouragement and advice. I also wish to thank Greg Kuny and Ann Eng at APPI for their thoughtful editorial work and Anne Barnes for her design of the cover and book.

Finally, I offer a word of gratitude to my wife, Nancy Butters, M.S.W., who patiently endured my many hours of solitary tapping at the keyboard.

Psychopharmacology is a complex and ever-changing field. No single work can do it justice. I hope that readers will feel free to contact me regarding errors, omissions, and other imperfections, of which, no doubt, there are many. Ars longa, vita brevis.

Ronald W. Pies, M.D.
Lexington, Massachusetts

CHAPTER

1

INTRODUCTION TO PHARMACODYNAMICS AND PHARMACOKINETICS

In essence, *pharmacodynamics* is what a drug does to your body; *pharmacokinetics* is what your body does to a drug. Understanding how psychotropic medications work is a much more complex task than we once believed. Whereas in years past, many antidepressants and antipsychotics were described solely in terms of their effects on specific neuronal receptors or biogenic amines, our present understanding suggests that more fundamental mechanisms of action are at work. We now have good evidence that many psychotropics actually alter neuronal function *at the level of the gene,* and that specific gene products, rather than superficial changes in receptors, are really the "business end" of a medication's clinical effects. While our understanding of drug metabolism has not deepened in quite the same way, it has at least broadened in recent years. Even as clinicians have struggled to master the subtleties of the cytochrome P450 (CYP) system, we have come to realize that cytochrome-based metabolism is merely one large piece of the puzzle. Now we must also contend with the burgeoning family of *glucuronidation* enzymes—not to mention interactions mediated by *P-glycoproteins.* Either of these topics—pharmacodynamics or pharmacokinetics—could easily take up an entire book. What follows is necessarily a brief introduction to these growing areas of investigation. The interested reader will find superbly detailed expositions in the chapters by Szabo et al. (2004) and DeVane (2004).

Pharmacodynamics

Pharmacodynamics is intimately tied to a drug's mechanism of action (MOA): how it brings about changes in the brain, or other systems, so as to produce its clinical effects. Pharmacodynamics also encompasses the ways by which a drug may cause unwanted *side effects,* such as dry mouth or orthostatic hypotension. In some cases, these side effects are merely extensions of a drug's therapeutic effect—for example, excessive daytime somnolence may be a by-product of a long-acting hypnotic's intended effects on sleep latency and duration.

In one sense, the MOA of many psychotropics has been the story of cellular receptors for various biogenic amines, such as norepinephrine, dopamine, and serotonin. In a deeper sense, this story is a bit misleading. Trying to fathom a drug's MOA by examining only its receptor effects is a bit like trying to understand a television program by putting your hand on the top of the TV to see if it's warm. Nevertheless, the story of pharmacodynamics properly begins with an understanding of neurotransmitters and receptor dynamics.

Ligands and Receptors

Any molecule that binds to a cellular receptor is termed a *ligand.* An *agonist* is a ligand that enhances some intrinsic activity of the receptor by *facilitating, or substituting for, the normal role of a particular endogenous ligand.* For example, benzodiazepines act as agonists at the benzodiazepine receptor, facilitating the action of the inhibitory neurotransmitter GABA (γ-aminobutyric acid) by enhancing chloride ion flow. An *antagonist* is a ligand that has no intrinsic activity but *blocks the action of an agonist.* Sometimes termed a *neutral antagonist,* this type of ligand may reestablish the "pre-agonist" status quo of the receptor, or it may keep an agonist from acting. Thus, flumazenil acts as an antagonist at benzodiazepine receptors by returning the chloride ion channel to its resting state; this drug is used clinically to counteract a benzodiazepine overdose. In contrast, an *inverse agonist* has the *opposite action of an agonist*—it actually counteracts or reverses some intrinsic activity of the receptor, for example, by leading to diminished chloride ion flow. (Chemicals called *beta-carbolines* may actually be anxiety-provoking by reversing the action of benzodiazepine-like ligands.) Finally, we have so-called *partial agonists,* whose action depends on the neurochemical environment. When the endogenous ligand—say, serotonin—is present in excess, a partial agonist behaves like an antagonist. When the endogenous ligand is in low supply, the partial agonist can "stand in" and act as an agonist—though sometimes with less intrinsic activity than the endogenous ligand. Buspirone, for example, is a partial agonist at postsynaptic serotonin$_{1A}$ (5-HT$_{1A}$) receptors.

Receptors located on presynaptic nerve endings may be described as *autoreceptors* and *heteroreceptors.* An autoreceptor is located on a neuron that produces the endogenous ligand for that particular autoreceptor—for example, a serotonergic autoreceptor must be located on a serotonin-producing neuron. In contrast, a heteroreceptor is present on a neuron that does *not* produce the neurotransmitter received by the heteroreceptor. For example, a heteroreceptor for serotonin may be located on a dopaminergic neuron. In this manner, one neurotransmitter can influence the activity or concentration of another—a critical MOA when we examine, for example, the antidepressant mirtazapine. Autoreceptors and heteroreceptors are critical components in the negative feedback loop that may reduce the firing rate of neurons or reduce the amount of neurotransmitter released by the neuron (Szabo et al. 2004).

Neurotransmitters and Signal Transduction

Neurotransmitters fall into three main categories: *amino acids, biogenic amines* (norepinephrine, serotonin, dopamine, and acetylcholine), and *peptides.* (There are also unusual neurotransmitters, such as the gas nitric oxide, that may play a role in some important neuropsychiatric functions.) There are probably hundreds of neurotransmitters or related chemical messengers in the central nervous system (CNS), and they interact in complex ways. For example, peptides (e.g., vasopressin) may work in tandem with biogenic amines and amino acids.

Neurotransmitters can affect neurons through two main receptor types: those linked to *ligand-gated channels* (ionotropic receptors) and those linked to *G-proteins.* The ligand-gated channels may be likened very roughly to rapidly swinging doors: they govern the momentary flux of ions, such as chloride, across the cell membrane. In contrast, the G-protein–linked receptors are more like relay stations, activating a much slower process. G-protein–linked receptors work via *secondary messenger* molecules, such as cyclic AMP (cAMP) and inositol trisphosphate. These messengers activate enzymes within the neuron called *protein kinases,* which, in turn, set in motion profound and enduring changes in the neuron. Specifically, the protein kinases lead to *phosphorylation of proteins*—a long-lasting chemical reaction that may alter both ion channel function (how readily the gates swing open) and, more important, *transcription of genetic material.* Phosphorylation of proteins and subsequent genetic transcription may underlie crucial processes such as *long-term memory,* as well as changes in the number or sensitivity (up- or down-regulation) of various neuronal receptors. Desensitization of certain serotonergic autoreceptors may play a critical role in the MOA of many antidepressants, as we shall see in Chapter 2 ("Antidepressants").

Transcription of genetic material proceeds via molecules called *tertiary messengers,* such as c-fos, which "turn on" various portions of nuclear DNA. DNA, in turn, is expressed via a similar molecule called *messenger RNA* (mRNA), which leads to production of various *nerve growth factors,* such as BDNF (brain-derived neurotrophic factor). There is good evidence that such growth factors are intimately involved in the MOA of both antidepressants and some mood stabilizers.

These complex processes are summarized in the greatly oversimplified diagram in Figure 1–1.

Amino acid neurotransmitters appear to work via ligand-gated channels. *Inhibitory* amino acid neurotransmitters, such as GABA and glycine, increase chloride ion flux into the neuron. These negatively charged ions hyperpolarize the already negatively charged cell and make it less likely to fire. In contrast, *excitatory* amino acid neurotransmitters, such as glutamate and aspartate, cause calcium or sodium ions to enter the cell. This flood of positively charged ions depolarizes the cell, causing it to fire. Excitatory amino acid receptors may be subclassified according to their corresponding agonists and antagonists or to the metabolic pathways they affect. For example, NMDA (*N*-methyl-D-aspartate) receptors and "metabotropic" receptors (which modify inositol phosphate metabolism) are two types of excitatory amino acid receptors.

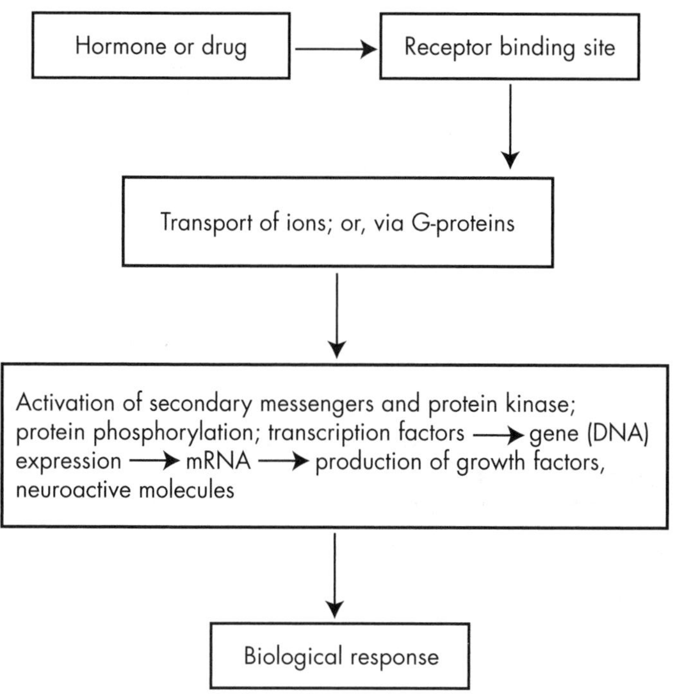

FIGURE 1–1. Drug mechanism of action (pharmacodynamics).

Source. Adapted from Cooper et al. 1996.

In contrast, most *biogenic amine* and *peptide* neurotransmitter receptors are not ligand-gated; rather, they are linked with G-proteins. These G-protein–linked receptors are not easily classified as excitatory or inhibitory; their actions are too complex and long-lasting to fit this dichotomy. (Acetylcholine acts on two classes of receptors—*muscarinic* and *nicotinic*—that are linked, respectively, to G-protein–coupled receptors and to ionotropic receptors.)

Finally, some hormones, such as glucocorticoids, attach to receptors located not in the cell membrane but in the *nucleus or cytoplasm* of the neuron. The hormone–receptor complex then binds to a specific portion of nuclear DNA. In this way, glucocorticoids can influence transcription of various genes. Notably, glucocorticoids appear to play an important role in some types of depression (Rothschild 2003).

Why such complexity? In the larger scheme of things, neurons need to be flexible—for example, they need to adapt to a rapidly changing set of metabolic needs. Neurons have accordingly evolved complex ways of balancing one neurotransmitter effect against another. For example, a neuron may have two types of receptors for norepinephrine on its surface—α_2 and β_2. Even though both receptors work via the enzyme adenylate cyclase, β_2 receptors lead to an *increase* in cAMP, whereas α_2 receptors lead to a *decrease* in cAMP (Cooper et al. 1996). The balance between these two opposing systems may allow the neuron to adapt in complex and subtle ways to the changing needs of the nervous system. At the same time, "breakdowns" at any step in the complex cascade could account for both emotional dysregulation and resistance to pharmacological treatment.

Pharmacokinetics

Pharmacokinetics comprises all bodily processes related to drug *absorption, distribution,* and *elimination* (DeVane 2004).

Absorption

Drug absorption—usually a passive process that occurs mainly in the small intestine—is an important factor in the drug's degree and onset of action. A poorly absorbed drug, for example, may not reach the so-called minimal effective concentration (MEC) in the blood required for clinical efficacy. A drug formulated as a "slow-release" or "extended release" agent may result in *delayed* absorption and a lower peak plasma level but may lead to an MEC similar to that of more rapidly acting formulations. This may be an advantage for some patients who are taking various antidepressants and mood stabilizers—for example, some slow-release formulations of lithium and selective serotonin reuptake inhibitors (SSRIs) lead to fewer gastrointestinal side effects than do regular formulations. Absorption of medications may sometimes be affected by factors such as food intake (which typically slows absorption) or gastric acidity.

Prior to distribution of a drug into the systemic circulation, a number of factors are involved in presystemic elimination (DeVane 2004), including the following:

1. Cytochrome enzyme activity in the intestinal epithelium, leading to localized metabolism of the parent compound.
2. A transmembrane pump known as P-glycoprotein (P-gp), which is expressed on the surface of intestinal cells. P-gp extrudes drugs from cells and returns them to the intestinal lumen, thus reducing systemic concentrations.
3. First-pass extraction of the drug as it passes from the small bowel into the portal circulation and the liver. Enzymes in the liver extract and metabolize a certain percentage of the parent compound, again reducing the concentration that reaches the systemic circulation.

Distribution

Distribution of the parent drug begins almost simultaneously with absorption into the systemic circulation. Distribution is an important factor in the onset of pharmacological response, after an *initial* dose (DeVane 2004; Greenblatt 1993). In large part, speed of distribution into the CNS is a function of a drug's *lipophilicity*—its tendency to penetrate and dissolve in fat. A drug with high lipophilicity, such as diazepam, has a very rapid onset of action after a single oral dose, as it quickly enters the CNS from the systemic circulation; however, there is also a "quick offset" of diazepam's clinical effect, as it rapidly moves out of the CNS into other adipose tissue in thighs, buttocks, and other parts of the body. Hence, for many drugs, after a single oral (or intravenous) dose, their onset and duration of action are governed mainly by their *distribution*—not their elimination half-life ($t_{1/2}\beta$). Failure to realize this may lead, for example, to the erroneous assumption that a *single* dose of diazepam will provide many hours of relief to a patient experiencing delirium tremens, owing to diazepam's long $t_{1/2}\beta$ (see Chapter 4, "Anxiolytics and Sedative-Hypnotics"). Eventually, an equilibrium is established between drug concentration in plasma, CNS, and other tissues. At that point, the drug's duration of action is more closely related to its $t_{1/2}\beta$; however, allowance must be made for drug that remains *bound to brain binding sites,* sometimes for many weeks.

In general, it is only *free drug* (i.e., drug unbound to plasma proteins) that can act at a target receptor in the CNS. The issue of protein binding has been much discussed and misunderstood and will be taken up again in later chapters. But in general, protein-binding issues are of relatively little enduring clinical significance, except to the extent that the interpretation of laboratory values is concerned. As Katzung (2001) notes, "Drug displaced from plasma protein will of course distribute throughout the volume of distribution, so that a 5% increase in the amount of unbound drug in the body produces at most a 5% increase in pharmacologically active unbound drug at the site of action" (p. 48). Fundamentally, the minimal importance of protein binding and displacement issues stems from the fact that the body is "an open system capable of eliminating unbound drug" quite rapidly (Katzung 2001, p. 48).

In this regard, it is important to remember that the steady-state (see next subsection) *concentration of free drug*—as distinguished from the *free fraction* of drug—is determined solely by 1) the *dose* and *dosing frequency* of the drug given, and 2) the drug's *clearance.* Clearance is the volume of blood per unit of time from which a drug is removed, often measured in mL/minute. Notice that protein binding does not enter into this equation at all (Greenblatt et al. 1982). *Aging,* however, is associated with reduced clearance of many drugs, owing to reduced hepatic metabolism and glomerular filtration rate and other factors (Jacobson et al. 2002).

Elimination

Elimination of most drugs, once in the systemic circulation, is primarily a function of renal and hepatic processes. The *elimination half-life* ($t_{1/2}\beta$) of a drug is essentially the time taken for drug concentration to decrease by one-half because of excretion and metabolic transformation. Actually, the $t_{1/2}\beta$ of a drug is related to both clearance (CL) and *volume of distribution* (V_d), according to the following formula (Katzung 2001):

$$t_{1/2}\beta = \frac{0.7 \times V_d}{CL}$$

It may be seen that if clearance of a lipophilic drug is reduced and volume of distribution (in adipose tissue) is increased—both of which may be true in elderly patients—the $t_{1/2}\beta$ of a drug may be increased substantially (Jacobson et al. 2002).

Steady state (SS) is a condition in which the rate of drug elimination is equal to the rate of drug administration, such that any resultant plasma levels are constant. SS is generally achieved in four to five half-lives for a given drug; conversely, when a drug is being discontinued, it takes about three to four half-lives for 90% of the drug to be eliminated. These principles become important when, for example, a drug must suddenly be discontinued. A drug with a very short $t_{1/2}\beta$—say, 8–10 hours—will be eliminated in just a couple of days (±26–33 hours), possibly exposing the patient to significant withdrawal effects. (This problem may occur when some antidepressants are suddenly stopped.) At steady state—assuming a constant total daily dose and clearance of agent—the *average* concentration of free drug will remain the same, regardless of the dosing interval. Thus, the *average* SS concentration for, say, nortriptyline will be the same, whether the drug is given as 150 mg in a single dose or as 50 mg in three divided doses. However, the "peaks and troughs" (fluctuations in plasma drug concentration) will be more pronounced with once-daily dosing (Katzung 2001).

Drug Metabolism

General Issues

Before discussing one important component of drug elimination—the CYP system—it is important to distinguish two types of metabolic processes. *Phase I* reactions include oxidative, reductive, and hydrolytic processes, leading to more polar, water-soluble molecules. Phase I reactions are largely dependent on hepatic function. In contrast, *phase II* metabolism occurs not only in the liver but also in the kidney, intestine, lungs, skin, prostate, and even the brain. *Glucuronidation* is one of the so-called phase II metabolic processes known collectively as *conjugation.*

With the exception of lithium and gabapentin, most drugs used in psychiatry are eliminated primarily via hepatic metabolism or via a combination of hepatic metabolism and extrahepatic glucuronidation. The *cytochromes* are a group of heme-containing enzymes found mainly in the endoplasmic reticulum of liver cells; however, cytochromes are also found in the bowel wall, kidneys, lungs, and even brain (Pies 2000). In the liver and bowel, the main function of the cytochromes is phase I (oxidative) metabolism of drugs—for example, hydroxylation and demethylation reactions, leading to more polar molecules that can be excreted in the urine or feces. The function of the cytochrome enzymes in lung and brain is not yet clear.

There are two main types of cytochrome enzymes: *steroidogenic* and *xeno-*

biotic. The latter group evolved as a kind of evolutionary defense mechanism that degraded plant toxins. Xenobiotic cytochrome enzymes mediate the biotransformation of most psychotropic drugs. The cytochrome enzymes are usually referred to as the cytochrome P450 (or CYP) system, where *450* refers to the wavelength of light absorbed by the pigment in the cytochromes. The CYP families are classified on the basis of amino acid sequence similarities (homology). In the designation CYP 2D6, the *2* refers to the enzyme *family; D*, to the *subfamily;* and *6,* to the individual *gene* coding for the enzyme.

Cytochrome Families

The CYP 3A4/5 family is the largest component of the CYP system, accounting for about 50% of oxidative drug metabolism. Many psychotropic drugs are metabolized via CYP 3A4, including tertiary tricyclics, triazolo-type benzodiazepines, sertraline, nefazodone, quetiapine, and risperidone (Table 1–1). Numerous nonpsychiatric medications are also substrates of 3A4, including several calcium channel blockers, erythromycin, steroid hormones, cyclosporine, and protease inhibitors. Enzyme activity in the intestinal epithelium (see discussion of presystemic elimination in "Absorption" subsection earlier in this chapter) is primarily via CYP 3A4, which may be inhibited by grapefruit juice and other 3A4 inhibitors.

The CYP 2D6 family is another clinically important CYP family, accounting for about 30% of oxidative metabolism. CYP 2D6 is responsible for the hydroxylation of all the tricyclic antidepressants (TCAs) and also metabolizes several SSRIs and antipsychotics. Many medications used in general medicine, including antiarrhythmic drugs, beta-blockers, and codeine, are also 2D6 substrates.

The CYP 1A2 system is involved in the metabolism of TCAs, mirtazapine, clozapine, olanzapine, and numerous nonpsychotropics (e.g., theophylline, caffeine, tacrine, phenacetin, and *R*-warfarin).

The CYP 2C family (subsuming 2C9 and 2C19) metabolizes several tricyclic agents, as well as citalopram, diazepam, barbiturates, phenytoin, and many agents used in general medicine.

Finally, other CYP families (e.g., CYP 2B and CYP 2E1) play a relatively small role in psychotropic drug metabolism; however, it is worth noting that *ethanol* is metabolized by the CYP 2E1 system, which also converts many substrates to potentially toxic free radicals.

TABLE 1–1. Selected substrates, inhibitors, and inducers of major cytochrome P450 enzymes

1A2	2C19	2C9	2D6	3A4
Substrates				
caffeine	amitriptyline	celecoxib	amitriptyline	alprazolam
clozapine	citalopram	diclofenac	amphetamine	amitriptyline
cyclobenzaprine	clomipramine	fluoxetine	aripiprazole	amlodipine
fluvoxamine	cyclophosphamide	flurbiprofen	clomipramine	aripiprazole
haloperidol	diazepam	fluvastatin	codeine	atorvastatin
imipramine	fluoxetine	glipizide	desipramine	buspirone
mexiletine	imipramine	ibuprofen	dextromethorphan	calcium channel blockers
mirtazapine	lansoprazole	irbesartan	donepezil	carbamazepine
naproxen	nelfinavir	losartan	flecainide	cerivastatin
olanzapine	omeprazole	naproxen	fluoxetine	chlorpheniramine
pentazocine	pantoprazole	phenytoin	fluvoxamine	clarithromycin
riluzole	phenytoin	piroxicam	haloperidol	clozapine
tacrine	sertraline	sertraline	imipramine	cyclosporine
theophylline	topiramate	sulfamethoxazole	lidocaine	diazepam
		tamoxifen	methadone	diltiazem
		tolbutamide	metoprolol	erythromycin
		torsemide	mexiletine	felodipine
		warfarin	mirtazapine	haloperidol
			nortriptyline	indinavir
			ondansetron	lovastatin
			oxycodone	methadone

TABLE 1–1. Selected substrates, inhibitors, and inducers of major cytochrome P450 enzymes *(continued)*

1A2	2C19	2C9	2D6	3A4
Substrates *(continued)*				
			paroxetine	midazolam
			propafenone	nefazodone
			propranolol	nifedipine
			risperidone	nisoldipine
			sertraline	pimozide
			tamoxifen	quetiapine
			thioridazine	quinidine
			timolol	quinine
			tolterodine	risperidone
			tramadol	ritonavir
			trazodone	saquinavir
			venlafaxine	sertraline
				sildenafil
				simvastatin
				tacrolimus
				tamoxifen
				trazodone
				triazolam
				verapamil
				vincristine
				ziprasidone

TABLE 1–1. Selected substrates, inhibitors, and inducers of major cytochrome P450 enzymes *(continued)*

1A2	2C19	2C9	2D6	3A4
Inhibitors				
cimetidine	cimetidine	amiodarone	amiodarone	amiodarone
fluoroquinolones	fluoxetine	fluconazole	chlorpheniramine	cimetidine
fluvoxamine	fluvoxamine	fluoxetine	cimetidine	clarithromycin
	ketoconazole	fluvastatin	clomipramine	erythromycin
	lansoprazole	fluvoxamine	fluoxetine	fluoxetine
	omeprazole	isoniazid	haloperidol	fluvoxamine
	paroxetine	metronidazole	indinavir	grapefruit juice
	sertraline	paroxetine	methadone	indinavir
	topiramate	zafirlukast	paroxetine	itraconazole
			perphenazine	ketoconazole
			quinidine	macrolide antibiotics
			ritonavir	nefazodone
			sertraline	nelfinavir
			terbinafine	ritonavir
				saquinavir
				troleandomycin

TABLE 1–1. Selected substrates, inhibitors, and inducers of major cytochrome P450 enzymes *(continued)*

1A2	2C19	2C9	2D6	3A4
Inducers				
carbamazepine	carbamazepine	chloral hydrate		carbamazepine
hydrocarbons (from smoking)	phenobarbital	phenobarbital		phenobarbital
rifampin	rifampin	rifampin		phenytoin
				rifabutin
				rifampin
				ritonavir
				St. John's wort

Note. The listing in this table is by no means exhaustive. Clinicians should always investigate the specific metabolic routes, inhibitors, inducers, and so forth for any given medication regimen, and check with a reliable pharmacy whenever an interaction is in doubt.

Source. Adapted and updated from Jacobson et al. 2002, which was prepared with consultation from David A. Flockhart, M.D., Ph.D.; new data obtained from Cozza et al. 2003.

A complete discussion of the CYP enzymes is well beyond the scope of this brief introduction; the reader is referred to the excellent and comprehensive text by Cozza and colleagues (2003). However, some of the principal substrates, inhibitors, and inducers of the CYP enzymes are shown in Table 1–1. It should be noted that many agents listed are substrates of more than one CYP pathway; the major metabolic routes for individual agents are discussed in subsequent chapters. The clinician should bear in mind that *induction* of the cytochromes requires protein synthesis and takes longer than *inhibition* of the CYP enzymes. Thus, the clinician should anticipate *delayed* effects on other medications when adding an inducer, but *rapid* effects (sometimes within a few days) when adding an inhibitor to a particular drug regimen (Pies 2000). Many of the clinical vignettes in subsequent chapters will explore these issues in detail.

Glucuronidation

Glucuronidation is becoming an increasingly important issue in pharmacokinetic research (Cozza et al. 2003; Liston et al. 2001). Numerous psychotropic medications undergo glucuronidation, including morphine, lorazepam, oxazepam, valproic acid, lamotrigine, and olanzapine. A variety of factors may affect glucuronidation, including age, sex, weight, certain disease states, and cigarette smoking (Liston et al. 2001). However, glucuronidation is much less affected by aging than are phase I processes—implying that in the elderly, drugs that undergo *only* glucuronidation (e.g., lorazepam, oxazepam) may sometimes be "safer" than those requiring the machinery of the CYP system (Jacobson et al. 2002).

Drug–Drug Interactions

As our knowledge of drug metabolism becomes increasingly complex, the clinician is faced with more and more questions regarding the significance of potential drug–drug interactions. Not every potential interaction signifies a clinically significant risk; indeed, the careful and astute clinician can sometimes take advantage of drug–drug interactions to use *less* of a given agent. So clinicians should be on guard and alert especially in the following situations (Pies 2000):

- When dealing with elderly or medically ill patients, particularly those with reduced hepatic or renal function
- When using agents at the higher end of the therapeutic dose range or when blood levels are approaching putatively "toxic" ranges (However, remember that "toxicity" is a clinical, not a laboratory, determination.)
- When one agent either is highly toxic or must be maintained within narrow blood level parameters (In either case, drug–drug interactions become more critical.)
- When two or more *inhibitors* of the same CYP system are being prescribed (Be alert for exaggerated psychotropic side effects due to agents metabolized by that system.)
- When a single powerful CYP inhibitor is used along with an agent that produces numerous side effects (Be especially concerned about pharmacokinetic interactions in this context.)
- When an *inhibitor* of a particular CYP metabolic pathway is stopped (Anticipate a *decrease* in drug levels of substrates for that pathway, along with possible loss of drug efficacy.)
- When a CYP *inducer* is stopped (Anticipate an *increase* in substrate drug levels for that pathway, along with possible new-onset side effects.)

Conclusion

We are just beginning to understand the fundamental mechanisms of action for most psychotropic medications. Already, we know that most work in a much more complex way than merely through their effects on neurotransmitter concentrations or receptor interactions. Many psychotropics affect the neuron—indeed, the entire organism—at the fundamental level of the gene.

The metabolism of psychotropic drugs—how they are broken down and eliminated—has critical implications for the patient's response, side-effect burden, and risk for drug–drug interactions. A knowledge of the various cytochrome pathways, as well as of glucuronidation, is becoming essential in the safe practice of psychiatry. Although the risk of drug–drug interactions can sometimes be exaggerated, it is important to know those circumstances in which patients are at high risk.

References

Cooper JR, Bloom FE, Roth RH: The Biochemical Basis of Neuropharmacology, 7th Edition. Oxford, England, Oxford University Press, 1996

Cozza KL, Armstrong SC, Oesterheld JR: Concise Guide to Drug Interaction Principles for Medical Practice: Cytochrome P450s, UGTs, P-Glycoproteins, 2nd Edition. Washington, DC, American Psychiatric Publishing, 2003

DeVane CL: Principles of pharmacokinetics and pharmacodynamics, in The American Psychiatric Publishing Textbook of Psychopharmacology, 3rd Edition. Edited by Schatzberg AF, Nemeroff CB. Washington, DC, American Psychiatric Publishing, 2004, pp 129–145

Greenblatt DJ: Basic pharmacokinetic principles and their application to psychotropic drugs. J Clin Psychiatry 54(suppl):8–13, 1993

Greenblatt DJ, Sellers EM, Koch-Weser J: Importance of protein binding for the interpretation of serum or plasma drug concentrations. J Clin Pharmacol 22:259–263, 1982

Jacobson SA, Pies RW, Greenblatt DJ: Handbook of Geriatric Psychopharmacology. Washington, DC, American Psychiatric Publishing, 2002

Katzung BG: Basic and Clinical Pharmacology, 8th Edition. New York, McGraw-Hill, 2001, pp 35–50

Liston HL, Markowitz JS, DeVane CL: Drug glucuronidation in clinical psychopharmacology. J Clin Psychopharmacol 21:500–515, 2001

Pies R: Mastering the cytochromes: a practical primer. J Psychiatr Pract 6:267–271, 2000

Rothschild AJ: The hypothalamic-pituitary-adrenal axis and psychiatric illness, in Psychoneuroendocrinology: The Scientific Basis of Clinical Practice. Edited by Wolkowitz OM, Rothschild AJ. Washington, DC, American Psychiatric Publishing, 2003, pp 139–163

Szabo ST, Gould TD, Manji HK: Neurotransmitters, receptors, signal transduction, and second messengers in psychiatric disorders, in The American Psychiatric Publishing Textbook of Psychopharmacology, 3rd Edition. Edited by Schatzberg AF, Nemeroff CB. Washington, DC, American Psychiatric Publishing, 2004, pp 3–52

CHAPTER 2

ANTIDEPRESSANTS

Overview

Drug Class

The class of agents termed *antidepressants* is a very heterogeneous group. The terminology applied to these agents can be quite confusing, since there is no universally acceptable term for the diverse agents that are *not* monoamine oxidase inhibitors (MAOIs). The term *heterocyclic* is widely used to describe all non-MAOIs, including the tricyclics and many newly introduced agents that have fewer or more than three "rings" (Ayd 1995). Actually, in most cases, it is the nature of the compound's "side chains"—not its cyclical structure—that strongly influences its biochemical function (Potter et al. 1995). We often speak of the SSRIs (selective serotonin reuptake inhibitors) as a homogeneous group, even though these agents differ in both structure and pharmacodynamic effect. The recent addition of newer agents with dual or atypical mechanisms of action, such as mirtazapine, makes classification even more complicated.

Although it makes sense to describe antidepressants (ADs) in terms of their neurotransmitter effects (see Table 2–1), even this classification will probably prove superficial as we learn more about the effects of ADs on neurotropic factors, secondary messenger systems, and gene products.

Indications

ADs, including tricyclics, heterocyclics, and MAOIs, are used in treating a wide variety of psychiatric disorders besides depression. However, their main indication is in the treatment of unipolar major depression and dysthymic disorder. The role of ADs in the treatment of bipolar disorder is a source of considerable controversy and will be taken up in some detail in this chapter and in Chapter 5 ("Mood Stabilizers").

Several serotonergic agents are also approved for the treatment of anxiety disorders, such as obsessive-compulsive disorder (OCD), generalized anxiety disorder (GAD), and posttraumatic stress disorder (PTSD). The tricyclic *clomipramine* has had U.S. Food and Drug Administration (FDA)–approved labeling for use in treating OCD for more than a decade, and MAOIs are occasionally used to treat panic disorder and OCD. Both tricyclics and, to some degree, serotonin reuptake inhibitors have been found useful in treating certain chronic pain disorders (e.g., diabetic neuropathy, fibromyalgia). Occasionally, some ADs are used in treating schizoaffective disorder, somatoform disorders, some personality disorders, eating disorders, chronic insomnia, and benzodiazepine withdrawal states. Agitated, disinhibited, or depressed patients with dementia may also benefit from certain ADs.

Mechanisms of Action

The precise mechanism or mechanisms underlying AD efficacy are not known. The old notion that ADs simply replenish one or more neurotransmitters is inadequate; most likely, ADs optimize the concentrations of several neurotransmitters—particularly serotonin (5-HT) and norepinephrine (NE)—and restore optimal pre- and postsynaptic receptor sensitivity. Some animal data suggest that depression may involve a state of supersensitive catecholamine receptors, secondary to decreased NE availability. ADs may work, in part, by "down-regulating" (reducing the number of) β-adrenergic receptors. Increased serotonin$_2$ (5-HT$_2$) binding sites have been found in the platelets and some brain regions of depressed/suicidal patients. Down-regulation of 5-HT$_2$ receptors seems to be a mechanism common to many ADs, but since electroconvulsive therapy (ECT) *increases* the density of 5-HT$_2$ receptors and is an extremely effective AD, it seems unlikely that 5-HT$_2$ down-regulation is causally related to AD effectiveness. ADs may also work, in part, by normalizing pathological neuroendocrine functions in depressed patients (e.g., hypercortisolemia due to excessive levels of corticotropin-releasing hormone) or by resetting aberrant circadian rhythms (e.g., decreased REM latency in many patients with major depression).

While all these theories have stimulated useful research, none has been consistently verifiable in animal or human models. Furthermore, many of the receptor changes noted above may actually be neuronal *adaptations* to the acute and subacute effects of ADs. The "real" mechanism of AD action probably involves changes below the level of the receptor, in which various secondary messengers ultimately lead to the production of new gene products. Recent interest has focused on the *neurotropic* effects of ADs, such as their ability to increase brain-derived neurotrophic factor (BDNF).

On the basis of the putative effects of ADs on brain biogenic amines, eight distinct but overlapping classes of ADs may be distinguished (Stahl 1998; see Table 2–1). Only bupropion and reboxetine avoid the serotonergic system. *Reboxetine* is a selective norepinephrine reuptake inhibitor (NRI) whose much-anticipated release in the United States remains uncertain at this time. The serotonin-norepinephrine reuptake inhibitor (SNRI) *duloxetine* has recently become available. *Atomoxetine* (Strattera)—another NRI—was introduced recently as the first nonstimulant approved for the treatment of attention-deficit/hyperactivity disorder (ADHD). In theory, atomoxetine could be useful in the treatment of depression, but recent controlled studies for this indication are lacking, and the drug does not have FDA-approved labeling for depression.

The MAOIs and the NaSSA (noradrenergic and specific serotonergic agent) mirtazapine are the only ADs that do not block the "reuptake" of the various monoamines. Instead, MAOIs block the *breakdown* of monoamines, and mirtazapine enhances the *release* of 5-HT and NE through α_2 autoreceptor (and heteroreceptor) antagonism.

Pharmacokinetics

ADs in general are absorbed from the small bowel; enter the portal blood; pass through the liver, where they undergo significant first-pass extraction and metabolism; and then enter the systemic circulation. ADs tend to be highly protein-bound and are highly lipophilic. Tricyclic antidepressants (TCAs) generally have elimination half-lives of 16–70 hours, but the $t_{1/2}\beta$ may be longer for protriptyline (Vivactil) and for any AD used in elderly patients.

Most of the SSRIs have a $t_{1/2}\beta$ in the range of 12 to 24 hours, with the exception of the much longer-acting fluoxetine.

ADs, like nearly all psychotropics, undergo extensive metabolism in the family of enzymes known as the cytochrome P450 (CYP) system. So-called *xenobiotic* CYP enzymes metabolize "foreign" biological substances, such as drugs and toxins, and are located in the endoplasmic reticulum of brain, liver, and bowel cells. (*Steroidogenic* CYP enzymes are located in the mitochondria of cells and are responsible mainly for the synthesis of steroids.) CYP enzymes in the liver and bowel wall carry out primarily *oxidative metabolism,* a process affecting many psychotropic agents, including the ADs. Many ADs are metabolized by CYP 2D6, 2C9/19, and 3A4; CYP 1A2 is involved mainly in TCA and fluvoxamine metabolism. Genetic polymorphism (variability) of the CYP enzymes may result in "poor" or "extensive" metabolizers in several racial groups—for example, about 8% of Caucasians show genetically based reduction of activity in the CYP 2D6 system (Cozza et al. 2003). Many psychotropic and "general medical" drugs also use the aforementioned CYP enzymes, and interactions with ADs are common (see subsection "Drug–Drug Interactions" later in this chapter).

Several studies suggest that therapeutic response to some TCAs may be related to plasma levels, and "therapeutic windows" (optimal dosage/plasma level ranges) have been postulated for several TCAs. The window for nortriptyline (roughly 50–150 ng/mL) is widely accepted. Plasma TCA levels may also be correlated with toxicity. Plasma levels seem to be far less useful with the SSRIs and other newer, non-TCA ADs, though grossly aberrant blood levels may point toward serious problems with compliance or metabolism.

Main Side Effects

Side effects of TCAs are of three main types, which overlap on a neurochemical level: cardiac/autonomic, anticholinergic, and neurobehavioral. *Cardiac/autonomic* side effects include orthostatic hypotension (secondary to α_1 receptor antagonism) and dizziness (α_1 and histamine receptor blockade properties); less commonly hypertension; tachycardia; and prolonged intracardiac conduction manifesting as prolonged QT intervals and sometimes "heart block." *Anticholinergic* side effects include dry mouth, urinary retention, blurry vision, constipation, confusion/memory impairment, and tachycardia. *Neurobehavioral* side effects include exacerbation of psychosis or mania, memory impairment (especially with highly anticholinergic agents), psychomotor stimulation (especially with desipramine and protriptyline), myoclonic twitches (including nocturnal myoclonus), tremors, and, rarely, extrapyramidal side effects (EPS). (Amoxapine may cause EPS and even, in rare cases, neuroleptic malignant syndrome because of its dopamine-blocking metabolite.) The effects of TCAs on seizure threshold are inconsistent, although high-dose clomipramine (and perhaps other tricyclics) appears to increase the risk of seizures through undetermined mechanisms (Edwards et al. 1986; Peck et al. 1983). Other side effects seen with TCAs (and other ADs) include significant sedation (especially with tertiary amines), weight gain, hepatic dysfunction, and sexual dysfunction (e.g., anorgasmia, impaired ejaculation).

The SSRIs (fluoxetine, sertraline, paroxetine, fluvoxamine, citalopram, and escitalopram) are less likely to cause anticholinergic and cardiac/autonomic side effects than are the TCAs; however, SSRIs are associated with frequent gastrointestinal (GI) side effects (nausea, diarrhea), headache, sexual dysfunction (sometimes associated with elevation in prolactin levels), insomnia, psychomotor agitation, and occasional extrapyramidal reactions. Less commonly, SSRIs may cause abnormal bleeding.

Newer agents such as nefazodone, venlafaxine, and mirtazapine have side-effect profiles that resemble those of the SSRIs but with some TCA-like effects as well—perhaps as a consequence of their complicated noradrenergic and serotonergic effects (see Table 2–1). Nefazodone and mirtazapine are quite sedating but are less likely than SSRIs to provoke sexual dysfunction (Montejo et al. 2001). Nefazodone recently received a "black box warning" secondary to rare cases of hepatic failure (approximately 1:250,000 patient-years). In the United States, shipments of nefazodone (Serzone) have been halted by the manufacturer, though generic versions apparently will remain available for some time (Mechcatie 2004).

Drug–Drug Interactions

As noted, most ADs have the potential for interacting with a wide variety of hepatically metabolized drugs, as well as with each other (Cozza et al. 2003). Both pharmacokinetic and pharmacodynamic interactions may occur. Fluoxetine, fluvoxamine, and paroxetine can significantly affect the metabolism of other non-SSRI ADs, leading to markedly elevated levels of some TCAs. SSRIs may also affect the metabolism of some antipsychotic agents (e.g., fluvoxamine substantially elevates olanzapine levels), barbiturates, triazolo-type benzodiazepines, and anticonvulsants. Pharmacodynamic interactions may also occur between SSRIs and various psychotropic agents (antipsychotics, buspirone, and lithium). A very serious and potentially fatal interaction may result from the combination of an MAOI with either an SSRI or some TCAs (especially imipramine or clomipramine). This lethal combination has resulted in a severe form of *serotonin syndrome.* Extreme caution should be used when such medications are prescribed together. MAOIs may also interact adversely with several antihypertensive agents (the specific effect—hypo- or hypertension—depends on the agent), opioids, and sympathomimetic amines. The SARI (serotonin antagonist reuptake inhibitor) nefazodone can inhibit the CYP 3A4 system and thus reduce the metabolism of triazolobenzodiazepines, quetiapine, ziprasidone, and many other substrates of this isoenzyme. Approximately 60%–70% of drugs depending on the CYP system are metabolized via the 3A4 isoenzyme.

Potentiating Maneuvers

Many patients with so-called treatment-resistant depression have actually received inadequate doses of ADs, achieved insufficient plasma levels, or taken the medication for too little time. Others have comorbid diagnoses (e.g., borderline personality disorder, substance use disorder, psychotic disorder) that diminish response to standard ADs. Numerous strategies may be used to augment the effects of ADs. One of the simplest techniques is to add another AD with a different mechanism of action (MOA). For example, combining an SSRI with bupropion may result in both enhanced serotonergic and dopaminergic/noradrenergic function, respectively. Alternatively, the addition of mirtazapine to venlafaxine should enhance release of 5-HT and NE while simultaneously inhibiting their reuptake.

Other approaches include the addition of lithium to a TCA or an SSRI. Although this may be the best-supported AD augmentation strategy, clinicians and patients may be reluctant to deal with lithium's side effects. *Thyroid hormone* or *psychostimulants* such as methylphenidate may also potentiate TCAs and SSRIs. The combination of a TCA (e.g., nortriptyline) and an SSRI (e.g., sertraline) may also benefit some patients with refractory depression, although pharmacokinetic and pharmacodynamic interactions may be problematic (e.g., elevated TCA levels, serotonin syndrome). MAOIs may be combined with TCAs (but not with SSRIs) in selected cases if the procedure is done carefully—for example, by beginning the two agents simultaneously, using very low doses of the MAOI, and avoiding imipramine or clomipramine, which have relatively large serotonergic effects.

When depression is accompanied by psychosis, the addition of an antipsychotic agent is usually necessary; indeed, AD treatment alone may lead to incomplete response or even worsening of the patient's condition. *Atypical antipsychotics* are now used in preference to older neuroleptics, and some atypicals may be effective AD augmenters even in cases of refractory but *nonpsychotic* major depression (Shelton et al. 2001). Pharmacokinetic interactions must be carefully considered with all combination strategies (e.g., avoiding an AD that strongly inhibits CYP 2D6 or 3A4 when the antipsychotic is a substrate of these pathways and could pose cardiovascular or other risks). In many cases of "psychotic depression," ECT is the treatment of choice (Fink 2003). This is especially true in cases involving severe inanition (e.g., refusal of food) or suicidality. However, ECT should not be inappropriately withheld from severely depressed patients in hopes of finding a pharmacological remedy.

Use in Special Populations

In elderly populations, the choice of AD is strongly influenced by comorbid medical conditions (e.g., cardiac disease) and the risk of drug–drug interactions (Jacobson et al. 2002). In general, the non-TCAs, including bupropion, venlafaxine, mirtazapine, and several of the SSRIs, are the ADs of choice in depressed elderly patients. Among the SSRIs, pharmacokinetic factors (e.g., strong inhibition of CYP 2D6 by fluoxetine and paroxetine) may influence choice of agent, particularly for elderly patients taking many concomitant medications. Weight loss and the syndrome of inappropriate antidiuretic hormone (SIADH) are potential side effects of SSRI treatment in the elderly (Goldstein et al. 1996). The elderly require special precautions when TCAs are used, even though TCAs may be highly effective (Jacobson et al. 2002). The elderly are especially sensitive to the anticholinergic and cardiovascular side effects of all TCAs, especially tertiary TCAs, and must be monitored carefully for postural hypotension, cardiac conduction abnormalities, and cognitive side effects. Elderly patients with ventricular arrhythmias and/or ischemic heart disease are generally not good candidates for TCAs (Glassman et al. 1993). Elderly patients with dementia may be severely affected by the anticholinergic effects of TCAs.

There are few well-designed, controlled studies of AD use in very young populations, in which placebo responsiveness may be very high. Among the SSRIs, only fluoxetine has been shown to be effective for treating major depression in both children and adolescents in double-blind, placebo-controlled studies (Emslie et al. 1997); however, other SSRIs may also be effective. Recent concerns about the safety of paroxetine, venlafaxine, and other serotonergic agents in younger patients are in need of validation. Several reports of apparent "sudden death" linked to desipramine use in children necessitate caution in prescribing TCAs in children.

The ADs as a group seem relatively safe in pregnancy, with little firm evidence of teratogenesis. Although, in some instances, it may be preferable to avoid AD use during the first trimester, the benefits of AD treatment during pregnancy sometimes outweigh the modest risks to the fetus. In some cases, ECT may be the treatment of choice. Several studies of fluoxetine in pregnancy suggest that it has very low teratogenicity, but it is correlated with a slight increase in miscarriage rate (possibly associated with depression itself). Other SSRIs also appear relatively safe during pregnancy.

Postnatal (postpartum) depression is often overlooked or undertreated and may be associated with significant morbidity and mortality. TCAs have been considered first-line therapy, but SSRIs, especially fluoxetine, have also been utilized (Altshuler et al. 2001). Controlled, comparative studies regarding the optimal treatment of postnatal depression are sorely lacking. Special concerns may arise when AD-treated mothers are breastfeeding, though this rarely poses major risks to the infant (Burt et al. 2001).

Tables

Drug Class

TABLE 2–1. Classification of antidepressants by putative neurotransmitter effects

Drug	Class	Mechanism of action
amitriptyline, nortriptyline, imipramine, desipramine	TCAs	Block reuptake of both 5-HT and NE
phenelzine, tranylcypromine, isocarboxazid	MAOIs (nonselective)	Inhibit enzymes (MAO-A, MAO-B) responsible for breakdown of 5-HT, NE, and DA
fluoxetine, paroxetine, fluvoxamine, sertraline, citalopram, escitalopram	SSRIs	Effect relatively selective inhibition of 5-HT reuptake (but have some effects on other neurotransmitters)
bupropion	NDRI (?)	? Inhibits the reuptake of NE and DA (DA > NE?)
trazodone, nefazodone	SARIs	Mainly antagonize 5-HT_2 receptors; nefazodone also modestly inhibits the reuptake of 5-HT, NE, and DA
mirtazapine	NaSSA	Antagonizes α_2 autoreceptors and heteroreceptors; also blocks 5-$HT_{2A/C}$ and 5-HT_3 receptors; stimulates 5-HT_1 receptors
reboxetine[a]	NRI	Selectively blocks NE reuptake
venlafaxine[b] (duloxetine, milnacipran[c])	SNRIs	Inhibit the reuptake of 5-HT and NE (and DA, depending on dose)

Note. ? = mechanism of action not well established. DA = dopamine; 5-HT = serotonin; 5-HT_1, 5-HT_2, 5-$HT_{2A/C}$, 5-HT_3 = serotonin receptors; MAOI = monoamine oxidase inhibitor; NaSSA = noradrenergic and specific serotonergic agent; NDRI = norepinephrine-dopamine reuptake inhibitor; NE = norepinephrine; NRI = norepinephrine reuptake inhibitor; SARI = serotonin antagonist reuptake inhibitor; SNRI = serotonin-norepinephrine reuptake inhibitor; SSRI = selective serotonin reuptake inhibitor; TCA = tricyclic antidepressant.

[a]Reboxetine's release in the United States remains uncertain as of this writing.

[b]Venlafaxine probably does not inhibit NE reuptake at a low-to-moderate dosage (e.g., < 300 mg/day).

[c]Expected to be released soon on U.S. market or being considered for development in the United States.

Source. Modified from Fava et al. 2003; Richelson 2003; Stahl 1998.

TABLE 2–2. Non-MAOI antidepressants: formulations, strengths, and usual maintenance dosage

Antidepressant	Tablet/capsule strengths and other formulations	Usual adult total daily dose range[a] (geriatric total daily dose[b])
amitriptyline (Elavil, Endep)	10, 25, 50, 75, 100, 150 mg	75–250 mg
amoxapine (Asendin)	25, 50, 100, 150 mg	200–300 mg
bupropion (Wellbutrin)	75, 100 mg	150–450 mg (75–225 mg)
bupropion SR (Wellbutrin SR)	100, 150, 200 mg (bid dosing)	150–400 mg (100–300 mg)
bupropion XL (Wellbutrin XL)	150, 300 mg (qd dosing)	150–450 mg (150–300 mg)
citalopram (Celexa)	10, 20, 40 mg Oral solution (10 mg/5 mL)	20–60 mg (10–40 mg)
clomipramine (Anafranil)	25, 50, 75 mg	50–200 mg
desipramine (Norpramin, Pertofrane)	10, 25, 50, 75, 100, 150 mg	75–250 mg
doxepin (Adapin, Sinequan)	10, 25, 50, 75, 100 mg Oral concentrate (10 mg/mL)	75–250 mg[c]
duloxetine[d]	20 mg	20–60 mg bid
escitalopram (Lexapro)	10, 20 mg Oral solution (5 mg/5mL)	10–20 mg (5–10 mg)
fluoxetine (Prozac)	10, 20, 40 mg 90-mg capsule (weekly dosing) Oral solution: 20 mg/5 mL	20–60 mg (5–40 mg)
fluvoxamine (Luvox)	25, 50, 100 mg	50–250 mg
imipramine HCl (Tofranil, Janimine)	10, 25, 50, 75, 100, 125, 150 mg	75–250 mg
maprotiline (Ludiomil)	25, 50, 75 mg	50–200 mg
mirtazapine (Remeron)	15, 30, 45 mg SolTabs: 15, 30, 45 mg	15–45 mg (7.5–30 mg)
nefazodone[e] (Serzone)	50, 100, 150, 200, 250 mg	200–500 mg
nortriptyline (Aventyl, Pamelor)	10, 25, 50, 75 mg	50–120 mg (10–100 mg[f])
paroxetine (Paxil)	10, 20, 30, 40 mg Suspension: 10 mg/5 mL	20–50 mg (5–40 mg)

TABLE 2–2. Non-MAOI antidepressants: formulations, strengths, and usual maintenance dosage *(continued)*

Antidepressant	Tablet/capsule strengths and other formulations	Usual adult total daily dose range[a] (geriatric total daily dose[b])
paroxetine CR (Paxil CR)	12.5, 25, 37.5 mg	25–75 mg (12.5–50 mg)
protriptyline (Vivactil)	5, 10 mg	20–45 mg
reboxetine[g]	—	8–10 mg (4–6 mg)
sertraline (Zoloft)	25, 50, 100 mg Oral solution: 20 mg/mL	50–200 mg (12.5–150 mg)
trazodone (Desyrel)	50, 100, 150, 300 mg	50–400 mg[h]
trimipramine (Surmontil)	25, 50, 100 mg	75–250 mg
venlafaxine (Effexor)	25, 37.5, 50, 75, 100 mg (bid or tid dosing)	75–375 mg (50–225 mg)
venlafaxine XR (Effexor XR)	37.5, 75, 150 mg (qd dosing)	75–225 mg (37.5–187.5 mg)

Note. CR = controlled release; MAOI = monoamine oxidase inhibitor; SR = sustained release; XL = extended release; XR = extended release.

[a]Upper limits of the therapeutic range may sometimes exceed those shown here (e.g., in extensive metabolizers). Medically ill patients (e.g., those with reduced hepatic or renal function) may require dosage reduction.

[b]Geriatric dosing is provided only for preferred or first-line agents in elderly patients (see Jacobson et al. 2002 for detailed information). Geriatric doses provided here are based on Jacobson et al. 2002, Kennedy 2001, and the author's clinical experience. Some geriatric patients will tolerate and/or require higher doses.

[c]While most references give similar total daily dose ranges for doxepin and other commonly used tricyclics, Janicak et al. (1993) note that "it is possible that doxepin is less potent than imipramine, and slightly higher doses may be necessary to achieve optimal benefit" (p. 228).

[d]Recently released in the United States.

[e]Labeling notes black box warning for hepatotoxicity. All but generic versions have been effectively taken off U.S. market.

[f]Nortriptyline is usually reserved for severe, refractory, or melancholic depression in elderly patients. With tricyclic antidepressants, plasma levels are important in determining the adequacy of dosage, with some elderly patients reaching therapeutic levels at lower daily doses than would younger patients.

[g]Not available in the United States.

[h]Trazodone is used most often nowadays as an aid to sleep in patients taking more stimulating antidepressants (e.g., fluoxetine), though controlled data are lacking for this use. Its antidepressant properties may not be fully realized until the dosage exceeds 300 mg/day, a dosage that causes a prohibitive degree of sedation for many patients and orthostatic hypotension in elderly patients.

TABLE 2–3. Monoamine oxidase inhibitors (MAOIs): tablet strengths and usual adult dosage

MAOI	Tablet strength, mg	Usual adult total daily dose, mg[a]
L-deprenyl (selegiline [Eldepryl])	5	10[b]
isocarboxazid (Marplan)	10	20–50
moclobemide (Manerix)[c]	100, 150	150–500
phenelzine (Nardil)	15	30–90
tranylcypromine (Parnate)	10	20–40

[a]Lower doses are often required in elderly or medically ill patients. Uppermost values of dosage ranges may exceed those shown here.
[b]L-Deprenyl loses its MAO-B selectivity at dosages above 10 mg/day but is more effective at higher dosages. A transdermal delivery system for use in depression is in phase III trials and may avoid tyramine sensitivity issues by circumventing MAO enzyme in the gut.
[c]Available in Canada but not in the United States.
Source. Data modified from Pies and Shader 2003.

TABLE 2–4. Relative monthly cost of selected antidepressants (low/middle therapeutic dosage range)

Agent (dosage[a])	Average wholesale price, (30-day supply)[b]
bupropion XL (300 mg/day)	$127.08 (brand) $96.28 (generic)
bupropion SR (300 mg/day)	$116.23 (generic)
citalopram (20 mg/day)	$85.50 (brand) $72.90 (generic)
escitalopram (10 mg/day)	$72.90
fluoxetine (20 mg/day)	$125.10 (brand) $80.00 (generic)
fluvoxamine (150 mg/day)	$154.00 (generic)
mirtazapine (30 mg/day)	$102.00 (brand) $84.00 (generic) $89.00 (SolTabs)
nortriptyline (75 mg/day)	$66.00
paroxetine (30 mg/day)	$98.64 (brand) $81.67 (generic)
paroxetine CR (37.5 mg/day)	$96.75
sertraline (100 mg/day)	$86.10
venlafaxine (125 mg/day)	$123.60 (brand) $111.30 (generic)

Note. Equivalent doses for duloxetine have not been worked out. The December 2004 average wholesale price cost for duloxetine is 40 mg/day, $190.50; 60 mg/day, $214.
CR=controlled release; SR=sustained release; XL=extended release.
[a]The dosages used are those that, in the author's clinical experience, are in the low-to-moderate end of the therapeutic range for the majority of patients. See letters by Gammon (1996) and Nemeroff (1996) for discussion of controversy regarding usually effective daily dose of sertraline.
[b]Based on average wholesale price information as of December 2004.

Indications

TABLE 2–5. "Off-label" and non–mood disorder indications for antidepressants

Drug or drug class	Indications	Comments
SSRIs/SNRIs	OCD	All SSRIs are probably useful in OCD; fluoxetine, fluvoxamine, paroxetine, and sertraline have FDA-approved labeling for adult OCD. Fluoxetine, fluvoxamine, and sertraline have FDA-approved labeling for use in children. Paroxetine has not been approved for use in pediatric OCD (see also warning about venlafaxine use in childhood depression[a]).
	Panic disorder	All SSRIs are probably useful; fluoxetine, paroxetine, and sertraline have FDA-approved labeling for panic disorder. Begin with small dose of SSRI to avoid overstimulation.
	PTSD	All SSRIs are probably useful, with superiority over placebo shown for fluoxetine, paroxetine, and sertraline. Paroxetine and sertraline carry FDA-approved labeling.
	GAD	SSRIs may be helpful; paroxetine and escitalopram have FDA-approved labeling. Venlafaxine, an SNRI, also has FDA-approved labeling for use in GAD.
	Social phobia	Preliminary data suggest most SSRIs are of benefit; sertraline, paroxetine (Paxil CR), and venlafaxine have FDA-approved labeling.
	Chronic pain syndromes	Modest documentation suggests efficacy for fluoxetine in treating migraine headache pain; diabetic neuropathy and other chronic pain states may respond to SSRIs. (Some patients develop headache as a side effect of SSRIs.)
	Personality disorders	Several small studies suggest efficacy for fluoxetine in treating patients with BPD (e.g., reduced impulsivity or aggression); one controlled study of fluvoxamine showed benefit for mood lability but not impulsivity and aggression.
	Eating disorders	Fluoxetine (60 mg/day) is helpful in the short-term management of binge-eating and purging in bulimia nervosa. Two uncontrolled studies show some efficacy of fluoxetine in treating anorexia nervosa patients.

TABLE 2–5. "Off-label" and non–mood disorder indications for antidepressants *(continued)*

Drug or drug class	Indications	Comments
SSRIs/SNRIs *(continued)*	Somatoform disorders	SSRIs may be useful in treating patients with BDD (fluoxetine) or hypochondriasis (paroxetine, fluoxetine), even if depression is not present. In BDD, a patient with the delusional subtype may respond to fluoxetine alone (without an antipsychotic).
	Insomnia	SSRIs are unreliable for initial insomnia (many patients feel overstimulated at bedtime); fluoxetine can lead to myoclonus and disrupted sleep architecture. When insomnia is part of major depression, SSRIs are helpful, at least in the first few months.
	Aggressive syndromes	Fluoxetine, sertraline, and other SSRIs are useful in treating patients whose aggression is associated with brain lesions.
	Dementia-related syndromes	SSRIs are useful in treating chronically agitated, aggressive dementia patients.
	PMDD	SSRIs have been found useful when administered during the luteal phase or continuously for PMDD. Sarafem (fluoxetine) has FDA-approved labeling for once-weekly dosing in treating PMDD; Paxil CR (paroxetine) and sertraline also have FDA-approved labeling for PMDD.
TCAs	OCD	Clomipramine was superior to nonserotonergic TCAs in a meta-analysis of 10 studies; clomipramine is the only TCA to have received FDA-approved labeling for OCD. Nortriptyline and desipramine are much less effective in treating OCD. Full response with CLOMIP may take >6 weeks.
	Panic disorder	In 7 studies, TCAs were superior to placebo (72% vs. 51%); imipramine is the most widely studied TCA, but efficacy has been reported with desipramine, nortriptyline, amitriptyline, and doxepin.

TABLE 2–5. "Off-label" and non–mood disorder indications for antidepressants *(continued)*

Drug or drug class	Indications	Comments
TCAs *(continued)*	PTSD	Open studies of TCAs have shown some benefits in treating patients with PTSD, but two double-blind controlled trials (using amitriptyline, desipramine) did not show substantial benefit in ameliorating core features of PTSD.
	GAD	Relatively low doses of imipramine may be useful in treating anticipatory anxiety, but the effects may not be evident for >1 month.
	Social phobia	No systematic data are available for TCAs.
	Chronic neuropathic pain syndromes	Amitriptyline, desipramine, doxepin, imipramine, and nortriptyline have all been reported to be useful, particularly in treating patients with diabetic or other peripheral neuropathy.
	Personality disorders	Generally poor response in patients with BPD; high potential for lethal overdose.
	Eating disorders	Imipramine and desipramine appear effective in the short term in reducing binge-eating/purging in patients with bulimia nervosa; long-term use carries risk of weight gain.
	Somatoform disorders[b]	Desipramine may be the treatment of choice for chronic pain associated with dysthymia. No specific pharmacological treatment of somatization disorder unless patient has concomitant depression—no convincing data on use of TCAs. Avoid tertiary TCAs in patients with hypochondriasis (poor tolerance of anticholinergic side effects).
	Insomnia	Low doses of doxepin or amitriptyline (e.g., 25–50 mg of either) may be useful in treating chronic insomnia (but use very cautiously in the elderly because of central anticholinergic side effects).

TABLE 2–5. "Off-label" and non–mood disorder indications for antidepressants *(continued)*

Drug or drug class	Indications	Comments
TCAs *(continued)*	Aggressive syndromes	Amitriptyline has been noted in a few reports to be useful in head-injured or encephalopathic patients; but patients with BPD may experience a worsening of symptoms with amitriptyline.
	Dementia-related syndromes	Imipramine and other TCAs may be effective in depressed Alzheimer's patients, but anticholinergic side effects may worsen cognitive symptoms.

Note. BDD=body dysmorphic disorder; BPD=borderline personality disorder; FDA=U.S. Food and Drug Administration; GAD=generalized anxiety disorder; OCD=obsessive-compulsive disorder; PMDD=premenstrual dysphoric disorder; PTSD=posttraumatic stress disorder; SNRI=serotonin-norepinephrine reuptake inhibitor; SSRI=selective serotonin reuptake inhibitor; TCA=tricyclic antidepressant.

[a]The FDA recently advised against the use of paroxetine in pediatric populations, owing to concerns about increased risk of suicidal ideation. The scientific basis for this concern remains, as of this writing, open to question. Also, Wyeth Pharmaceuticals (August 22, 2003) has advised against use of Effexor and Effexor XR in children and adolescents, owing to increased suicidal ideation and self-injurious behaviors when compared with subjects receiving placebo. In any event, the efficacy of venlafaxine in depressed children has not been clearly established in randomized, double-blind, controlled studies.

[b]Includes DSM-III-R somatoform pain disorder (American Psychiatric Association 1987) and DSM-IV pain disorder (American Psychiatric Association 1994).

Source. Agras 1995; Ayd 1995; Blumer 1987; Denys et al. 2004; Dewan and Pies 2001; Gelenberg 2003; Janicak et al. 1993; Kline et al. 1993; Phillips 1991; Phillips et al. 2002; Physicians' Desk Reference 2004; Potter et al. 1995; Rinne et al. 2002; Shader 1994; Silver 1995; Taylor 1995; Tollefson 1995; Trestman et al. 1995; Yudofsky et al. 1995; Zajecka 1995.

Mechanisms of Action

TABLE 2–6. Neurotransmitter effects of selected antidepressants

Agent	NE	5-HT	DA
amitriptyline	+++	++++	–
bupropion[a]	+	0	+
desipramine	+++++	+++	–
citalopram	–	+++++	0
duloxetine	++++	++++++	+
fluoxetine	++	+++++	–
mirtazapine[b]	++	++	0
nefazodone[c]	++	++	++
nortriptyline	++++	+++	–
paroxetine	+++	++++++	+
reboxetine	++++	–	–
sertraline[d]	+	++++++	+++
venlafaxine[e]	+	++++	+/–

Note. 0 = no effect; – = minimal; + to ++++++ = increasing level of potency; +/– = minimal except at very high dosage. Magnitudes of effects shown are only approximations and are not precisely translatable into binding affinity measures (K_i), as provided by Richelson 2003. Magnitude of effects also may depend on dose.

DA = dopamine; 5-HT = serotonin; NE = norepinephrine.

[a]The mechanism of action of bupropion remains unclear. While some animal and human data support a dopaminergic and/or noradrenergic effect, some animal models do not show dopaminergic effects (see Dong and Blier 2001). Noradrenergic effects may actually be due to a metabolite (Richelson 2003).

[b]Mirtazapine does not work via inhibition of reuptake (transporter blockade), but rather via autoreceptor and heteroreceptor effects.

[c]Nefazodone mainly antagonizes 5-HT_2 receptors, while showing modest blockade of 5-HT, NE, and DA reuptake.

[d]SSRIs have variable effects on DA, perhaps decreasing DA levels in some brain regions. However, sertraline has substantial DA reuptake inhibition compared with the other SSRIs—a feature that may have implications for its apparently beneficial effects on cognitive function in some patients.

[e]NE and DA effects probably occur only at dosages >250 and 350 mg/day, respectively. At low-to-moderate dosages, 5-HT effects predominate.

Source. Demitrack 2002; Ereshefsky et al. 1996; Richelson 2003; Schatzberg and Cole 1991; Sherman 1996.

TABLE 2–7. Effects of reuptake blockade and receptor antagonism

Neurotransmitter/receptor	Possible clinical implications/side effects
Blockade of reuptake at synapse	
NE	Antidepressant effect (venlafaxine) Tremors, jitteriness, tachycardia, sweating
5-HT	Antidepressant effect (SSRIs) Gastrointestinal side effects, sexual dysfunction, decreased appetite, variable effects on anxiety, risk of 5-HT syndrome
DA	Psychomotor activation, antiparkinsonian effect; possible worsening of mania, psychosis; sexual arousal, activation of "reward" pathways
Antagonism of receptors or autoreceptors	
5-HT_1 autoreceptors	Inhibition (normally) of neuron firing rate by 5-HT acting on 5-HT_{1A} receptors on neuronal cell body; inhibition (normally) of 5-HT release by $5\text{-HT}_{1B/D}$ receptors on nerve terminal; conversely, increased firing rate or increased 5-HT release resulting from antagonism or down-regulation of 5-HT_{1A} or $5\text{-HT}_{1B/D}$ autoreceptors, respectively
5-HT_2 receptors	? Probable antidepressant effect (cf. nefazodone) ? Antipsychotic effect (cf. atypical antipsychotics) ? Counteracting of sexual dysfunction, anxiety, insomnia
Histaminic (H_1) receptors	Sedation, weight gain, potentiation of CNS depressants, transient cognitive impairment
Muscarinic (cholinergic) receptors	Dry mouth, blurry vision, constipation, urinary retention, tachycardia, cognitive impairment
α_1-Adrenergic receptors	Postural hypotension, dizziness, reflex tachycardia, impaired ejaculation, priapism (cf. trazodone)
α_2 (Presynaptic)–adrenergic autoreceptors	Antagonism of autoreceptors (which normally mediate negative feedback of NE on presynaptic neuron), leading to increased NE release from presynaptic neuron (cf. yohimbine, mirtazapine); may have antidepressant effects but may increase anxiety (e.g., yohimbine)

Note. CNS = central nervous system; DA = dopamine; 5-HT = serotonin; NE = norepinephrine; SSRI = selective serotonin reuptake inhibitor.

Source. Blier 2003; Preskorn 1994; Richelson 1994; Segraves 1989.

TABLE 2–8. Effects of serotonin (5-HT) receptor stimulation

Receptor stimulated	Postulated effect/side effect
5-HT_{1A}	Anxiolytic, antidepressant action (cf. buspirone, which is a partial agonist at postsynaptic 5-HT_{1A} receptors, and mirtazapine, which has selective agonist activity at 5-HT_{1A} receptors)
5-HT_2	Anxiety, insomnia, sexual dysfunction (cf. SSRI side effects)
5-HT_3[a]	Nausea, gastrointestinal problems

Note. SSRI = selective serotonin reuptake inhibitor.
[a]Receptors in brain stem and gut.
Source. Stahl 1997a, 1997b.

Pharmacokinetics

TABLE 2–9. Pharmacokinetics of selected antidepressants

Drug/ metabolite	$t_{1/2}$ of parent compound and main active metabolites	Main route(s) of elimination/ CYP metabolism	Degree of inhibition by parent compound/metabolite on CYP			
			3A4	2D6	1A2	2C9/19
bupropion (Wellbutrin)	8–24 hours	2B6 (plus several other pathways)	—	++	—	—
hydroxybupropion[a]	~20 hours	?	?	?	?	?
citalopram (Celexa)	35 hours	2C19, 3A4 (some 2D6)	—	+/– to +	+/– to +	+/– to +
duloxetine (Cymbalta)	8–17 hours	2D6, 1A2	+/–	+	+/–	+/–
escitalopram (Lexapro)	27–32 hours	2C19, 3A4 (some 2D6)	—	+/–	—	—
fluoxetine (Prozac)	2–4 days	2D6 (also 2C, 3A4) (NonL)	+ to ++	+++	+	++ (2C19>2C9)
norfluoxetine	7–10 days	2D6 (also 2C, 3A4)	++ to +++	+++	+	++ (2C19>2C9)
fluvoxamine (Luvox)	15–19 hours	1A2, 2D6	++	+	+++	++ (2C19>2C9)

TABLE 2–9. Pharmacokinetics of selected antidepressants *(continued)*

Drug/ metabolite	$t_{1/2}$ of parent compound and main active metabolites	Main route(s) of elimination/ CYP metabolism	Degree of inhibition by parent compound/metabolite on CYP			
			3A4	2D6	1A2	2C9/19
imipramine (Tofranil)	11–24 hours	2D6 (hydroxylation) 1A2, 3A4 (demethylation)	—	+	—	+
desmethylimipramine[b]	12–24 hours	2D6 (hydroxylation)	—	+	—	—
mirtazapine (Remeron)	20–40 hours	1A2, 3A4, 2D6	—	—	—	—
nefazodone (Serzone)	3 hours	3A4 (NonL)	+++	+	—	—
hydroxynefazodone/ triazoledione[c]	3 hours/18–33 hours	?	?	?	?	?
nortriptyline (Pamelor)	18–44 hours	2D6 (hydroxylation)	—	+	—	—
paroxetine (Paxil)	21–24 hours	2D6 (NonL)	+	+++	+	+
sertraline[d] (Zoloft)	25–32 hours	2C9 (also 3A4, 2C19, 2D6)	++	+	+	+

TABLE 2–9. Pharmacokinetics of selected antidepressants *(continued)*

Drug/ metabolite	$t_{1/2}$ of parent compound and main active metabolites	Main route(s) of elimination/ CYP metabolism	Degree of inhibition by parent compound/metabolite on CYP			
			3A4	2D6	1A2	2C9/19
desmethylsertraline	60–75 hours	2C9 (also 3A4, 2C19, 2D6)	+	+/–	+/–	+/–
venlafaxine (Effexor)	5 hours	2D6	+/–	+	+/–	—
O-desmethylvenlafaxine	11 hours	3A4	?	?	?	?

Note. —=None or none reported; ?=insufficient data; +/–=minimal degree; +=modest degree; ++=significant degree; +++=substantial degree. CYP=cytochrome P450; NonL=nonlinear pharmacokinetics (implies that dosage increase may lead to higher-than-expected increase in plasma levels and/or clinical effect, particularly at higher dose ranges); otherwise, all metabolism shown is linear; $t_{1/2}$=half-life.

[a]One of three active metabolites.

[b]A metabolite of imipramine, also marketed as an antidepressant, desipramine.

[c]The compound m-CPP (*m*-chlorophenylpiperazine), which is a significant metabolite of trazodone, is a negligible metabolite of nefazodone. m-CPP may be anxiogenic in some patients and is metabolized by CYP 2D6. Strong inhibitors of CYP 2D6 may increase levels of m-CPP, with potential anxiogenic effects.

[d]At high dosages (>200 mg/day), sertraline is a potent CYP 2D6 inhibitor.

Source. Ciraulo et al. 1995b; Cozza et al. 2003; DeVane 1995; Drug Facts and Comparisons 1995; Gelenberg 1995; Goff and Baldessarini 1995; Golden et al. 1995; Ketter et al. 1995; Nemeroff et al. 1995–1996; Pollock et al. 1996; Preskorn 1996; Tollefson 1995.

TABLE 2–10. Pharmacodynamic and pharmacokinetic profiles of newer antidepressants

Drug	Pharmacodynamics	Pharmacokinetics	Comments/Special considerations
fluoxetine (Prozac)	Moderate noradrenergic activity in addition to 5-HT reuptake blockade	Nonlinear pharmacokinetics; longest $t_{1/2}$ of SSRIs; active metabolite (norfluoxetine); parent compound and metabolite strong CYP 2D6 and moderate CYP 3A4 inhibitors	Generic available; more data showing safety in pregnancy than for other SSRIs; reduced risk of withdrawal symptoms if discontinued, but takes longer to “wash out”; nervousness may be more common than with other SSRIs Dose increase leads to disproportionate rise in blood levels; significant drug interactions due to CYP inhibition
sertraline (Zoloft)	Greater dopaminergic activity than with other SSRIs; slightly noradrenergic	Moderate $t_{1/2}$ + active metabolite (desmethylsertraline); parent compound and metabolite both modest CYP 2C, 2C19, and 3A4 inhibitors	More data suggesting overall safety in breastfeeding than for other SSRIs; in theory, might be more helpful than other SSRIs in patients with Parkinson’s disease, but no controlled data; dopaminergic effects suggest caution in deciding whether to use in patients with mania/psychosis Less overall CYP inhibition than with some SSRIs; may mean fewer drug–drug interactions

TABLE 2–10. Pharmacodynamic and pharmacokinetic profiles of newer antidepressants *(continued)*

Drug	Pharmacodynamics	Pharmacokinetics	Comments/Special considerations
paroxetine (Paxil)	Potent 5-HT reuptake blockade; most potent inhibitor of NE transporter among SSRIs; modest to moderate anticholinergic effects (more so in vitro than in vivo)	Nonlinear pharmacokinetics; no active metabolites; strong CYP 2D6 inhibitor; modest inhibitor of other CYP enzymes	Not clear if NE effects confer therapeutic advantage; weight gain often reported, but not clear if gain is greater than with other SSRIs; some patients may experience dry mouth, other anticholinergic effects; withdrawal syndrome may be more common than with some other SSRIs Sometimes recommended for bipolar depression (American Psychiatric Association 2002), but few controlled, comparative data available to support preference Dose increase leads to disproportionate rise in blood levels; significant drug interactions due to CYP inhibition

TABLE 2–10. Pharmacodynamic and pharmacokinetic profiles of newer antidepressants *(continued)*

Drug	Pharmacodynamics	Pharmacokinetics	Comments/Special considerations
citalopram (Celexa) escitalopram (Lexapro)	Selective and potent 5-HT reuptake inhibitor; virtually no effects on NE, DA reuptake; no anticholinergic effects	Very little inhibition of major CYP enzymes	Clinical advantages of 5-HT selectivity not clear (e.g., some patients may need multiple neurotransmitter effects; lack of anticholinergic effects may be advantage) May be useful for medical and geriatric patients taking multiple medications Minimal drug interactions from citalopram's effect on CYP enzymes, but agents that inhibit 2C19, 3A4 may raise blood levels of both citalopram and escitalopram Somewhat fewer side effects with escitalopram vs. citalopram
fluvoxamine (Luvox)	Potent and selective 5-HT reuptake blockade; very little effect on other neurotransmitters	Nonlinear pharmacokinetics; strong CYP 1A2 inhibition; moderate CYP 3A4, 2C19 inhibition	Generic available; has FDA-approved labeling for OCD in all age groups (but not clearly superior to other SSRIs for OCD) Nausea more common than with other SSRIs Dose increase leads to disproportionate rise in blood levels; may increase blood levels of several CYP 1A2 substrates (e.g., olanzapine)

TABLE 2–10. Pharmacodynamic and pharmacokinetic profiles of newer antidepressants *(continued)*

Drug	Pharmacodynamics	Pharmacokinetics	Comments/Special considerations
venlafaxine (Effexor)	Serotonergic effects at lower dosages, modest noradrenergic effects at higher dosages (>250 mg/day)	Has active metabolite (*O*-desmethylvenlafaxine); short $t_{1/2}$ (±14 hours for parent compound and metabolite)	Described as "dual action" agent, but has very limited noradrenergic effects at dosages<250 mg/day; some data indicating benefits in treatment-refractory depression GI side effects common with high doses, rapid dose escalation (XR formulation somewhat better tolerated); monitor blood pressure at high dosages (>225 mg/day, less in elderly); short $t_{1/2}$ may mean higher risk of withdrawal syndrome than with most newer agents

TABLE 2–10. Pharmacodynamic and pharmacokinetic profiles of newer antidepressants *(continued)*

Drug	Pharmacodynamics	Pharmacokinetics	Comments/Special considerations
bupropion (Wellbutrin)	Dopaminergic activity; mild noradrenergic activity; essentially no serotonergic or anticholinergic effects	Unusual metabolic route (via CYP 2B6); two active metabolites; strong CYP 2D6 inhibition	Rare weight gain or sexual side effects; stimulating effects may be limiting factor for some patients, useful in others Useful in smoking cessation; often recommended in bipolar depression (on the basis of limited data) Useful in geriatric and medical patients owing to benign cardiovascular profile, lack of anticholinergic, sedative side effects Relatively contraindicated in patients with eating or seizure disorders, but at lower doses, seizure risk comparable to that of other antidepressants (SR formulation may decrease seizure risk relative to regular formulation) Can increase blood levels of SSRIs, other CYP 2D6 substrates

TABLE 2–10. Pharmacodynamic and pharmacokinetic profiles of newer antidepressants *(continued)*

Drug	Pharmacodynamics	Pharmacokinetics	Comments/Special considerations
mirtazapine (Remeron)	Increases both 5-HT and NE via auto/heteroreceptor blockade; 5-HT_2, 5-HT_3 blockade, but increased 5-HT_{1A} receptor–mediated transmission; little effect on muscarinic receptors, moderate histaminergic (H_1) blockade	Very little CYP enzyme inhibition	Weight gain, sedating (possibly less at higher doses, owing to increased noradrenergic effects); fewer GI, sexual side effects than most SSRIs No significant effects on hemostasis reported (vs. SSRIs) Few drug interactions due to inhibitor effect on CYP enzymes
nefazodone (Serzone)	Serotonergic, 5-HT_2 blockade	Nonlinear pharmacokinetics; strong CYP 3A4 inhibitor	Quite sedating (may have benign effects on sleep architecture); weight gain, sexual side effects rare compared with SSRIs; orthostasis and dizziness common; occasional visual abnormalities; black box warning regarding hepatic failure, but such events very rare (1 per 250,000 patient-years) Dose increase leads to disproportionate rise in blood levels; interactions with triazolobenzodiazepines, quetiapine, antifungals, steroids, and other CYP 3A4 substrates

Note. CYP=cytochrome P450; DA=dopamine; FDA=U.S. Food and Drug Administration; 5-HT=serotonin; GI=gastrointestinal; NE= norepinephrine; OCD=obsessive-compulsive disorder; SR=slow release; SSRI=selective serotonin reuptake inhibitor; $t_{1/2}$=half-life; XR=extended release.

Source. A. Rajparia, M.D., personal communication, February 25, 2004; American Psychiatric Association 2002; Cozza et al. 2003; Golden et al. 2004; Herr and Nemeroff 2004; Shim and Yonkers 2004; Thase and Sloan 2004.

TABLE 2–11. Putative optimal plasma levels for tricyclic antidepressants

Agent	Optimal plasma level (ng/mL)	Comments
amitriptyline (parent compound)	80–150	Results conflicting regarding linear, curvilinear, or no relationship to efficacy
desipramine (as single agent)	>125 or between 110 and 160	Unclear whether relationship is linear or curvilinear
imipramine[a]	>225	Linear relationship in adults
nortriptyline[b]	50–150	Better predictor of antidepressant response in patients taking amitriptyline

[a]Includes its metabolite, desipramine.
[b]A metabolite of amitriptyline.
Source. Arana and Hyman 1991; Janicak et al. 1993.

Main Side Effects

TABLE 2–12. Side-effect profiles of commonly used antidepressants[†]

Drug	Anticholinergic effects (blurry vision, dry mouth, constipation)	Sedation/ drowsiness	Insomnia/ agitation	Orthostatic hypotension	Cardiac arrhythmia	GI distress/ diarrhea	Weight gain[a]
amitriptyline (Elavil)	4	4	0.5	4	3	0.5	4
bupropion (Wellbutrin)	0	0.5	2	0	0.5	1	0
citalopram (Celexa)[b]	0.5	0.5	0.5	0	0	1.5	0
desipramine (Norpramin)	1	1	1	2	3	0.5	1
doxepin (Sinequan)	3	4	0.5	3	2	0.5	3
fluoxetine (Prozac)	0	0.5	2	0	0.5	3	0
clomipramine (Anafranil)	3	3	0.5	3	3	0.5	3
trimipramine (Surmontil)	2	3	0.5	2	2	0.5	3
imipramine (Tofranil)	3	3	1	4	3	1	3
mirtazapine (Remeron)	0.5–1[c]	4	0.5	0.5	0	0	4
nefazodone (Serzone)	0.5	0.5	0	2	0.5	2	0.5
nortriptyline (Pamelor)	1	2	0.5	1	2	0.5	2
paroxetine (Paxil)	2	0.5	1	0	0.5	3	0–0.5

TABLE 2–12. Side-effect profiles of commonly used antidepressants[†] *(continued)*

Drug	Anticholinergic effects (blurry vision, dry mouth, constipation)	Sedation/ drowsiness	Insomnia/ agitation	Orthostatic hypotension	Cardiac arrhythmia	GI distress/ diarrhea	Weight gain[a]
sertraline (Zoloft)	0	0.5	1	0	0.5	3	0
venlafaxine (Effexor)	0.5	0.5	2	0	0.5	3	0

Note. 0 = virtually none; 0.5 = minimal; 1 = modest; 1.5 = moderate; 2 = significant; 3 = moderately high; 4 = high. GI = gastrointestinal.

[†]Because postmarketing clinical experience with duloxetine (Cymbalta) as compared with older antidepressants is still limited, relative values for side effects are not listed. Given duloxetine's low affinity (in vitro) for muscarinic, adrenergic, and histaminic receptors, one would predict relatively low rates of anticholinergic side effects, hypotension, sedation, and weight gain. However, clinical studies with this agent find that common side effects (occurring in >5% of patients) include nausea, dry mouth, constipation, decreased appetite, fatigue, and somnolence (Physicians' Desk Reference Concise Prescribing Guide 2004). Head-to-head comparisons of duloxetine versus other antidepressants and placebo are needed.

[a]Anecdotal and naturalistic experience has shown that some patients—often after an initial period of weight loss—may gain substantial weight with fluoxetine, paroxetine, and perhaps other selective serotonin reuptake inhibitors (SSRIs) (see Gelenberg 1997; Sachs and Guille 1999). However, some weight gain may represent "regain" of weight lost as a result of the depression itself. Randomized, controlled studies of SSRIs generally do not demonstrate significant weight gain; however, one study did show increased risk with paroxetine (Fava et al. 2000).

[b]Side effects are generally similar for escitalopram (Lexapro), though some studies indicate slightly reduced GI side effects with escitalopram (vs. citalopram).

[c]Mirtazapine, though lacking strong anticholinergic effects, has prominent *antihistaminic* effects that are associated with both sedation and weight gain. Some reports and clinical experience suggest that higher dosages (>15 mg/day) are associated with *less* sedation and weight gain, perhaps as a result of increased noradrenergic effects.

Source. Data based on the DHHS clinical practice guideline *Depression in Primary Care* (Depression Guideline Panel 1993); Physicians' Desk Reference 2004; Preskorn 1995; and the author's clinical experience. *All values are merely rough guidelines and may vary according to dose, duration of treatment, and age of patient.*

TABLE 2–13. Side effects of tricyclic vs. selected nontricyclic antidepressants (% of patients reporting, placebo adjusted)

Side effect	Imipramine[a]	Bupropion	Fluoxetine	Nefazodone	Paroxetine	Sertraline	Venlafaxine	Mirtazapine
Dry mouth	50.0	9.2	3.5	12.0	6.0	7.0	11.0	10.0
Constipation	26.5	8.7	1.2	6	5.2	2.1	8.0	6.0
Nausea	3.5	4.0	11.0	11	16.4	14.3	26	0
Diarrhea	1.0	−1.8	5.3	1.0	4.0	8.4	1.0	0
Sexual dysfunction[b]	>15.0	1.0	>15.0	5.0	>20.0	>15.0	>18.0	>12.0
Neurobehavioral								
Drowsiness	25.5	0.3	5.9	11.0	14.3	7.5	14.0	36.0
Insomnia	8.0	5.3	6.7	2.0	7.1	7.6	8.0	0
Nervousness	20.0	13.9	10.3	—	4.9	4.4	12.0	0
Headache	2.0	3.5	4.8	3.0	0.3	1.3	1.0	0

Note. — indicates that drug effect was less than or equal to effect of placebo.

[a]For imipramine, figures represent average of imipramine–placebo difference based on two studies (Branconnier et al. 1983; Dunbar et al. 1991).

[b]Reports of sexual dysfunction vary greatly with the type and number of questions asked. Studies using both placebo controls and structured questionnaires are very rare. Figures cited are proportional *estimates* based on several studies and typical placebo responses, not on direct comparisons with placebo. Figures probably represent underestimates of the actual prevalence of sexual dysfunction (Hallward and Ellison 2001; Montejo et al. 2001).

Source. Physicians' Desk Reference 2004; Preskorn 1995, 1999.

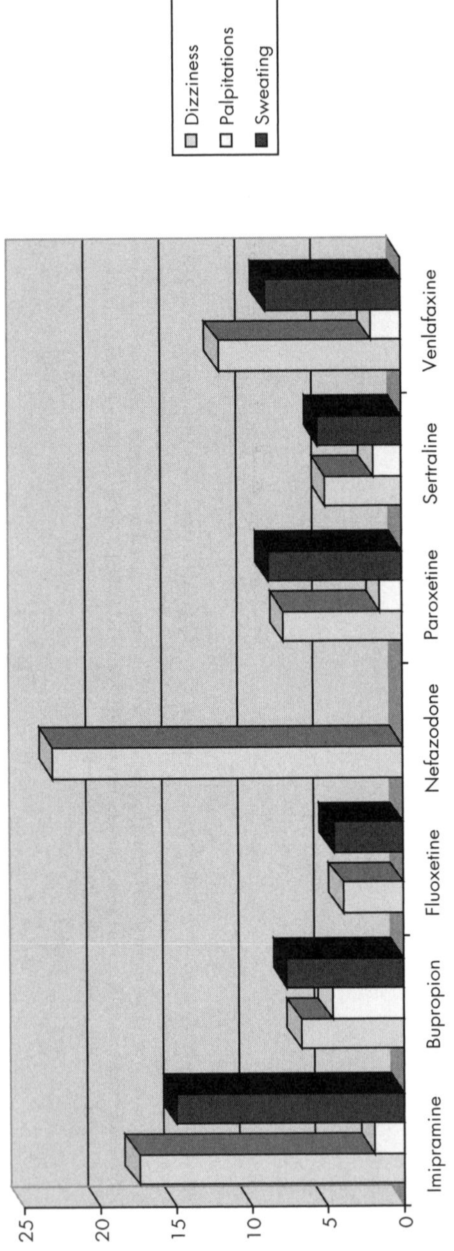

FIGURE 2–1. Cardiac and autonomic side effects of selected antidepressants.
Source. Data from Preskorn 1995.

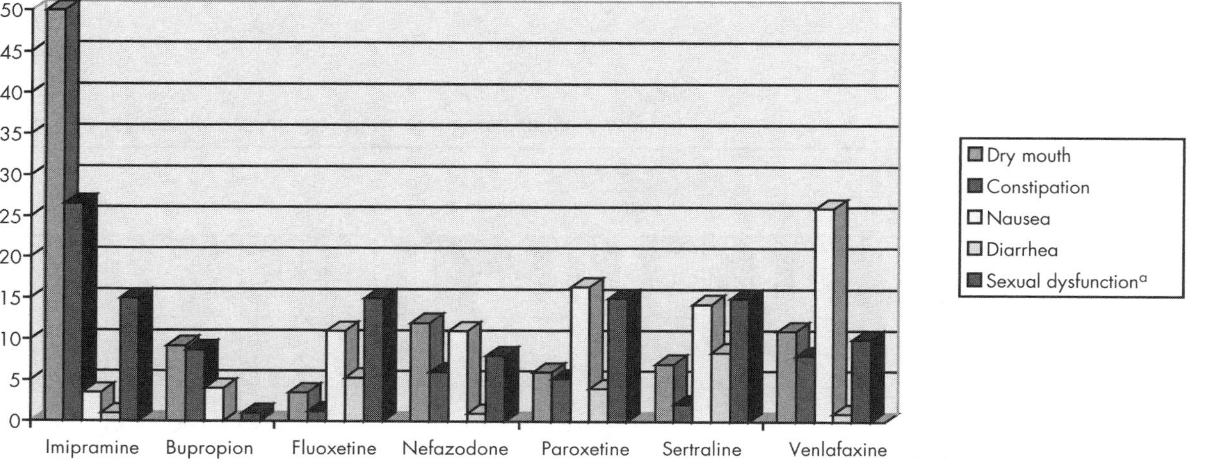

FIGURE 2–2. Gastrointestinal and sexual side effects of selected antidepressants.

[a]Percentages probably represent underestimate because most studies used inadequate assessment tools.

Source. Data from Preskorn 1995.

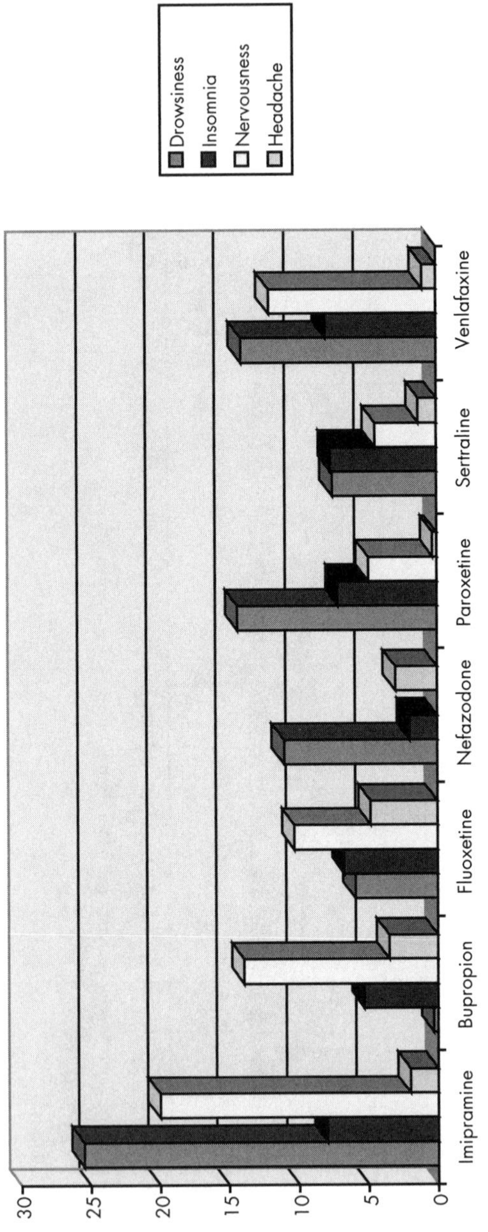

FIGURE 2–3. Neurobehavioral side effects of selected antidepressants.

Source. Data from Preskorn 1995.

TABLE 2–14. Some comparative side effects of selective serotonin reuptake inhibitors (placebo-adjusted %)

Side effect	Fluoxetine	Sertraline	Paroxetine	Escitalopram	Citalopram	Fluvoxamine
Headache	4.8	1.3	0.3	<placebo	<placebo	2.0
Nervousness	10.3	4.4	4.9	<placebo	1.0	7.0
Insomnia	6.7	7.6	7.1	5.0	1.0	11.0
Drowsiness	5.9	7.5	14.3	4.0	8.0	14.0
Fatigue	5.6	2.5	10.3	3.0	2.0	8.0[a]
Diarrhea	5.3	8.4	4.0	3.0	3.0	4.0
Nausea	11.0	14.3	16.4	8.0	7.0	26.0
Constipation	1.2	2.1	5.2	2.0	<placebo	2.0
Dry mouth	3.5	7.0	6.0	1.0	6.0	4.0

Note. Note that percentages are not derived from head-to-head comparisons.

[a]Asthenia.

Source. Physicians' Desk Reference 2004; Preskorn 1995; for escitalopram, product labeling insert (Forest Pharmaceuticals 2003).

TABLE 2–15. Basic management of antidepressant side effects

Side effects	Management strategies
Anticholinergic side effects	Reduce dose Wait for tolerance Consider sugar-free candies, "artificial saliva," fluoride lozenges, drops for dry mouth (*Note:* dry mouth predisposes to dental caries) Increase fluid and fiber; ? try bulk-forming agents for constipation Consider bethanechol 10–50 mg tid–qid Consider pilocarpine solution for dry mouth, blurry vision
Cardiovascular side effects	
Orthostatic hypotension from TCAs	Switch to less hypotensive agent Warn and instruct patients about orthostasis (e.g., rising slowly) Ensure ample fluid intake Consider support stockings (e.g., TED), abdominal binder for orthostasis Consider supplemental NaCl (1–3 g/day), small doses of caffeine; consider fludrocortisone (0.1–0.3 mg/day) in refractory cases
Sinus tachycardia, conduction delays, arrhythmias with TCAs	Consider dosage reduction, splitting dose, "watchful waiting" for tachycardia (may be helpful) Obtain pretreatment and follow-up ECG, which are now standard of care for all patients taking TCAs[a] Presence of new conduction delay (e.g., second-degree heart block) is usually contraindication to continued use of agent
Hypertension with venlafaxine	Monitor blood pressure Reduce venlafaxine dosage
Hypotension with MAOIs	Monitor blood pressure periodically (hypotension can occur after several weeks of MAOI treatment) Use strategies similar to those for TCAs
Hypertensive crisis with MAOIs	Instruct patient to avoid tyramine and other pressor substances; give written list of foods and medications to avoid to patient

TABLE 2–15. Basic management of antidepressant side effects *(continued)*

Side effects	Management strategies
Excessive sedation (daytime somnolence, psychomotor slowing)	"Start low, go slow" with dose Wait to see if tolerance develops Consider change to less sedating agent Give drug in divided or mostly bedtime dosing Add small amount of caffeine, psychostimulant,[b] or bupropion Add modafinil 100–400 mg/day (?) (controlled data lacking[c])
Insomnia	Rule out hypomania/mania, mixed states, worsening of underlying mood or anxiety disorder, akathisia, and nocturnal myoclonus due to antidepressant Wait for tolerance to develop Administer all medication in morning Add trazodone (25–300 mg qhs) if insomnia is due to SSRI (common approach, but not based on controlled studies; trazodone may have cardiac and other side effects) Add benzodiazepine (especially for nocturnal myoclonus) or zolpidem (5–10 mg qhs) Add low dose of gabapentin (100–400 mg hs) (based largely on anecdotal data) Add low dose of sedating TCA (amitriptyline, clomipramine) if insomnia is due to SSRI (but note TCAs may cause nocturnal myoclonus) Consider change to nefazodone or mirtazapine if insomnia is associated with SSRI

TABLE 2–15. Basic management of antidepressant side effects *(continued)*

Side effects	Management strategies
Agitation/"jitteriness"	Rule out worsening of depression, anxiety, akathisia, hypomania/mania, and mixed states. "Start low, go slow" (especially with SSRIs, venlafaxine, bupropion) Wait for tolerance to develop Reduce dose Switch to less activating agent (e.g., mirtazapine) Add benzodiazepine or gabapentin Add beta-blocker (e.g., propranolol 10–20 mg bid) if no medical contraindication

Note. ECG = electrocardiogram; MAOI = monoamine oxidase inhibitor; SSRI = selective serotonin reuptake inhibitor; TCA = tricyclic antidepressant; TED = thromboembolic diseases.
[a]While some clinicians and textbooks continue to advocate baseline ECGs only for patients over age 40 or for those with known cardiac conditions, the evolving standard of care points toward baseline (and follow-up) ECGs for *all* patients taking TCAs. As Stoudemire et al. (1995) noted, "A prolonged Q-T interval presents a relative contraindication to [TCA] treatment because of the hazard of malignant ventricular arrhythmias…prolonged Q-T intervals may…occur on a congenital basis and present problems in using TCAs. Such patients may not be symptomatic and may only be detected on a routine ECG" (p. 784).
[b]*Caution:* There is a theoretical risk of hypertension with concomitant MAOI.
[c]Anecdotal support only (Teitelman 2001).
Source. McElroy 1995; Pies and Shader 2003.

TABLE 2–16. Selected co-prescribed agents for antidepressant-induced sexual dysfunction

Agent	Mechanism of action in sexual dysfunction	Initial dosage	Selected risks/ side effects[a]
bupropion	Increased dopaminergic (and noradrenergic?) tone	75 mg qd or 1–2 hrs PTSA	Hypertension, increased seizure risk
methylphenidate	Increased dopaminergic (and noradrenergic?) tone	5–10 mg PTSA	Overstimulation, palpitations, tachycardia, potential abuse
cyproheptadine	Antagonism of 5-HT receptors	4–12 mg/day or PTSA	Sedation, dry mouth; may ↓ antidepressant effect
yohimbine	Increased NE outflow	5.4–10.8 mg qd or PTSA	Increased anxiety; hypertension; may aggravate opioid withdrawal; ? efficacy in females (not well studied)
sildenafil	Increased nitric oxide	50 mg PTSA	Hypotension, other cardiovascular side effects, drug interactions
bethanechol	Increased cholinergic tone	25–50 mg qd or PTSA	Diarrhea, autonomic side effects; numerous medical contraindications

Note. 5-HT=serotonin; NE=norepinephrine; PTSA=prior to sexual activity.
[a]List of side effects is *not* exhaustive: consult *Physicians' Desk Reference* (2004) for details.
Source. Hallward and Ellison 2001.

Drug–Drug Interactions

TABLE 2–17. Drug–drug interactions with tricyclic antidepressants (TCAs)

Drug added to TCA	Interaction
Anticholinergic agents	Urinary retention, constipation, dry mouth, dry eyes, blurry vision
Cimetidine, neuroleptics, SSRIs, oral contraceptives, isoniazid, acetaminophen, chloramphenicol, verapamil, quinidine, epinephrine, disulfiram, methylphenidate, methadone	Increased TCA blood levels, potential toxicity
Concomitant sympathomimetic use	Hypertension
Coumarin anticoagulants	Prolonged bleeding
Guanethidine, clonidine	Reduced antihypertensive effect
L-Dopa	Increased agitation Decreased plasma level of antidepressants
MAOIs	CNS toxicity, hyperpyrexia, serotonin syndrome (greatest risk is with MAOI plus clomipramine, imipramine, and perhaps desipramine; see Table 2–19)
Phenytoin, barbiturates, carbamazepine, phenylbutazone, rifampin, doxycycline	Decreased level/effect of antidepressants
Quinidine, procainamide	Prolonged cardiac conduction
Sedatives, tranquilizers (including benzodiazepines)	CNS depression

Note. CNS = central nervous system; MAOI = monoamine oxidase inhibitor; SSRI = selective serotonin reuptake inhibitor.

Source. Ciraulo et al. 1995a; Krishnan et al. 1996; Pies and Weinberg 1990.

TABLE 2–18. Some drugs used in clinical practice that may interact with selective serotonin reuptake inhibitors (SSRIs) and related antidepressants

Drug class/agent	Possible interaction effect	Possible mechanism of interaction
Antiarrhythmics (flecainide, propafenone, mexiletine)	↑ Blood level of antiarrhythmic	Inhibition of CYP 2D6 (which metabolizes antiarrhythmics) by SSRIs (especially paroxetine, fluoxetine)
Antibiotics (clarithromycin, erythromycin, ciprofloxacin)	↑ Levels of some antidepressants (sertraline, nefazodone, citalopram)	Inhibition of CYP 3A4 by antibiotics
Anticoagulant (warfarin)	↑ *S*-Warfarin levels in presence of fluvoxamine, perhaps other SSRIs	Inhibition of CYP 2C9 (which metabolizes *S*-enantiomer of warfarin) by fluvoxamine
Anticonvulsants (carbamazepine, oxcarbazepine, divalproex)	Variable and complex interactions: for example, 1. CBZ may ↓ some SSRI levels, whereas OXCB may ↑ them 2. SSRIs may ↑ CBZ levels 3. Concomitant use of valproate and fluoxetine may ↑ levels of both	1. "Pan-inducer" such as CBZ enhances drug metabolism and ↓ SSRI blood levels (OXCB may inhibit CYP 2C19, thus ↑ levels of some SSRIs) 2. Nefazodone and some SSRIs may inhibit CYP 3A4, ↑ CBZ or OXCB levels 3. DVPX may inhibit CYP 2D6 and other CYP enzymes involved in SSRI metabolism; fluoxetine may inhibit CYP 2C9/19, which is partly involved in DVPX metabolism

TABLE 2–18. Some drugs used in clinical practice that may interact with selective serotonin reuptake inhibitors (SSRIs) and related antidepressants *(continued)*

Drug class/agent	Possible interaction effect	Possible mechanism of interaction
Antidepressants (e.g., TCAs)[a]	Potentially both pharmacodyamic and pharmacokinetic interactions (e.g., 5-HT syndrome, ↑ blood levels of TCAs in presence of some SSRIs). Possibly fatal 5-HT syndrome when MAOIs combined with SSRIs	Combined serotonergic effects at level of the CNS, gut; inhibition of TCA or other antidepressant metabolism by SSRI (e.g., paroxetine, fluoxetine ↑ levels of desipramine)
Antifungals (ketoconazole, itraconazole)	↑ Blood level of some SSRIs, other newer agents (citalopram, sertraline, nefazodone)	Inhibition of metabolism of SSRIs and nefazodone via CYP 3A4
Antipsychotics	↑ Blood levels of some antipsychotics (e.g., fluoxetine/haloperidol, fluvoxamine/olanzapine) Possible ↑ EPS with coprescription of an SSRI	Inhibition of CYP 2D6 (fluoxetine, paroxetine) and 1A2 (fluvoxamine) by some SSRIs, leading to ↑ blood levels of haloperidol and risperidone (both 2D6 substrates) and olanzapine (1A2 substrate) ↑EPS may be a result of ↓ DA function due to SSRI
Benzodiazepines (BZDs)	↑ BZD blood levels and CNS effects	Variable inhibition of CYP 2C and 3A4 (which metabolize several BZDs, such as diazepam and alprazolam) by fluoxetine, fluvoxamine, and sertraline

TABLE 2–18. Some drugs used in clinical practice that may interact with selective serotonin reuptake inhibitors (SSRIs) and related antidepressants *(continued)*

Drug class/agent	Possible interaction effect	Possible mechanism of interaction
Calcium channel blockers (nifedipine, verapamil, diltiazem)	↑ Blood levels, cardiac effects of calcium channel blockers with some SSRIs and with nefazodone	Inhibition of calcium channel blocker metabolism by SSRI and nefazodone via CYP 3A4
"Herbal" or over-the-counter agents (St. John's wort, ginkgo), grapefruit juice	↑ Bleeding risk with SSRI + ginkgo; possible 5-HT syndrome with St. John's wort, but also potential for ↓ SSRI level; possible ↑ SSRI blood levels with grapefruit juice	Impairment of platelet function by SSRIs and ginkgo; St. John's wort has serotonergic effects, but also induces CYP 3A4; inhibition of 3A4 in gut by grapefruit juice
Narcotic analgesics (codeine, pentazocine, tramadol, methadone)	Possible ↓ codeine effect with paroxetine, fluoxetine[b]; possible ↑ methadone levels with fluvoxamine; possible 5-HT syndrome with tramadol and SSRIs	Possible reduction in conversion of codeine to active morphine by SSRI inhibition of CYP 2D6[b]; possible ↓ metabolism of methadone by fluvoxamine via CYP 3A4; possible ↑ serotonergic effects of tramadol and/or inhibition of its metabolism by SSRIs via 2D6

TABLE 2–18. Some drugs used in clinical practice that may interact with selective serotonin reuptake inhibitors (SSRIs) and related antidepressants *(continued)*

Drug class/agent	Possible interaction effect	Possible mechanism of interaction
Protease inhibitors (ritonavir, saquinavir) and NNRTIs (efavirenz, delavirdine)	Possible 5-HT syndrome with SSRI use; ↑ SSRI levels with protease inhibitors, NNRTIs; in theory, ↓ SSRI levels after *longer exposure* to ritonavir	Initial inhibition of CYP 2D6, 3A4 by ritonavir; but after days or weeks, possible *induction* of 3A4 by this agent Potent inhibition of CYP 3A4 by NNRTIs

Note. This table should not be construed as an exhaustive list of drug–drug interactions. See Cozza et al. 2003; Sandson 2003 for details. CBZ = carbamazepine; CNS = central nervous system; CYP = cytochrome P450; DA = dopamine; DVPX = divalproex; EPS = extrapyramidal side effects; 5-HT = serotonin; MAOI = monoamine oxidase inhibitor; NNRTI = non-nucleoside reverse transcriptase inhibitor; OXCB = oxcarbazepine; TCA = tricyclic antidepressant.

[a]Some antidepressant combinations may have therapeutic benefits (e.g., combination of mirtazapine and SSRI may mitigate some sexual and other SSRI side effects and augment antidepressant effect.

[b]The importance of this interaction has recently been questioned in several studies (see Cozza et al. 2003, pp. 333–334 for discussion).

Source. Bezchlibnyk-Butler and Jeffries 2000; Cozza et al. 2003.

TABLE 2–19. Drug–drug interactions with monoamine oxidase inhibitors (MAOIs)

Drug added to MAOI	Interaction
Atropine compounds	Increased anticholinergic effects
Fenfluramine	Confusional state (? hyperserotonergic effect)
Guanethidine, reserpine, clonidine	Reversal of antihypertensive effect; reserpine + MAOI may lead to hypomania
Insulin	Dangerous hypoglycemia
L-Dopa	Hypertension when used with nonselective or MAO-A–selective MAOI; appears to be safe with selective MAO-B inhibitor (selegiline 10 mg/day)
Meperidine, fentanyl	Toxic brain syndrome/serotonin syndrome, ANS collapse, death; codeine safer but not risk-free
Methadone	Minimal interaction, but needs careful monitoring
Methyldopa	CNS excitation, hypertension
Morphine	Hypotension
Other antihypertensive agents	Hypotension
Other MAOIs, sympathomimetic agents,[a] and tyramine	Hypertensive crisis when used concomitantly
Phentermine	Hypertensive reaction
Succinylcholine + phenelzine	Phenelzine may reduce cholinesterase levels, leading to increased levels of succinylcholine and prolonged apnea during ECT; tranylcypromine does not seem to have this effect
Sumatriptan	Increased sumatriptan effects
Thiazide diuretic	Increased risk of hypotension
TCAs (especially imipramine, clomipramine), SSRIs, buspirone, other serotonergic agents, dextromethorphan	Hyperserotonergic syndrome, severe confusional states, coma possible

Note. ANS = autonomic nervous system; CNS = central nervous system; ECT = electroconvulsive therapy; SSRI = selective serotonin reuptake inhibitor; TCA = tricyclic antidepressant.
[a]Including ephedrine, phenylephrine, phenylpropanolamine, dopamine, amphetamines.
Source. Ayd 1995; Creelman and Ciraulo 1995; Krishnan et al. 1996; Pies and Weinberg 1990.

TABLE 2–20. Food restrictions for patients taking conventional monoamine oxidase inhibitors (MAOIs)

Type of food	Avoid entirely	Probably safe in moderation
Cheese, dairy products	All matured or aged cheese; casseroles made with these cheeses (all cheeses except those in "safe" column)	Fresh cottage cheese, cream cheese, ricotta cheese, processed cheese slices All fresh milk products (including sour cream, yogurt, ice cream) if stored properly
Meat, fish, poultry	Aged/cured meats (e.g., fermented/dry sausage, pepperoni, salami, mortadella, summer sausage); improperly stored meat, fish, poultry; pickled herring	All fresh/properly refrigerated packaged or processed meat, fish, poultry
Fruits, vegetables	Broad bean pods; overripe figs; banana peel; ? fava beans[a]	All fruits (including banana pulp) and vegetables (except those listed in "avoid" column)
Alcoholic beverages	All tap beers; ? red wine,[a] ? bottled/canned beer[a]	Vodka, gin, white wine, canned or bottled beer, including nonalcoholic type (no more than one bottle or can per day)
Miscellaneous	Marmite concentrated yeast extract, sauerkraut, soy sauce and other soybean condiments, tofu	Brewer's yeast, breads, soy milk

[a]Some disagreement in published literature. Patients are generally best advised to err on the side of caution because identical foods and beverages vary widely in tyramine content from region to region.

Source. Gardner et al. 1996.

TABLE 2–21. The serotonin syndrome: differential diagnosis

	Serotonin syndrome	NMS	Malignant hyperthermia	Lethal (pernicious) catatonia	Central anticholinergic syndrome
Core symptoms	*Variable temperature elevation* (to 37.4°C–42.5°C) Mental status changes *Hypomania* Restlessness Myoclonus Hyperreflexia Diaphoresis *Shivering/teeth chattering* Tremor Diarrhea Incoordination	Hyperthermia Severe muscle rigidity (usually "lead pipe") Diaphoresis Delirium Muteness Incontinence Rhabdomyolysis *Autonomic instability (fluctuating blood pressure, pallor/flushing)* Tremulousness Tachycardia Tachypnea Extrapyramidal symptoms *Most common temporal sequence: mental status change → rigidity → autonomic → hyperthermia*	Hyperthermia (core temperature >41°C) Muscle rigidity Ischemia Hot skin *Mottled cyanosis* *Hypotension* Rhabdomyolysis	Hyperthermia Muscle rigidity Diaphoresis Delirium *Extreme hyper-activity* (often early in syndrome) or stupor *Psychotic prodrome* *Mutism* *Posturing* *Stupor alternating with excitement* Hypertension Tremulousness	Hyperthermia *Decreased sweating* Hot, *dry skin* Dilated, *sluggish pupils* Tachycardia *Constipation* *Urinary retention* Confusion Impaired memory Delirium Hallucinations

TABLE 2–21. The serotonin syndrome: differential diagnosis *(continued)*

	Serotonin syndrome	NMS	Malignant hyperthermia	Lethal (pernicious) catatonia	Central anticholinergic syndrome
Laboratory findings	No specific findings	*Elevated CPK levels,* WBC, LFTs; myoglobinuria	*Disseminated intravascular coagulation* *Respiratory/ metabolite acidosis, hyperkalemia, hypermagne-semia*	No specific findings	No specific findings
Causes/ mechanisms	Activation of 5-HT_{1A} receptors in brain stem, spinal cord; enhancement of overall 5-HT neurotransmission. Most commonly due to interaction between MAOI and serotonergic agent (L-tryptophan, SSRI); but may occur with any serotonergic drug	Presumed: blockade of dopaminergic pathways in basal ganglia and hypothalamus; also may result from sudden withdrawal of DA agonist. ? May be precipitated by lithium ? Low serum levels of iron	Inherited disorder; triggering anes-thetic (halothane, methoxyflurane) causes calcium release from sarco-plasmic reticu-lum, leading to activation of myosin ATPase, heat production	Manic and depressed mood states; schizophrenia (also secondary to infection, metabolic, other medical disorders)	Blockade of central and peripheral muscarinic receptors (due to, e.g., tricyclic or phenothiazine)

TABLE 2–21. The serotonin syndrome: differential diagnosis *(continued)*

	Serotonin syndrome	NMS	Malignant hyperthermia	Lethal (pernicious) catatonia	Central anticholinergic syndrome
Management	Discontinue suspected agent; use supportive measures (cooling blanket for hyperthermia); propranolol, methysergide, cyproheptadine may help	Use supportive measures (cooling); stop neuroleptic; no clear treatment of choice, but DA agonists (bromocriptine 5 mg tid), dantrolene, ECT may help	Dantrolene sodium 1 mg/kg via rapid intravenous infusion; 100% O_2; sodium bicarbonate; external cooling	Some recommend ECT as treatment of choice (within first 5 days); lorazepam 1–2 mg po or im up to qid also useful; neuroleptics generally best withheld	Remove offending agent; physostigmine usually not indicated (? unless cardiac arrhythmia is present)

Note. *Italics* show features that help differentiate syndromes. Some authors believe that neuroleptic malignant syndrome and lethal catatonia are closely related syndromes.

CPK=creatine phosphokinase; DA=dopamine; ECT=electroconvulsive therapy; 5-HT=serotonin; LFT=liver function test; MAOI=monoamine oxidase inhibitor; SSRI=selective serotonin reuptake inhibitor; WBC=white blood cell count.

Source. Ayd 1995; Castillo et al. 1989; Fink 1996; Fink et al. 1993; Jenkins et al. 2001; Pearlman 1986; Petersdorf 1991; Sternbach 1991; Theoharides et al. 1995; Velamoor et al. 1995.

TABLE 2–22. Serotonin syndrome

Symptom	**Patients reporting symptoms, % (*N*=38)**
Confusion	42
Hypomania	21
Restlessness	45
Myoclonus	34
Hyperreflexia	29
Diaphoresis	26
Shivering	26
Tremor	26
Diarrhea	16
Incoordination	13

Source. Sternbach 1991.

Potentiating Maneuvers

TABLE 2–23. Agents used to potentiate or augment antidepressants

Agent	Rationale/Comments
Antipsychotics	Almost always necessary in treatment of psychotic depression; olanzapine may augment fluoxetine in nonpsychotic, refractory unipolar major depression. One open-label study found ziprasidone augmentation useful in treating SSRI-resistant major depression. *Caution:* Some antidepressants may inhibit the clearance of various antipsychotics.
Buspirone	At high dosages (>50 mg/day), buspirone has antidepressant properties; may be useful as an augmenting agent for ongoing tricyclic or SSRI treatment. (However, buspirone, a partial 5-HT agonist, can in some cases undermine the effects of SSRIs.)
Dopaminergic agonists (e.g., pergolide, pramipexole)	Augmenting dopaminergic function may be necessary in some patients with atypical depression or in those taking SSRIs (who may have reduced dopamine in some brain regions).
Estrogen	Data are not yet conclusive, but estrogen may augment central noradrenergic and/or serotonergic activity. Could be used in refractory cases after other augmentation agents have failed; may have role in perimenopausal depression.
Lithium	Probably enhances serotonergic function. Lithium augmentation is sustained and may reduce relapse rate. Response to lithium augmentation may be within the first week, but it usually takes longer.
Psychostimulants (e.g., methylphenidate)	May enhance dopaminergic function, reduce drowsiness, counteract sexual side effects of SSRIs. One small, open study suggests acceleration of response to citalopram in depressed elderly patients (mean dosage of methylphenidate = 12 mg/day).
Modafinil	Uncontrolled data suggest possible augmenting effect when combined with SSRIs. Possible risk of manic switch with high doses.

TABLE 2–23. Agents used to potentiate or augment antidepressants *(continued)*

Agent	Rationale/Comments
Thyroid hormone (usually T_3)	Some depressed patients have subclinical hypothyroidism (e.g., normal T_3, T_4, slightly elevated TSH levels). Even euthyroid patients, however, may benefit. T_3 may be better than T_4 for unipolar depression. T_4 may be better as mood stabilizer in rapid-cycling bipolar disorder. Optimal dosage of T_3 is 15–25 μg/day. Most data in unipolar depression involve addition of T_3 to a tricyclic; only a few case reports suggest efficacy when T_3 is added to SSRIs. Avoid thyroid augmentation in patients with atrial fibrillation, coronary artery disease, osteoporosis.

Note. 5-HT = serotonin; SSRI = selective serotonin reuptake inhibitor; T_3 = triiodothyronine; T_4 = thyroxine; TSH = thyroid-stimulating hormone.

Source. Charney et al. 1995; Joffe 2001; Lavretsky et al. 2003; Markovitz and Wagner 2003; Menza et al. 2000; O'Reardon 2004; Shelton et al. 2001.

TABLE 2–24. Psychostimulants and related agents: main features

Medication	Duration of clinical effects, hours	Dosage[a]	Comments
Methylphenidate			
Short-acting			
Ritalin	3–4	5–30 mg bid	Methylphenidate
Focalin	3–4	2.5–10 mg bid	Dexmethylphenidate
Methylin	3–4	5–30 mg bid	Methylphenidate
Intermediate-acting			
Ritalin SR	4–8[b]	20–60 mg qam	Continuous release
Metadate ER	4–8[b]	20–60 mg qam	Continuous release
Methylin ER	4–8	20–60 mg qam	
Long-acting			
Concerta	12	18–56 mg qam	Osmotically controlled release; provides initial bolus, with peak at 1–2 hours, then continuous release, with peak at about 7 hours; mimics tid dosing of standard methylphenidate
Metadate CD	8	20–60 mg qam	Bead delivery system for biphasic release; mimics bid dosing; peaks at about 1.5 and 4.5 hours after dosing
Ritalin LA	8–12	20–60 mg qam	Mimics bid dosing of standard methylphenidate; bead delivery system
Amphetamine			
Short-acting			
Dexedrine	3–5	5–20 mg bid	Dextroamphetamine
Dextrostat	3–5	5–20 mg bid	Dextroamphetamine

TABLE 2–24. Psychostimulants and related agents: main features *(continued)*

Medication	Duration of clinical effects, hours	Dosage[a]	Comments
Amphetamine *(continued)*			
Intermediate-acting			
Adderall	4–8	5–30 mg bid or 5–60 mg qam	Mixed salt of L- and D-amphetamine
Long-acting			
Dexedrine Spansules	5–8	20 mg qam	Initial bolus, then continuous release; beads
Adderall XR	8–12	5–30 mg qam	Mixed salt of L- and D-amphetamine; immediate- and delayed-release beads; mimics bid dosing of Adderall
Nonstimulants			
Atomoxetine	May act via long-term effects on brain despite short $t_{1/2}$ of 3 hours	0.5–1.2 mg/kg per day (40–80 mg/day) (either as single dose or bid regimen)	Not considered a stimulant and not classified as controlled substance; however, "mood swings," excitation have been reported; works as selective norepinephrine reuptake inhibitor; substrate of CYP 2D6 (subject to drug interactions)

Note. CYP = cytochrome P450; $t_{1/2}$ = half-life.

[a]Dosages and dosing schedules have been derived from the literature on treatment of attention-deficit/hyperactivity disorder (ADHD) and are not necessarily applicable when psychostimulants are used as adjuncts in mood disorders. In general, dosages for adjunctive treatment of depression tend to be about 50% of those used in ADHD.

[b]Less predictable because of wax matrix.

Source. Modified from Carlat 2003b; Oesterheld et al. 2003; Physicians' Desk Reference 2004; Rosenblatt and Rosenblatt 2003; Witcher et al. 2003.

Use in Special Populations

TABLE 2–25. Selection of nontricyclic antidepressants for patients with special needs or comorbid conditions

Comorbidity	Preferred agents[a]	Rationale
"Atypical" features (hypersomnia, hyperphagia)	Bupropion, fluoxetine, venlafaxine	Bupropion, fluoxetine may be more "alerting"; fluoxetine, other SSRIs may decrease carbohydrate craving. Venlafaxine is generally less sedating than other agents, does not appear to promote weight gain.
Cardiac disease	SSRIs, bupropion *Possibly* nefazodone[b] (watch for CYP 3A4 interactions, orthostatic hypotension), venlafaxine (may ↑ diastolic BP); mirtazapine (some concern about ↑ cholesterol, occasional PVCs, bradycardia with mirtazapine)	SSRIs, bupropion, venlafaxine, mirtazapine have minimal effects on cardiac conduction; rarely associated with arrhythmias. Monitor vitals, and use cautious dosing with these agents.
Obesity	Bupropion, fluoxetine (? other SSRIs)	SSRIs may decrease carbohydrate craving. *Note:* Fluoxetine may cause unwanted weight loss in the elderly; conversely, mirtazapine may promote some weight gain in cachectic elderly patients. One study in overweight women found bupropion useful as a weight loss agent—but caution if combined with other antidepressants (may affect blood levels of either agent).

TABLE 2–25. Selection of nontricyclic antidepressants for patients with special needs or comorbid conditions *(continued)*

Comorbidity	Preferred agents[a]	Rationale
Diabetes mellitus	Bupropion, venlafaxine, SSRIs; *possibly* nefazodone[b]	Little effect on blood glucose level (bupropion, venlafaxine) or hypoglycemic effect (SSRIs).
ADHD	Bupropion, venlafaxine	Some data suggest efficacy in ADHD.
Nicotine dependence	Bupropion	May help with smoking cessation.
Bulimia	Fluoxetine	Best-studied SSRI for this condition.
Severe insomnia with comorbid depression	Mirtazapine; nefazodone[b]	Both agents are sedating, given at bedtime; nefazodone has no adverse effects on normal sleep architecture.
Parkinson's disease	TCAs; ? SSRIs; ? bupropion	Anticholinergic effects of TCAs may be helpful; SSRIs may be well tolerated but, in a few patients, may decrease dopamine and worsen EPS. In theory, bupropion's dopaminergic effects may be useful, but data are mixed.
Seizure disorder	Desipramine, SSRIs, MAOIs	Lower seizure threshold less than do others; avoid bupropion, maprotiline, clomipramine (relatively high incidence of seizures at dosages >250 mg/day).
Peptic ulcer disease	TCAs (e.g., doxepin)	Blockade of histamine H_2 receptor reduces gastric acid.
Respiratory (pulmonary) disease	SSRIs (most data with sertraline)	May reduce anxiety and dyspnea; little effect on pulmonary functions.
Sexual dysfunction	Bupropion, nefazodone,[b] mirtazapine	Very rarely associated with sexual dysfunction; may ameliorate it in patients taking SSRIs.

TABLE 2–25. Selection of nontricyclic antidepressants for patients with special needs or comorbid conditions *(continued)*

Comorbidity	Preferred agents[a]	Rationale
Angle closure glaucoma	SSRIs, bupropion, nefazodone[b]	Lack of anticholinergic effects; avoid TCAs.
Anxiety disorder	SSRIs, nefazodone[b]	SSRIs useful for panic disorder, OCD, ? generalized anxiety. Preliminary data suggest nefazodone may be helpful for panic attacks.

Note. ADHD=attention-deficit/hyperactivity disorder; BP=blood pressure; CYP=cytochrome P450; EPS=extrapyramidal side effects; MAOI=monoamine oxidase inhibitor; OCD=obsessive-compulsive disorder; PVC=premature ventricular contraction; SSRI=selective serotonin reuptake inhibitor; TCA=tricyclic antidepressant.

[a]Based mainly on anecdotal and open studies.

[b]Despite nefazodone's favorable pharmacodynamic profile, the black box warning of hepatotoxicity renders nefazodone a second-line agent for most patients. All but generic versions of nefazodone have been discontinued in the United States and Canada.

Source. Apter and Kushner 1996; Charney et al. 1995; Cole et al. 1996; Gadde et al. 2001; Glassman et al. 1993; Goodnick et al. 1995; Harnett 2001; Jacobson et al. 2002; Smoller et al. 1998.

TABLE 2–26. Antidepressant dosing in children and adolescents

Agent	Initial dose range (mg)	Target dosage (mg/kg per day)	Schedule
Fluoxetine[a]	10–20 qam	0.25–0.70	qd–bid
Paroxetine[b]	5–10 qam	0.25–0.70	qd–bid
Sertraline	12.5–50 qam	1.5–3.0	qd–bid
Citalopram	10 qam	0.25–0.70	qd
Escitalopram	5 qam	0.125–0.35	qd
Venlafaxine (extended-release)	25–37.5 qam	1.0–3.0	qd–bid
Mirtazapine	7.5–15 qhs	0.2–0.4	qhs or bid
Nefazodone[c]	25–50 bid	4.0–8.0	bid
Bupropion (slow-release)	50–100 qam	2.0–4.0	qd–bid

[a]Has U.S. Food and Drug Administration (FDA)–approved labeling for treatment of depression in children and adolescents.

[b]The FDA has recently recommended against use of paroxetine (Paxil) in children and adolescents.

[c]Labeling notes black box warning for hepatotoxicity. All but generic versions have been effectively taken off U.S. market.

Source. Adapted from Bostic et al. 2003.

Questions and Answers

Drug Class

Q. Are any of the antidepressants (ADs) formulated for intramuscular or intravenous use? Is there any experience with the latter for treatment of depression or other conditions?

A. Intramuscular preparations are available for amitriptyline, imipramine, and doxepin. A long-acting, injectable form of imipramine (imipramine pamoate) is also available. These intramuscular formulations may sometimes be useful in medically ill patients (see subsection "Use in Special Populations" in "Overview" section of this chapter). Clomipramine is available in intravenous form and, in Europe, has been used to treat both obsessive-compulsive disorder (OCD) and major depression. At least for OCD, the data suggest that intravenous clomipramine may reduce symptoms more quickly than oral clomipramine and (surprisingly) is better tolerated (Koran et al. 1997). A recent study using intravenous citalopram found that it was effective and well tolerated in patients with refractory OCD (Pallanti et al. 2002).

Indications

Q. What factors are considered in choosing a particular AD for a given patient?

A. Since all ADs are roughly equal in efficacy, the choice of agent depends on the patient's personal, medical, and symptomatic profile. *Past response* to a particular agent is an important concern—for example, demonstration that a patient had an excellent response to agent A in the past is a compelling reason to use agent A for the index episode. To some degree, the *response of a family member* may be useful—for example, if a first-degree relative has responded well to agent A, this agent may be a good choice for the patient, all other factors being equal. The patient's *age and associated medical conditions* are critical factors in choosing an AD. Thus, the elderly are usually not good candidates for highly sedating, anticholinergic agents, such as tertiary tricyclics. The presence of a *cardiac conduction abnormality, urinary retention,* or *narrow angle-*

glaucoma would also be a relative contraindication for use of a tricyclic antidepressant (TCA). A patient's known or presumed *suicide risk* is an important factor, since the TCAs are much more toxic in overdose than most newer agents, such as the selective serotonin reuptake inhibitor (SSRIs). Among the TCAs, desipramine appears to have higher toxicity in overdose. The *symptom picture of the patient's depression*, while not relevant to the ultimate benefits of AD treatment, may influence the choice of agent, based on the patient's comfort during the first few weeks of treatment. Thus, a more sedating/anxiolytic agent (e.g., mirtazapine) may *initially* be preferable to more "activating" agents (e.g., desipramine or bupropion) for depressed patients with severe insomnia, anxiety, and agitation. (Bupropion seems to have less robust benefits for anxiety and agitation.) *Cost* is also an important consideration for many patients. The tablet-for-tablet cost of TCAs is much less than that for newer agents; however, the *cost-effectiveness* of the newer agents may be greater in the long run because of the greater likelihood of serious adverse reactions requiring urgent care, more frequent plasma level monitoring, and the somewhat higher dropout rate for the TCAs. Nevertheless, the overall number of patients completing treatment with TCAs versus SSRIs is relatively similar (Nelson 1994), and the choice of agent must remain a highly individualized decision involving all of the above factors (Pies 1995). Finally, concomitant medications also play an important role in treatment selection, since many of the AD agents are involved in drug–drug interactions.

Q. When does a patient with unipolar major depression need to be maintained indefinitely on an AD?

A. Around 75% of individuals who suffer a first episode of major depression will go on to have multiple episodes (Greden 1995–1996). The more episodes a patient has, the more the clinician can expect the patient to have, and the closer together these episodes will occur. Episodes also tend to be longer lasting and more severe over the course of the patient's lifetime (Greden 1995–1996; Post 1994). Greden (1995–1996) believes that the best rule of thumb for the clinician is "Three strikes and you're on"—that is, with three or more episodes of major depression, the patient should remain "on" AD indefinitely. This strategy will reduce the recurrence rate for most patients. In contrast, around 75% of untreated patients with recurrent major depression will relapse within a year after discontinuing medication. Of course, the decision to maintain a patient on ADs must be based on informed consent, in which *all* the relevant factors—for example, actual benefit from medication; medication side effects; degree of incapacity when not taking medication—are carefully considered. Finally, highly recurrent major depression should always raise a question of covert bipolar disorder (Ghaemi 2003).

Q. Is there an AD of first choice in treating patients with borderline personality disorder (BPD)?

A. It could be argued that the indications for *any* psychotropic in treating BPD are questionable, based on the most rigorous studies (see Cornelius et al. 1993; Zanarini and Silk 2001). Long-term success is apparently quite limited with the use of ADs in BPD patients, although many reports suggest short-term improvement in some BPD symptoms. On the other hand, amitriptyline may actually *worsen* behavioral dyscontrol in some BPD patients. Monoamine oxidase inhibitors (MAOIs) may be helpful in some BPD patients whose symptoms fit Klein's description of "hysteroid dysphoria" (high rejection sensitivity, histrionic when not depressed, frequent abuse of diet pills/stimulants, hypersomnic/lethargic when depressed); however, the risks associated with the misuse of MAOIs are significant, and some BPD patients will "test out" the dangers of, for example, tyramine-rich foods. Since many BPD patients have symptoms that also fit the criteria for posttraumatic stress disorder (PTSD), the SSRIs may make sense, given that serotonergic agents seem to ameliorate some symptoms of PTSD. Impulsivity and aggression, as often seen in BPD, are probably mediated by low serotonergic function, and it would seem reasonable that SSRIs would reduce these aspects of BPD. However, a recent double-blind, placebo-controlled, randomized trial of fluvoxamine for 6 weeks (followed by a blind half-crossover for 6 weeks, and an open follow-up for another 12 weeks) was conducted with 38 nonschizophrenic, nonbipolar female patients with BPD (Rinne et al. 2002). Fluvoxamine, but not placebo, produced a robust and long-lasting *reduction in rapid mood shifts*. However, somewhat surprisingly, no difference between the fluvoxamine and placebo groups was observed in the effect on impulsivity and aggression scores. Further randomized studies with other SSRIs are clearly needed.

Q. Can any AD be used in treating patients with OCD, and if so, are certain types better?

A. ADs that lack serotonergic properties have little effect in the treatment of OCD. Thus, the recommended first-line agents for OCD are the SSRIs (and clomipramine, though this is less commonly used). All the SSRIs except citalopram have FDA-approved labeling for use in OCD, although citalopram appears to have efficacy as well (Pallanti et al. 2002).

A highly noradrenergic TCA such as desipramine is not likely to be effective in OCD, though it may be effective for comorbid major depression (which often accompanies OCD). Bupropion has also not been shown to be effective in OCD (Zajecka 1995). A case report from Zajecka and colleagues (1990) found that venlafaxine had anti-obsessional effects in a patient with coexisting major depression and OCD. Another case report from Grossman and Hollander (1996) found venlafaxine useful in treating a man with OCD with no comorbidity whose symptoms had been refractory to paroxetine. Rauch and colleagues (1996) reported the successful use of venlafaxine in a small group of OCD patients; however, minor side effects (especially nausea) were common, and a "troublesome" withdrawal syndrome developed in four patients whose venlafaxine was tapered and discontinued over a period of 4–14 days. Nefazodone has not been systematically tested in OCD, though a case report noted emergence of obsessive symptoms in a depressed patient whose depression had actually responded to nefazodone (Sofuoglu and DeBattista 1996). Remember that OCD requires a different dosage and/or time course than major depression; namely, higher doses of ADs for longer periods of time may be necessary in patients with OCD (Taylor 1995).

Q. Can ADs be used in treating patients with panic disorder (PD), and if so, do they all work equally well?

A. SSRIs have been shown, in several studies, to be effective for PD and are now considered first-line treatments. All SSRIs are probably useful; fluoxetine, paroxetine, and sertraline have FDA-approved labeling for PD. Imipramine and MAOIs such as phenelzine are the "old standbys" and are the ADs most thoroughly studied for use in PD. Other TCAs, such as desipramine, nortriptyline, clomipramine, and amitriptyline, have been found to be effective in a limited number of studies, but there are few comparative data (Taylor 1995). In contrast, bupropion does *not* seem to have robust antipanic properties (Zajecka 1995).

Some early anecdotal data suggest that both venlafaxine and nefazodone are effective antipanic agents, and nefazodone seems useful in the reduction of generalized anxiety and agitation when compared with imipramine (Zajecka 1995). However, nefazodone (as the brand Serzone) is no longer being produced or marketed in the United States. AD agents are not effective for PD acutely (e.g., to abort an attack already under way) and may actually worsen both generalized and panic-type anxiety when first administered. Some data suggest that the final target dose of an SSRI may need to be higher in PD than in depression (Sutherland and Krishnan 2001). It is important, however, to *begin* with a *small* dose of an SSRI (or imipramine)—for example, 2.5–5.0 mg of fluoxetine (or 10 mg of imipramine), with very gradual upward titration—in order to avoid overstimulation.

Q. What is the role of ADs in treating patients with mixed anxiety-depressive (MAD) states?

A. Most of the available ADs have demonstrated some degree of benefit in MAD states, though controlled studies of well-defined patients with MAD are lacking (Zajecka 1995). SSRIs, MAOIs, and nefazodone may be especially effective in MAD patients, though large-scale controlled studies are lacking. The presentation of some patients with "atypical depression" clearly overlaps with that of MAD patients, though the definition of "atypical" has varied widely in the literature (Pies 1988). Nevertheless, there is a strong clinical impression that MAOIs may be superior to TCAs for atypical depression with prominent anxiety (Zajecka 1995).

Q. Are the MAOIs especially effective in treating patients with "atypical depression"?

A. The term *atypical depression* has had many meanings over the years. Ironically, patients with "atypical" features, variously defined, are quite common in clinical practice (see Pies 1988; Pies and Shader 2003). While one meaning of "atypical depression" has, indeed, included marked anxiety or panic attacks, that is not the sense in which the term is used in DSM-IV-TR (American Psychiatric Association 2000); there, the specifier "with atypical features" applies to patients who show a) mood reactivity (i.e., mood brightens in response to positive events) and b) two or more of the following: significant weight gain or hyperphagia; hypersomnia; "leaden paralysis"; and a long-standing pattern of interpersonal rejection sensitivity. These criteria were heavily influenced by the research of the "Columbia Group" (see Quitkin et al. 1988) and differ somewhat from the clinical features of the "anxious, phobic" patients described in some early British studies (e.g., West and Dally 1959).

Though some studies have shown MAOIs to be superior to TCAs in treating anxious depressive patients, most of the "pro-MAOI" data stem from studies of patients who met the Columbia criteria for atypical depression and who underwent treatment with either imipramine or the MAOI phenelzine. The Columbia criteria may identify, as Davidson (1992) noted, "a type of depression which is somewhat unresponsive to imipramine, although the effects of imipramine would still appear to outweigh those of placebo" (p. 347). Some authors have erroneously concluded from these limited data that MAOIs "don't work" for patients with "typical" depression (e.g., patients with major depression and melancholic features), although there is little evidence for this view (Giller et al. 1984). In short: MAOIs appear more effective for some atypically depressed patients, though these persons are not necessarily those with MAD, and may also be effective for patients whose symptoms do not meet the criteria for atypicality.

Q. Are ADs useful in treating patients with dysthymic disorder?

A. Yes, though there have been only a few controlled studies of "pure" dysthymia in which ADs were used. Overall, both imipramine and the SSRIs were superior to placebo (Harrison and Stewart 1995). In one large, multicenter study (N=416) of early-onset dysthymic disorder, imipramine and sertraline were shown to be similarly effective, and both were more effective than placebo (Kocsis et al. 1994). The sertraline group had a significantly lower rate of discontinuation (due to side effects) than did the imipramine group (25% vs. 51%). In an open study of primary dysthymia using a dichotomy developed by Akiskal (1983) and colleagues, Ravindran and colleagues (1994) found fluoxetine effective in patients with the *subaffective,* but not the character spectrum, subtype of dysthymia (77% vs. 25% response rate). The subaffective dysthymic patients are essentially those with some melancholic features and a family history of mood disorders. The character spectrum patients are those who show significant character pathology, drug/alcohol abuse, and a family history of alcoholism and personality disorder more so than mood disorder. One interpretation of this study is that the more dysthymic patients resemble patients with "classic" major depression, the better their response to an SSRI. Some patients labeled as being "dysthymic" may also respond to MAOIs (Harrison and Stewart 1995). The response of dysthymic patients to SSRIs may take as long as 6–16 weeks. This protracted response time was confirmed by a German study (Albert and Ebert 1996) in which fluvoxamine was administered to patients with pure dysthymia who had not responded to 6 weeks of a TCA followed by 6 weeks of fluvoxamine. The patients kept taking fluvoxamine for another 10 weeks at the maximum dosage (300 mg/day). By week 8 of fluvoxamine treatment, only 11% were responders. But by week 16, 53% of the refractory patients had responded, as determined by Hamilton Rating Scale for Depression scores. There was no control group, so conclusions are tentative. However, it seems prudent to extend AD trials in patients with refractory dysthymia well beyond the usual 6 weeks deemed adequate for major depression. Recently, in a single-blind randomized clinical trial (Browne et al. 2002), 707 adults with DSM-IV dysthymic disorder, with or without past and/or current major depression, were randomized to treatment with either sertraline alone (50–200 mg), interpersonal therapy (IPT) alone, or sertraline and IPT combined. Sertraline or sertraline plus IPT was more effective than IPT alone after 6 months. Over the long term (2 years), all three treatments were reasonably effective, but sertraline and sertraline plus IPT were more effective than IPT alone.

Mechanisms of Action

Q. What is the role of serotonin (5-HT) receptors in the mechanism of ADs?

A. Although the story is incomplete, it seems likely that serotonergic *autoreceptors* are intimately involved in the mechanism of action (MOA) of SSRIs and some other serotonergic ADs. Initially, SSRIs increase synaptic levels of 5-HT in specific brain regions. However, serotonergic neuron firing activity actually *decreases* at first, owing to activation of 5-HT_{1A} autoreceptors on the cell body—the "brake pedal" that normally reduces presynaptic 5-HT release. This may account for the "lag phase" of several weeks prior to AD response (Blier 2003). After a few weeks, these same autoreceptors may become "desensitized," and the serotonergic neuron firing rate returns to normal. With ongoing treatment, it appears that other autoreceptors on *nerve terminals*—$5\text{-HT}_{1B/D}$ autoreceptors—also become desensitized, leading to a net increase in 5-HT function in the system. Thus, the reuptake blockade that gives SSRIs their somewhat inappropriate name may not be the "real" MOA of these agents (which probably occurs at the level of the gene, as discussed below). Finally, recent research points to genetic variation (polymorphism) in the 5-HT transporter gene as a factor in response to the SSRI citalopram (Arias et al. 2003).

Q. Do SSRIs affect other neurotransmitters (or neurotransmitter tracts) besides 5-HT?

A. Yes. In fact, the most recent data, based on cloned human monoamine transporter studies (Richelson 2003), suggest that the term *selective serotonin reuptake inhibitor* is inappropriate. As shown in Table 2–6, sertraline has prominent *dopaminergic* effects (comparable to those of methylphenidate), and paroxetine demonstrates strong *noradrenergic* reuptake blockade. Somewhat paradoxically, venlafaxine—often called an "SNRI" (serotonin-norepinephrine reuptake inhibitor)—may actually function as an SSRI at dosages less than 300 mg/day. Furthermore, SSRIs may indirectly *reduce the firing rate of norepinephrine (NE) neurons* in the locus coeruleus, probably via GABAergic interneurons. This effect appears to be mediated by 5-HT_{2A} receptors (Blier 2003). In theory, SSRIs might lead to anxiolytic effects, since excessive NE activity in the locus coeruleus has been implicated in panic disorder; however, this same reduced NE activity may "undercut" some SSRI's AD effects in a subset of patients (Blier 2003). Again, the term *selective serotonin reuptake inhibitor* is misleading. This highlights a principle that is becoming increasingly important in neuropharmacology: the interdependence of neurotransmitter systems. It is doubtful, on a neurochemical level, that there are "pure" effectors of only one neurotransmitter system among the available ADs.

Q. Some postmortem data suggest that in major depression, there may be pathological "up-regulation" of 5-HT_2 receptors in the brain (Fava 2003). Do ADs work by altering this receptor?

A. Although 5-HT_2 receptors appear to be involved in both the etiology of depression and AD effects, it is not clear that 5-HT_2 receptors are causally involved in the antidepressant action of most ADs. Thus, down-regulation of 5-HT_2 receptors seems to be a common mechanism of TCAs and SSRIs. But since electroconvulsive therapy (ECT) may *increase* the density of 5-HT_2 receptors (in rodent studies) and is an extremely effective AD, it seems unlikely that 5-HT_2 down-regulation per se is necessary for AD effectiveness (Leonard 1996). On the other hand, *antagonism* of the aforementioned 5-HT_{2A} receptor—as seen with most atypical antipsychotics and with the AD *nefazodone*—may reduce the inhibitory effect of serotonergic neurons on noradrenergic neurons (Blier 2003). This action could have indirect AD effects in some patients. Nefazodone also produces modest 5-HT, NE, and dopamine reuptake blockade (Richelson 2003).

Q. What is the role of noradrenergic and dopaminergic function in the MOA of ADs?

A. In animal studies, chronic AD treatment leads to decreased activity and density of cortical β adrenoreceptors, increased density of cortical α_1 adrenoreceptors, and decreased functional activity of cortical α_2 autoreceptors (Leonard 1996). These autoreceptors normally exert an inhibitory influence on NE "outflow," analogous to the role of 5-HT_{1A} autoreceptors in reducing presynaptic 5-HT release. It is difficult to subsume all these changes under a simple "increase" or "decrease" model of noradrenergic function; rather, these changes, if applicable in humans, seem to indicate a subtle reconfiguring of noradrenergic function, perhaps favoring a net increase in noradrenergic activity. Chronic AD treatment also leads to decreased functional activity of dopamine autoreceptors in rat brain cortex, implying a net increase in dopaminergic function (Leonard 1996). Blockade of the dopamine transporter with, for example, nefazodone, sertraline, or methylphenidate is usually associated with increased motivation and psychomotor activity and, in some cases, mania or psychosis (Richelson 2003).

Q. Mirtazapine seems to work via an atypical MOA. How does it differ from, say, venlafaxine?

A. Mirtazapine is the only AD that affects both 5-HT and NE via a "non-reuptake" MOA; in contrast, for example, to paroxetine and venlafaxine, which inhibit reuptake of both 5-HT and NE (Richelson 2003). Instead, mirtazapine antagonizes the α_2 adrenoreceptor, which normally reduces NE outflow; thus, mirtazapine "releases" the noradrenergic neuron from its autoreceptor, leading to increased NE outflow. By antagonizing α_2 *heteroreceptors* located on serotonergic nerve terminals, mirtazapine also leads to increased 5-HT output. Since mirtazapine blocks 5-HT_2 and 5-HT_3 receptors, its serotonergic effect is more selectively directed at 5-HT_{1A} receptors, the activation of which is thought to have AD and perhaps anxiolytic effects. Moreover, the lack of 5-HT_2 and 5-HT_3 activation seems to reduce typical serotonergic side effects, such as sexual dysfunction and gastrointestinal (GI) complaints.

Q. Are there ADs now under development that work via new monoamine-based biochemical mechanisms?

A. Several agents now being tested (e.g., idazoxan and mianserin) act as α_2 adrenoreceptor antagonists. As noted in the "Overview" of this chapter (see subsection "Mechanisms of Action"), antagonism of this autoreceptor leads to enhanced noradrenergic outflow from the presynaptic neuron. In addition to the already-available SNRI, other SNRIs such as duloxetine, are also being developed. Some data suggest these agents may be more effective than SSRIs in achieving remission from depression. Milnacipran is another SNRI that is being tested in the United States for treatment of fibromyalgia (Stahl and Grady 2003) and could find its way into the AD market. Milnacipran appears to have equivalent reuptake inhibition for both NE and 5-HT, with few antimuscarinic or antihistaminic effects. It is effective as an AD at dosages of 50–100 mg/day (Morishita and Arita 2003). Selective NRIs, including reboxetine and atomoxetine, are not currently used as ADs in the United States, though reboxetine is available in Europe as an AD. Stahl and Grady (2003) note that atomoxetine should have AD properties, either as monotherapy or in combination with other ADs; however, in the United States, it is now marketed only for use in treating ADHD. Other monoamine-based agents being investigated as ADs include 5-HT_{1A} partial agonists (e.g., gepirone); 5-HT_{1D} antagonists; reversible inhibitors of MAO-A (RIMAs) (e.g., befloxatone); and transdermal selegiline (an MAOI with selectivity for MAO-A in low doses), which is administered as a patch and does not require the usual MAOI dietary restrictions.

Q. Is there any readily available way to predict, from some biochemical test, which patients will respond to serotonergic versus noradrenergic ADs?

A. The short answer is no. Attempts have been made to relate differential drug response to factors such as urinary MHPG (3-methoxy-4-hydroxyphenylglycol, a metabolite of NE); cerebrospinal fluid levels of 5-HIAA (5-hydroxyindoleacetic acid, a 5-HT metabolite); or the ratio of serum tryptophan to other amino acids. These attempts have generally foundered, with too much variability in the results to prove clinically useful (Charney et al. 1995). Thus, selection of an AD is based primarily on the factors discussed in the "Overview" section of this chapter (see subsection "Indications").

Q. Are there ADs under investigation that have *non*–monoamine-based MOAs?

A. Several agents that antagonize glucocorticoid receptors (e.g., mifepristone) or corticotropin-releasing factor are under investigation (Belanoff et al. 2001). Peptides called *neurokinins,* such as substance P, have also been of great interest. Some, but not all, preliminary studies have found that antagonists to the receptors for substance P (NK_1 receptors) have AD properties (Stahl and Grady 2003). At present, however, these strategies are not clinically feasible.

Q. Are there ways of "speeding up" the MOA of ADs?

A. The question of speeding up the MOA of ADs remains unsettled (Pies 1997). Despite claims of some new "dual action" ADs, there are few data showing that any such agent has a faster onset of action of *clinical significance,* when compared with standard tricyclic agents or SSRIs. (Standard ADs usually require 3–6 weeks for significant therapeutic effects.) *Statistically* significant improvement on mood rating scales should not be considered synonymous with *clinically* significant improvement! "Pushing" the dose of the SNRI venlafaxine to high levels during the first week of treatment *may* accelerate response in some patients, but the accompanying GI side effects often make this strategy counterproductive, in the author's experience. Studies have used the β adrenoreceptor antagonist pindolol to reduce the "lag time" and/or to potentiate the AD effects of various SSRIs (Artigas et al. 1994). Pindolol apparently acts as an antagonist at the 5-HT_{1A} autoreceptor, thereby increasing serotonergic outflow from the presynaptic neuron. However, pindolol is neither selective nor specific for this autoreceptor (Skolnick 2002). Clinical experience and controlled studies with pindolol have yielded equivocal results. Large-scale, controlled studies will be needed to confirm pindolol's putative accelerating or augmenting effects in depression (Leonard 1996; Skolnick 2002).

Q. Are there AD MOAs more "fundamental" than simply affecting monoamine receptors or concentrations?

A. Almost certainly. We know that most monoamine-based ADs stimulate a "cascade reaction" involving G-proteins, cyclic AMP (cAMP), and an enzyme called protein kinase A (Skolnick 2002). Duman and colleagues (1997) have hypothesized that chronic AD treatment leads (via protein kinase A) to activation of a transcription factor called cAMP response binding protein (CREB). CREB, in turn, increases levels of messenger RNA coding for a nerve growth factor called *brain-derived neurotrophic growth factor* (BDNF) in the hippocampus. The "protective" effect of BDNF on serotonergic and dopaminergic neurons—and BDNF's ability to dampen excitatory *N*-methyl-D-aspartate (NMDA) receptor function—may be the ultimate MOA of a variety of ADs (Skolnick 2002). In effect, ADs probably "work" by turning on portions of the neuron's genetic machinery, which in turn produces salutary nerve growth factors.

Pharmacokinetics

Q. What happens to AD metabolism in various age groups?

A. As a broad generalization, neonates have relatively low rates of hepatic metabolism, whereas children have very high rates. Rates of metabolism in older adolescents and young adults are not far from those in the neonatal range, and elderly patients may have reduced metabolism for at least some ADs (Nemeroff 1995–1996). With respect to specific cytochrome families, it appears that whereas CYP 1A2 and 3A4 activity does decline with age, CYP 2D6 activity does not (Jacobson et al. 2002). However, in the elderly, much depends on the particular agent. Demethylation of tertiary amines—for example, conversion of amitriptyline to nortriptyline—is reduced in the elderly (Dubovsky 1994), whereas metabolism of desipramine seems minimally affected by age

(Dunner 1994; von Moltke et al. 1993). (Decreased renal function, however, may lead to higher levels of desipramine's hydroxylated metabolite.) Nortriptyline metabolism seems largely unaffected by age in elderly patients without concurrent medical illness (Dunner 1994; von Moltke et al. 1993); but again, one would expect levels of its hydroxylated metabolite to increase if renal excretion were reduced. Fluoxetine metabolism does not seem to be markedly affected by aging, though more information is needed regarding its metabolite, norfluoxetine (von Moltke et al. 1993). In contrast, paroxetine metabolism does seem to be reduced in the elderly, with therapeutic plasma levels achieved at about half the young adult dosage (10 mg/day vs. 20 mg/day) (Dunner 1994). Steady-state pharmacokinetics of venlafaxine does not seem to be altered in healthy elderly subjects; however, clearance of desmethylvenlafaxine may be about 15% less in those over age 60, probably because of slightly decreased renal function (G. Magni, quoted in "Venlafaxine" 1993).

Q. What is known about the metabolic pathways for bupropion metabolism?

A. Bupropion is hydroxylated by a very minor cytochrome P450 family, CYP 2B6, which accounts for less than 1% of CYP activity; however, alternate pathways may include 1A2, 2C9, 3A4, and others. Recently, it has become clear that bupropion is a potent inhibitor of the CYP 2D6 system (Cozza et al. 2003).

Q. Is it necessary to "taper off" ADs prior to discontinuing them, and if so, does the $t_{1/2}$ of the agent influence the rate of tapering?

A. As a general rule, it is rarely wise to stop any psychotropic suddenly, except in cases of severe drug toxicity, anaphylactic reaction, or another life-threatening condition arising from the agent's use. Most ADs may be discontinued over brief periods of time (3–7 days) without serious withdrawal reactions. However, with highly anticholinergic ADs, especially when used in high doses, rapid discontinuation of the drug can lead to a "cholinergic rebound" syndrome, characterized by hypersalivation, diarrhea, urinary urgency, abdominal cramping, and sweating. Some authorities (e.g., Schatzberg and Cole 1991) advise a tapering schedule no more rapid than 25–50 mg q 2–3 days for TCAs. Should GI symptoms develop during TCA withdrawal, treatment with propantheline bromide (15 mg tid prn) is recommended. (It may be just as useful to restart the TCA at a low dosage, e.g., amitriptyline 15–25 mg/day.) In general, sudden discontinuation of any psychotropic with a short $t_{1/2}$ is associated with more rapid, if not more intense, withdrawal symptoms than would be seen with longer-acting agents. Most of the TCAs have similar half-lives, in the range of 24 to 70 hours. Therefore, likelihood of withdrawal symptoms may depend more on how anticholinergic the TCA is, and how high the dose was at the time of discontinuation. Among the SSRIs, fluoxetine has a markedly longer $t_{1/2}$ than do the other agents in this class (see Table 2–9). In theory, sudden discontinuation of fluoxetine should not pose a high risk of withdrawal symptoms, and clinical experience generally confirms this. Sertraline has a shorter $t_{1/2}$ than fluoxetine (roughly 25–32 hours vs. 2–4 days, respectively), but sertraline's metabolite, desmethylsertraline, has modest clinical activity and a $t_{1/2}$ of about 60–75 hours. This may act as a "buffer" against withdrawal symptoms to some extent. In contrast, rather severe withdrawal reactions have been reported even with relatively gradual discontinuation of paroxetine, which has a $t_{1/2}$ of only 21–24 hours and no active metabolites. Such reactions may present as a flulike syndrome characterized by nausea, vomiting, fatigue, myalgia, vertigo, headache, and insomnia (Barr et al. 1994). These symptoms have occurred even when paroxetine was tapered over 7–10 days. Venlafaxine-induced withdrawal has been treated with fluoxetine, probably owing to the latter's long-lasting serotonergic action (Giakas and Davis 1997).

Q. What are the effects of hepatic and renal disease on the pharmacokinetics of ADs? What are the risks of hepatotoxicity with ADs?

A. Hepatic damage leads to reduced first-pass extraction of most psychotropic drugs, with resultant higher plasma levels of the parent compound after oral administration. TCAs such as amitriptyline and imipramine will be less readily demethylated to nortriptyline and desmethylimipramine, respectively, when hepatic damage is significant (e.g., in severe cirrhosis). This may result in more side effects related to the parent compounds, such as sedation or hypotension. SSRIs undergoing demethylation—for example, fluoxetine to norfluoxetine, or sertraline to desmethylsertraline—will also be affected by significant hepatic dysfunction. In cirrhotic patients, the mean $t_{1/2}$ of fluoxetine may increase from 2–4 days to 7.6 days, and of norfluoxetine, from 7–10 days to 12 days or longer (Physicians' Desk Reference 2004). The clearance of sertraline is also decreased in cirrhotic patients. Even though paroxetine has a short $t_{1/2}$ and no active metabolites, increased plasma levels can occur in patients with severe hepatic impairment (Physicians' Desk Reference 2004). Hepatotoxicity is associated with the MAOIs isocarboxazid (no longer available in the United States) and phenelzine; tranylcypromine is less hepatotoxic. Recently, nefazodone recently received a black box warning secondary to hepatotoxicity (Physicians' Desk Reference 2004), although severe liver damage appears to be very rare.

With respect to renal impairment, it appears that mild to moderate renal disease has little impact on AD pharmacokinetics. However, severe renal impairment may increase plasma levels of virtually all ADs. In particular, *water-soluble metabolites* of ADs (e.g., 11-hydroxynortriptyline, *O*-desmethylvenlafaxine) may show reduced excretion in cases of significant renal dysfunction.

Q. How do alterations in plasma binding proteins change the clinical effects of ADs?

A. Reduced hepatic production of plasma binding proteins is often said to produce increased levels of "free drug" and, thus, more side effects. But while changes in binding proteins can affect the measurement of *total drug* (free plus bound) and the *free fraction* (percent of unbound drug), the *absolute* amount of free drug (free drug concentration) is a function of *drug dosage* and *elimination,* not the amount of binding proteins (see Greenblatt et al. 1982 for a thorough explanation of this much-confused topic). In practice, changes in binding proteins usually affect the *therapeutic* and *toxic ranges* for a given agent, not the patient's "real" exposure to the unbound drug (see subsection "Vignettes/Puzzlers" for a clinical example).

Q. Should ADs be taken with or without food?

A. In general, food intake and timing is not a very important factor in the efficacy of AD therapy. However, sertraline plasma levels may be higher if sertraline is taken with food, whereas nefazodone levels may be decreased (Nemeroff 1995–1996).

Q. When is monitoring of plasma levels (therapeutic drug monitoring) of ADs necessary or useful?

A. For the most part, only nortriptyline has demonstrated a strong relationship between a well-defined plasma level and therapeutic efficacy, although data exist for other TCAs (see Table 2–11). Most of the newer agents—for example, SSRIs, bupropion, and nefazodone—have not yet been studied sufficiently to generate such correlations. Nevertheless, obtaining plasma levels (i.e., therapeutic drug monitoring) of ADs can be important in the following circumstances (Arana and Hyman 1991; Ayd 1995):

- To assess the patient's compliance
- To confirm that the patient is a rapid or slow hepatic metabolizer
- To monitor changes in AD levels when other hepatically metabolized agents are coadministered (e.g., an SSRI is added to ongoing TCA therapy)
- To help confirm the clinical diagnosis of drug toxicity
- To document, prior to terminating a trial, that adequate plasma levels have been attained
- To justify an unusually low or high AD dosage

This last point is relevant when, for example, it requires 350 mg/day of, say, desipramine to achieve a plasma level of 110 ng/mL, which represents the lower end of the putative therapeutic range.

Main Side Effects

Q. What are the relative rates of AD-induced seizures among the various tricyclic and nontricyclic agents?

A. In general, the ADs are not highly "epileptogenic." In one study in which the mean follow-up period was 28 months, the overall incidence of seizures during imipramine or amitriptyline therapy was approximately 0.5% in non-epileptic patients; thus, the cumulative *yearly* incidence of seizures during TCA therapy would be estimated at approximately 0.2% (Lowry and Dunner 1980). Some data indicate a seizure rate of around 0.45% for imipramine, at effective doses, whereas clomipramine is associated with a seizure incidence of about

1.5% (Rosenstein et al. 1993). Among the commonly used TCAs, amitriptyline may be more likely to aggravate seizures (Edwards et al. 1986). While standard-formulation (immediate-release [IR]) bupropion at high dosages (>450 mg/day) may have a greater likelihood of inducing seizures than do other ADs, a 102-site study of bupropion-IR at dosages of up to 450 mg/day showed an overall incidence of seizures of 0.36%—an incidence interpreted as comparable to that of other ADs (Johnston et al. 1991). Moreover, a large, open-label surveillance study of more than 3,000 patients treated with sustained-release bupropion (bupropion-SR), at dosages of up to 300 mg/day, found a cumulative seizure rate of only about 0.1% over 1 year (Dunner et al. 1998). Maprotiline (Ludiomil), a rarely used AD, does appear to have a higher risk of inducing seizures than do the TCAs.

The SSRIs appear to have an approximately 0.2% incidence of seizures (Johnston et al. 1991), which is somewhat lower than the incidence for TCAs (Rosenstein et al. 1993). One uncontrolled study suggested that fluoxetine actually had *anticonvulsant* effects in a small group of patients with complex partial seizures (Favale et al. 1995); these patients were also maintained on their usual anticonvulsants, however. MAOIs also seem to have a lower risk than do TCAs (Rosenstein et al. 1993).

Although there is less postmarketing information regarding nefazodone and venlafaxine, it appears that both agents have a low rate of associated seizures. During clinical trials with nefazodone, the overall incidence of seizures was only 0.04%; however, patients with a history of seizures had been excluded from these studies (Bristol-Myers-Squibb data on file with company). In a similar population treated with venlafaxine, premarketing testing showed a seizure rate of 0.26% (8/3,082) (D.L. Albano, Wyeth-Ayerst Laboratories, personal communication, February 22, 1996). This rate was found to be comparable to the rate of seizures seen in the placebo group, and less than that for comparator drugs, including imipramine, trazodone, clomipramine, fluoxetine, and amitriptyline. Premarketing clinical trials with mirtazapine reported only one seizure among the 2,796 patients treated, but there are no controlled studies of this drug in patients with a seizure history (Physicians' Desk Reference 2004). It is important to keep in mind that postmarketing reports do not necessarily establish a cause-and-effect relationship between the index drug and the occurrence of a seizure.

Predisposing factors for AD-related seizures appear to include history of personal or familial seizure disorder, abnormal pretreatment electroencephalogram (EEG), postnatal brain damage, cerebrovascular disease, head trauma, sedative or alcohol withdrawal, and multiple concomitant medications (Lowry and Dunner 1980; Rosenstein et al. 1993). Seizure risk for most ADs appears to increase with dose and/or blood level (Rosenstein et al. 1993) and is especially high after an overdose. In summary, all ADs, with the exceptions of maprotiline, clomipramine, and perhaps high-dose bupropion, have a relatively low rate of associated seizures.

Q. Do SSRIs affect hemostasis?

A. Several case reports have implicated several SSRIs (e.g., fluoxetine, fluvoxamine, and paroxetine) in abnormal bleeding (Aranth and Lindberg 1992; Ottervanger et al. 1994), but the frequency of this reaction is unknown. Abnormal bleeding has been attributed to SSRI-induced depletion of platelet 5-HT and may be associated with *normal* values for platelet count, prothrombin time, and partial thromboplastin time (Ottervanger et al. 1994). In a case–control study, de Abajo and colleagues (1999) found an increased risk of upper GI bleeding associated with serotonergic ADs, and such a reaction is especially likely (12 times the expected rate) if the patient is also taking a nonsteroidal anti-inflammatory drug (NSAID) (Dalton et al. 2003). Hyperserotonemia can also cause dilated capillaries or telangiectasia, possibly leading to ecchymoses without hemostatic defect. One case report found vitamin C (500 mg/day) to be helpful for SSRI-related bleeding (Tielens 1997).

Q. What are the main side effects of mirtazapine (Remeron)?

A. The most common side effects are somnolence, increased appetite, weight gain, and dizziness. SSRI-like side effects (nausea, insomnia, sexual dysfunction) seem to be minimal (Kehoe and Schorr 1996).

Q. What is the risk of agranulocytosis with mirtazapine, and how should it be managed?

A. Preclinical experience with mirtazapine indicated that agranulocytosis occurred in 2 of 2,796 patients, leading the manufacturer to estimate the risk as roughly 1.1 per 1,000. (One of the two patients had a rare autoimmune disease, so it is not clear that this incidence will hold up in clinical studies.) While the manufacturer advises informing the patient of this risk, no specific guidelines for blood monitoring are given. The package insert does state that "if a patient develops a sore throat, fever, stomatitis or other signs of infection, along with a low WBC count, treatment with Remeron should be discontinued and the patient...closely monitored" (Physicians' Desk Reference 2004). However, postmarketing experience has generally not supported a substantial risk of agranulocytosis with this agent.

Q. What are the side-effect profiles of the two new ADs reboxetine and duloxetine?

A. While clinical experience is limited with these agents, studies to date suggest that both agents are generally well tolerated. Duloxetine may be associated with limited hypertension, withdrawal symptoms after discontinuation, and urinary retention—a profile that is characteristic of SNRI agents (Stahl and Grady 2003). Some preliminary data suggest that duloxetine may be associated with reduced rates of sexual dysfunction compared with SSRIs (Schatzberg 2003); however, clinical experience has repeatedly cast doubt on such claims once structured assessment of sexual dysfunction has been carried out (Hallward and Ellison 2001). Reboxetine, with its specific noradrenergic effects, may be associated with increased heart rate, urinary hestitancy, constipation, sweating, and insomnia (Arana and Rosenbaum 2000).

Q. Can ADs induce hypomania/mania or "rapid cycling" in bipolar patients? If so, what is the best strategy to use in treating depressed bipolar patients?

A. Although described in 30%–70% of bipolar patients, *antidepressant-induced mania* (AIM) remains a source of great controversy (Bowden and Goldberg 2003; Goodwin and Jamison 1990). Little is known about which bipolar patients are most susceptible to AIM or rapid cycling (more than four major mood episodes per year) and at what period in their course of illness they are most susceptible (Coryell et al. 2003; Goldberg and Whiteside 2002). Furthermore, some recent nonrandomized and randomized controlled studies have questioned the association between AD use and either AIM or rapid cycling in bipolar populations (Altshuler et al. 2003; Coryell et al. 2003). In contrast, a naturalistic study by Ghaemi and colleagues (2000) found that AD use was associated with a worsened course of bipolar illness, including new-onset or worsening of rapid cycling. Most researchers agree that there are "risk factors" for AIM and/or rapid cycling (Altshuler et al. 1995; Goldberg and Whiteside 2002), such as the following:

- A strong family and personal history of AD-induced mania or cycle acceleration
- A history of numerous AD exposures
- Substance abuse
- Early age at onset of mood symptoms and/or treatment

The revised APA Guideline for Treatment of Bipolar Disorder recommends that ADs generally be employed for short periods, and always with a mood stabilizer (American Psychiatric Association 2002). Goldberg and Whiteside (2002), among others (Coryell et al. 2003), have questioned this stringency, citing high suicide rates in bipolar depression, a significant risk for depression relapse once treatment with ADs is ended, and a paucity of empirical information on pro-cycling risks versus AD benefits. The conventional wisdom is that *nontricyclic* ADs, such as the SSRIs and bupropion, have a reduced risk of causing AIM, compared with the TCAs. However, not all studies have supported this differential risk (Goldberg and Whiteside 2002). Indeed, rates of AIM with bupropion may vary from 11% to nearly 50% (Fogelson et al. 1992; Sachs et al. 1994). (In the author's experience, low-dose bupropion—sometimes as little as ¼ of a 75-mg tablet of bupropion per day—may be effective and well tolerated in some depressed bipolar II patients, in combination with divalproex.) SSRIs have been advocated, on the basis of very limited data, as *monotherapy* for bipolar II disorder (Amsterdam et al. 1998); however, randomized controlled studies using appropriate measures of mania/hypomania have not been performed.

Recently, the FDA approved the anticonvulsant lamotrigine for the maintenance treatment of adults with bipolar I disorder. The data suggest that lamotrigine's effects are more robust in bipolar depression than in mania/hypomania/mixed episodes (Bowden et al. 2003). This issue is discussed in detail later in this handbook (see Chapter 5, "Mood Stabilizers"). Lamotrigine may offer a reasonable way out of the dilemma of AD use in bipolar depression. **The bottom line:** Avoid ADs in all bipolar patients if clinically feasible, and use ADs very carefully when clinically necessary, in conjunction with a mood stabilizer.

Q. How do older and newer ADs compare with respect to sexual side effects?

A. AD-induced sexual dysfunction (AISD) contributes to both noncompliance with medication and decreased quality of life. AISD may take the form of decreased libido; erectile dysfunction; delayed orgasm; anorgasmia; impaired or painful ejaculation; penile or clitoral anesthesia; and penile or clitoral priapism. AISD tends to be more common with the TCAs (particularly clomipramine), SSRIs, MAOIs, and venlafaxine. Trazodone is disproportionately associated with priapism, although this occurs in only about 1 in 6,000 male patients. Curiously, when priapism does occur, it often occurs at dosages of *less* than 150 mg/day, and during the first month of treatment (Golden et al. 1995; Thompson et al. 1990).

Although head-to-head prospective studies are rare, one large (*N*=1,022) prospective study found that within the SSRI group, paroxetine, citalopram, and venlafaxine were associated with the highest rates of sexual side effects (Montejo et al. 2001). Rates of sexual dysfunction with these three agents, assessed by means of a structured questionnaire, exceeded 65%. However, even the most benign among the SSRIs—fluoxetine—came in at 58%. With mirtazapine, there was a quantum leap downward, to about 24%; with nefazodone, only an 8% rate of sexual dysfunction occurred (Montejo et al. 2001).

Q. What are the best strategies for managing AISD?

A. Management actually begins *before* prescribing medication, by means of a thorough sexual history (regarding, e.g., predepression and pretreatment sexual functioning). General management includes careful questioning about specific sexual problems (which patients may be reluctant to discuss); careful differential diagnosis (e.g., sexual dysfunction may be an integral part of major depression or may be secondary to medical illness); and dosage reduction, if clinically feasible. "Watchful waiting," in hopes that AISD will spontaneously remit, is usually not successful (Montejo et al. 2001). "Drug holidays" run the risk of undermining treatment and/or producing AD withdrawal effects. If AISD persists, switching to bupropion, mirtazapine, or nefazodone, or adding an agent to enhance sexual function, is an appropriate strategy (Hallward and Ellison 2001). Case reports have noted success with the addition of yohimbine (5.4–16.2 mg/day), bupropion (75–150 mg/day), trazodone (50–200 mg/day), bethanechol (10–50 mg tid to qid), cyproheptadine (4–12 mg qhs), amantadine (100–300 mg/day), or buspirone (15–60 mg/day); and low doses of D-amphetamine (McElroy 1995). However, the use of cyproheptadine, a 5-HT antagonist, has sometimes been associated with recurrence of depression or decreased efficacy of concomitant SSRI treatment (Feder 1991b). Recent studies in males suggest that adding sildenafil may counteract SSRI-related sexual dysfunction, and some data indicate that women with AISD may also benefit from sildenafil (Hallward and Ellison 2001). Some pros and cons of these strategies are found in Table 2–16.

Q. What is the mechanism for SSRI-induced "apathy," and how is this side effect best managed?

A. It has been observed that after a period of weeks or months, some patients taking SSRIs develop a syndrome of apathy, loss of initiative, lack of emotional responsiveness, or (less commonly) "disinhibition" (Hoehn-Saric et al. 1991). While this "frontal lobe syndrome" has been reported with fluoxetine and fluvoxamine, it can occur with the other SSRIs, in the author's experience. In the case reported by Hoehn-Saric and colleagues (1991), this syndrome was associated with decreased cerebral blood flow in the frontal lobes and neuropsychological changes associated with frontal lobe impairment; clinical manifestations disappeared about a month after discontinuation of fluoxetine. While the mechanism underlying these "frontal lobe" symptoms is unclear, it is possible that 5-HT's ability to decrease dopaminergic tone in some brain regions (Roth and Meltzer 1995) may be involved. In the author's experience, the use of the dopaminergic agent methylphenidate (10–20 mg/day) may help restore normal mood and affect in some patients with this syndrome, but controlled studies of this intervention are lacking.

Q. With respect to TCA toxicity in an overdose, which is more useful: a TCA plasma level or an electrocardiogram (ECG)?

A. Some patients with relatively low plasma TCA levels may still have complete heart block; conversely, some patients with high TCA plasma levels (e.g., >400 ng/mL) show no cardiac arrhythmias. Thus, an ECG is the more relevant and useful test in an overdose situation (Nemeroff 1995–1996), with a QRS duration of >0.10 seconds being a particularly useful index of toxicity (Janicak et al. 1993). Nevertheless, TCA plasma levels in excess of

1,000 ng/mL are associated with increased cardiac and neurological morbidity (Janicak et al. 1993).

Drug–Drug Interactions

Q. What are the most serious drug–drug interactions with TCA and non-TCA antidepressants?

A. Drug–drug interactions that may be serious and/or life-threatening include the following (see also Tables 2–17, 2–18, and 2–19):

1. *Combination of MAOI and SSRI,* which may lead to severe serotonin syndrome (fever, myoclonus, confusion, coma) and death
2. *Combination of MAOI and meperidine (Demerol),* which may lead to fatal hyperthermia and serotonin syndrome (Dextromethorphan may also be dangerous in combination with an MAOI)
3. *Combination of MAOI and sympathomimetic, such as amphetamine,* which may provoke a hypertensive reaction
4. *Combination of MAOI and TCA,* which also provokes a serotonergic syndrome (less commonly, a hypertensive reaction)

Potentially dangerous reactions may also result from a combination of some SSRIs and TCAs, which may lead to markedly increased levels of the TCA, and from the combination of a TCA with a type 1A antiarrhythmic agent such as quinidine, which can lead to dangerous conduction abnormalities.

Despite the risks associated with these various combinations, certain cases of refractory depression may warrant such polypharmacy. Thus, when carefully controlled and monitored, TCAs may be combined with MAOIs, and SSRIs with TCAs (see subsection "Potentiating Maneuvers" in the "Overview" section of this chapter). However, MAOIs should *not* be used with SSRIs.

Q. What are the pharmacokinetic "risks" of combining ADs with antipsychotics and anticonvulsants? Which combinations are safest?

A. Complex interactions often occur when hepatically metabolized psychotropics are combined. This is even more likely to occur when one agent is metabolized by a cytochrome pathway that is strongly inhibited (or induced) by the other agent (Pies 2000).

As a rule, TCAs increase plasma levels of some antipsychotic agents—for example, imipramine and nortriptyline increase chlorpromazine levels. SSRIs show considerable variability in their effects on the cytochromes (see Table 2–9). Fluoxetine impairs the metabolism of haloperidol and virtually any other psychotropic using the CYP 2D6 pathway. Similarly, fluvoxamine (a substantial inhibitor of CYP 1A2) may elevate plasma levels of olanzapine or clozapine (Cozza et al. 2003).

Older neuroleptics such as haloperidol, thiothixene, perphenazine, and chlorpromazine may potently inhibit metabolism in CYP 2D6, thus elevating levels of TCAs, SSRIs, and other ADs metabolized by this system (Ciraulo et al. 1995a; Cozza et al. 2003). When TCAs and phenothiazine-type antipsychotics are given together, higher plasma levels of both types of agent often occur, leading to increased sedation, anticholinergic effects, and perhaps cardiac toxicity due to quinidine-like effects. Atypical antipsychotics are generally not potent cytochrome P450 inhibitors, though clozapine and risperidone may inhibit CYP 2D6 to some degree (Cozza et al. 2003); in theory, these agents could raise blood levels of ADs metabolized by CYP 2D6.

Anticonvulsants may affect the metabolism of some ADs (Ciraulo et al. 1995a). Carbamazepine tends to be an enzymatic inducer, leading to reduced levels of nearly all psychotropics—especially those metabolized by CYP 3A4. Valproate tends to inhibit metabolism of other psychotropics via effects on CYP 2D6 and 2C9 and glucuronidation, but it usually has no major pharmacokinetic interactions with newer ADs (Cozza et al. 2003). Lamotrigine is not a potent cytochrome P450 inhibitor or inducer and thus would not be expected to alter AD levels significantly; however, sertraline may substantially *increase* lamotrigine levels, probably via inhibition of glucuronidation (Cozza et al. 2003; Kaufman and Gerner 1998).

Q. What drugs used in general and internal medicine are likely to have pharmacokinetic interactions with ADs?

A. Since many such drugs use the same cytochrome systems as do ADs, there is significant potential for interaction (see Tables 2–17 and 2–18). Analgesics such as acetaminophen, ibuprofen, naproxen, and codeine; calcium channel blockers; beta-blockers; corticosteroids; androgens; estrogens; and macrolide antibiotics—all may interact with ADs metabolized via CYP 1A2, 2C19, 2C9, 2D6, and 3A3/4. Other agents that may interact with ADs include theophylline, barbiturates, omeprazole, coumadin, quinidine, tamoxifen, and ketoconazole (Ereshefsky 1996; Ereshefsky et al. 1996). ADs with potent CYP 2D6 inhibition (e.g., fluoxetine, paroxetine) may elevate blood levels of antiarrhythmic agents such as mexiletine and encainide (Cozza et al. 2003). Recently, paroxetine was found to reduce conversion of tamoxifen to its active, antineoplastic metabolite—a step apparently requiring CYP 2D6 activity (Stearns et al. 2003).

Q. Can foods or beverages interact pharmacokinetically with ADs?

A. *Grapefruit juice* appears to be a significant inhibitor of CYP 3A3/4 and may increase plasma levels of clomipramine and its metabolite, desmethylclomipramine (Oesterheld and Kallepalli 1997). In principle, other ADs metabolized via this cytochrome system (e.g., nefazodone), as well as triazolam, calcium channel blockers, and other drugs, could be affected by unusually high intake of grapefruit juice. The CYP 1A2 system may be induced by broccoli, brussel sprouts, and charcoal-broiled foods.

Potentiating Maneuvers

Q. What constitutes an adequate duration of trial for an AD?

A. The notion that we can reach final conclusions about an AD's efficacy after 4 weeks is probably wrong, with 5–6 weeks being closer to the minimum time needed to know whether a drug will work. Some patients will continue to show improvement while taking an AD up to 12 weeks after beginning treatment (Gorman 1995). Geriatric patients sometimes require up to 12–16 weeks to show a full response (Wise 1995). In practical terms, however, if a patient shows absolutely no improvement after 3–4 weeks—despite adequate doses and/or AD plasma levels (for TCAs)—it is the author's practice to switch to another agent. If the patient has had a *partial* response to the first agent after 3–4 weeks, it may be reasonable simply to "wait"—on the premise that a full response might be seen with an additional week or two. However, if a patient is still in significant distress even after a partial response by week 3, it is the author's usual practice to try an augmentation strategy at that point.

Q. Are TCAs or other ADs more effective for severe depression than SSRIs?

A. Randomized, prospective controlled studies that would answer this question are in short supply. Although there is modest evidence that TCAs may be more effective in severe melancholic depression in the elderly (Roose et al. 1994), the majority of studies have not established any overall superiority of the TCAs when compared with the SSRIs (Nierenberg 1994). In the author's experience, however, a TCA will often be effective in older patients who have failed trials on more than one SSRI.

With respect to newer ADs, Phillips and Nierenberg (1994) reported a 40% response rate with venlafaxine treatment in patients who failed other treatments, including MAOIs and ECT. Similarly, one 8-week open study (Fava et al. 2001) found that about half of patients with major depression that was previously refractory to several SSRIs showed significant improvement when switched to mirtazapine. Newer SNRIs, such as duloxetine, may prove to be as effective as the older TCAs, though this has not been investigated in randomized controlled trials in populations with refractory depression. Some evidence suggests that venlafaxine and duloxetine produce numerically higher remission rates than other, "single-action" ADs, such as fluoxetine (Goldstein et al. 2002); however, these data have been called into question. Carlat (2004), for example, points out that researchers in some studies of response and remission rates with duloxetine use unconventional statistical methods to arrive at their conclusions. Clinical experience conjoined with more probing statistical analysis will need to be the final arbiters.

Q. In refractory major depression, when is it appropriate to *potentiate* an ongoing AD, as opposed to *switching* to another class of agent?

A. There are no randomized, prospective controlled studies (to date) *directly* comparing these strategies. Thus, most of the advice given on this question is derived from clinical experience and a few studies examining success rates in depressed patients switched from one agent to another ("crossover monotherapy"). Keller (1995) suggested that crossover monotherapy for treatment-resistant depression may have advantages over the use of combination treatments. With crossover monotherapy (e.g., switching a patient with treatment-resistant depression from a TCA to a SSRI or vice versa), there is reduced risk of drug–drug interactions and (usually) reduced expense, compared with augmentation therapy.

Keller (1995) presented preliminary results of two such crossover studies involving patients with "double depression" (major depression plus dysthymia) ($n=341$) and chronic major depression ($n=294$). Keller and his colleagues found that of the 198 patients for whom data were available, only about 27% had actually undergone an adequate trial of an AD (defined as at least 150 mg/day of imipramine or its equivalent for at least 4 consecutive weeks) prior to the study. In phase I (lasting 12 weeks), patients were randomly assigned to either sertraline or imipramine in a 2:1 ratio. Among those who completed the 12-week acute treatment phase, responders to either drug continued on the same drug in double-blind fashion for 16 weeks. Nonresponders to either drug were "crossed over" to the other drug, also in double-blind fashion (phase II). Results of the first (12-week) phase showed that slightly over 60% of patients who completed this phase were responders to either treatment, suggesting that even patients with chronic depression are responsive to adequate medication. With respect to phase II—the crossover from one agent to the other—results indicated that sertraline treatment of imipramine nonresponders was both effective and well tolerated. Similarly, imipramine treatment of sertraline nonresponders was also effective—though less so than sertraline treatment of imipramine nonresponders. In the Keller et al. study, imipramine was not as well tolerated as sertraline. Interestingly, the response to crossover medication was inversely proportional to the initial drug response—in effect, *the worse the response to the first drug, the more likely the response to the second (crossover) medication.*

There are fewer studies of crossover from an SSRI to a TCA. One such study, by Peselow et al. (1989), investigated the use of imipramine in patients who had not responded to paroxetine and found a 73% response rate after 6 weeks of imipramine treatment (see Thase and Rush 1995 for a full discussion of these studies).

In summary, rather than using an augmenting agent, the clinician may find it worthwhile, in some patients with treatment-resistant depression, first to change from one AD class to another. In the author's experience, this strategy makes sense primarily in patients who have had poor or minimal response to the first agent (cf. Fava 2000). Indeed, Quitkin and colleagues (1996) suggested two chronological guidelines. First, a switch should be made if there is very little or no improvement after 4 weeks of AD therapy—a situation that occurs in about 10% of the patients who receive AD treatment. Second, if there is minimal improvement initially, and if further improvement ceases after 5 weeks of continuous treatment, a switch to another agent generally should be made. However, it may take up to 10 weeks to achieve full therapeutic response in patients with long-standing depression, such as chronic dysthymic disorder.

Q. What about changing from one SSRI to another SSRI in a patient with treatment-resistant depression?

A. Four studies (using varying methods) have looked at this question and reached somewhat different conclusions. In the main, however, the change from one SSRI to another *does* make sense in many patients with treatment-resistant depression, at least up to a point (Gelenberg 1996). Brown and Harrison (1995) found that 72% of fluoxetine-intolerant outpatients ($n = 113$) responded to sertraline and were generally able to tolerate it (only 10% had adverse reactions). Conversely, Apter and Birkett (1995) found that around 63% of outpatients who had failed treatment with sertraline (because of a lack of effect or intolerable side effects) responded well to fluoxetine, with only one patient dropping out because of an adverse event.

Zarate and colleagues (1996) came to a less positive conclusion in their retrospective review of 39 inpatients sequentially treated with fluoxetine and sertraline. They found that of 31 inpatients with major depression or bipolar depression treated with sertraline, only 42% were judged to have had an adequate response; of those, only 26% continued to do well at follow-up. Of 21 patients who had discontinued fluoxetine because of intolerable side effects, 43% also discontinued sertraline because of side effects. Twelve (75%) of 16 patients who had side effects during sertraline treatment had the *same* side effects as when taking fluoxetine (including allergic-type reactions). Zarate et al. concluded that if a patient has not done well while taking fluoxetine, there is only a modest benefit in changing to sertraline. Looking at the Zarate et al. data from a different perspective, we can say that at least one in four fluoxetine nonresponders may do quite well when taking sertraline.

Finally, in an open study of 55 patients with major depression who had failed a trial with one of the SSRIs, Joffe and colleagues (1996b) found that 28 of the 55 had a marked or complete AD response to a second SSRI.

In toto, these data support the utility of switching from one SSRI to another, even though some patients will have similar side effects with each agent. This approach of switching to another SSRI is consistent with the differing pharmacodynamic profiles of the SSRIs (see Table 2–10). However, in the author's experience, a patient who has had absolutely no response to two or three full SSRI trials rarely responds to yet another SSRI. At that point, trying an agent with different chemical properties (e.g., bupropion, mirtazapine) may make more sense.

Q. How effective is the addition of a TCA to an SSRI, or vice versa?

A. Most studies of TCA–SSRI combinations have been open-label, and most have involved fluoxetine, sertraline, desipramine, and nortriptyline. Thus, sweeping conclusions regarding this strategy are inappropriate. Price and colleagues (2001) cited both positive and negative studies using such combinations and cautioned that, in some cases, "patients who appear to respond in these circumstances are responding to the new agent, rather than to the combination" (p. 205). The potential for both pharmacodynamic and pharmacokinetic interactions (e.g., serotonin syndrome) must also be kept in mind. If this strategy is used, a "start low, go slow" approach is indicated, with careful monitoring of the patients for side effects. At this time, citalopram or escitalopram might be the SSRI of choice for this combined strategy, given the minimal inhibitory effects of these agents on the cytochrome system; however, controlled study of this question is sorely lacking.

Q. Can SSRIs be combined with bupropion in treating patients with refractory depression?

A. Large-scale, controlled studies of this combination are not available, but a few case reports suggest that this combination may be safe and effective. In one such case, a woman whose depression had been refractory to both paroxetine alone (with intolerable sedation at a dosage of 50 mg/day) and bupropion alone (with significant agitation at 300 mg/day) responded well to a combination of paroxetine 30 mg/day and bupropion 225 mg/day—with reduction in the aforementioned side effects (Marshall and Liebowitz 1996). (It should be noted also that her concomitant obsessive-compulsive symptoms improved along with the depression.) A second case series reported the efficacy of sertraline combined with bupropion in treating refractory depression (Marshall et al. 1995). Keep in mind that, since the metabolic pathway of bupropion is not well defined, it is possible that some SSRIs increase plasma levels of bupropion (and those of its metabolite, hydroxybupropion); in theory, this could increase seizure risk at higher bupropion doses. Indeed, there are now several case reports of anxiety and neurotoxicity (e.g., myoclonus, delirium) following use of combined fluoxetine and bupropion (Hopkins 1996). The pharmacodynamic mechanism of bupropion's efficacy is not known, though noradrenergic effects and dopaminergic effects are likely. Finally, since bupropion is a substantial inhibitor of CYP 2D6 (Cozza et al. 2003), blood levels of SSRIs that are metabolized via this pathway may be elevated.

Q. Can psychostimulants be used to potentiate the effects of SSRIs?

A. Stoll and colleagues (1996) presented five cases of major depression in which methylphenidate (10–40 mg/day) was used, in open trials, to augment fluoxetine or paroxetine. Self-reported symptom reduction occurred rapidly in all cases, with few adverse effects. The authors discussed the possibility that methylphenidate and other psychostimulants reverse the dopamine-depleting effect of the SSRIs. Metz and Shader (1991) also reported the effectiveness of the combination of fluoxetine and pemoline in several cases of refractory major depression.

Q. Can modafinil be useful as an augmenting agent in refractory depression?

A. Very few controlled studies of modafinil as an augmenting agent have been undertaken, but one case series and one open study suggest that modafinil may be useful and well tolerated as an augmenting agent (Markovitz and Wagner 2003; Menza et al. 2000). In the open study ($N=27$), Global Assessment of Functioning Scale scores improved significantly when modafinil (200–400 mg/day) was used to augment treatment with SSRIs or venlafaxine. One recent randomized, placebo-controlled study (DeBattista et al. 2003) investigated modafinil as adjunctive therapy in partial responders with major depression. Although modafinil was useful in reducing fatigue and sleepiness during the first 2 weeks of use, it did not surpass placebo in reducing depression scores on the Hamilton Rating Scale for Depression. AD–modafinil combination treatment generally appears to be well tolerated, though modafinil's *inhibitory* effects on CYP 2C19 and its *inducing* effects on CYP 3A4 could alter plasma levels of some ADs (Cozza et al. 2003). There are also anecdotal reports of possible exacerbation of psychosis or mania with modafinil (Narendran et al. 2002). In short, further controlled studies are needed to establish modafinil's utility in treating patients with unipolar or bipolar depression.

Q. How effective is lithium in combination with TCAs or SSRIs in treating patients with refractory depression? How is it prescribed?

A. Textbooks often point to lithium augmentation as a robust strategy in treating patients with refractory depression; however, lithium's efficacy as an augmenting agent has not been shown in all studies. Several studies suffer from retrospective analysis, uncontrolled design, or inadequate dose/duration of treatment (Nierenberg et al. 2003; O'Reardon 2004). One recent placebo-controlled trial (Nierenberg et al. 2003) found lithium augmentation of nortriptyline ineffective in patients who had failed multiple trials of ADs. These patients had a mean of two previous failed trials, and lithium blood levels during the 6-week study were in the lower end of the therapeutic range (about 0.6 mEq/L). Some open data support the efficacy of lithium as an augmenter of SSRIs, but studies are limited.

It is not clear whether once-daily administration of lithium is as effective as divided doses, or how long to continue lithium augmentation (Boyer and Bunt 2001). Some clinical experience suggests that effective lithium augmentation requires blood levels of 0.6 mEq/L or higher for at least 4 weeks (O'Reardon 2004), but not all data support a dose–plasma level response. It has also been suggested that lithium is useful in augmenting serotonergic, but *not* noradrenergic, ADs (Bschor and Bauer 2004). Comparative, controlled studies are clearly needed.

Q. Can MAOIs be potentiated with either TCAs or stimulants, such as methylphenidate? What about combining MAOIs with lithium in treating patients with refractory depression?

A. The combination of an MAOI and a TCA is somewhat controversial, primarily because of the paucity of controlled outcome studies and the theoretical risk of the serotonin syndrome (Pies and Shader 2003). In general, this combination should be used only after other potentiation strategies and/or ECT have failed; nevertheless, when carried out properly, an MAOI–TCA combination may be safe and effective for appropriately selected patients (Ayd 1995). Among this group are patients with highly refractory anxious, phobic, and somatized ("atypical") depressions who do *not* have a history of hypomania, mania, or psychosis (Ayd 1995). Some data implicate imipramine, clomipramine, and perhaps desipramine as the most likely TCAs to interact adversely with an MAOI, so these agents should be avoided (Ciraulo et al. 1995a). The best approach to MAOI–TCA cotherapy is to begin both agents simultaneously, using small doses of each; or to add a small amount of the MAOI (e.g., 5 mg/day of tranylcypromine) to ongoing TCA treatment (Pies and Shader 2003). TCAs should *never* be added to an ongoing MAOI regimen (Ciraulo et al. 1995a).

Despite theoretical concerns about hypertensive reactions, MAOIs have been successfully combined with pemoline (Fawcett et al. 1991) in treating patients with treatment-resistant depression. Methylphenidate may also be combined with an MAOI, though some patients may experience orthostatic hypotension, restlessness, or hypomania (Ayd 1995; Feighner et al. 1985). MAOIs may be combined with lithium in patients with refractory depression. In general, this combination seems to be well tolerated, though some patients may become tremulous or hypomanic. There have been two case reports of dyskinetic movements associated with this combination (Ayd 1995).

Q. What is the role of benzodiazepines (BZDs) in the adjunctive treatment of depression?

A. Although BZDs are sometimes used during the initiation of AD therapy—particularly for very agitated or insomniac depressed patients whose primary AD is a more "stimulating" type—they have a rather limited role in the long-term treatment of depression. Indeed, BZDs may sometimes exacerbate depression, although this effect does not appear to be common (Smith and Salzman 1991). Summing up the available data, Joffe and colleagues (1996a) concluded, "Benzodiazepines decrease nonspecific symptoms of depression such as insomnia, agitation, and anxiety, but do not have specific or intrinsic AD effects and do not have an enduring therapeutic benefit" (p. 29) (but see Chapter 3, "Antipsychotics," regarding alprazolam as an AD).

Use in Special Populations

Q. What are the special needs of depressed patients with cancer and other medical illnesses?

A. Major depression may be seen in roughly 5%–15% of cancer patients—a prevalence higher than the prevalence in the general population (6%) but probably no higher than that seen in comparably ill medical patients with other diagnoses (Derogatis et al. 1983; Pies 1996). Depressive symptoms vary along a continuum of severity in cancer patients, ranging from no depression at all in more than 40% of cancer patients to mild, moderate, or severe symptoms in the remainder (Derogatis et al. 1983; Massie and Holland 1990). Massie and Holland (1990) suggest that the following features should prompt consideration of a psychiatric consultation: depressive symptoms that last longer than a week; worsening course of depressive symptoms; and depressive symptoms that interfere with the patient's ability to function or to cooperate with treatment.

The tertiary TCAs (e.g., amitriptyline, doxepin) or trazodone may be especially useful for depressed cancer patients with significant agitation and insomnia. Less-sedating secondary amine tricyclics (e.g., desipramine, nortriptyline) may be more useful in lethargic patients or those at risk for anticholinergic side effects (see below).

There is no convincing evidence, however, that one type of AD is more effective than another in the long-term treatment of cancer patients. Newer, nontricyclic agents—particularly the SSRIs—may be of use in depressed cancer patients with significant orthostatic hypotension or cardiac conduction abnormalities, but the side-effect profiles of the SSRIs are not always suitable for cancer patients. ADs may be used as analgesic adjuncts in managing cancer-related pain, and appear to be effective for pain relief even in the absence of clinical depression. Cancer patients, like most elderly patients, generally require lower total therapeutic dosages of TCAs (roughly 50–100 mg/day), perhaps as a consequence of altered drug metabolism and absorption (Massie and Holland 1990). (However, plasma levels of the TCAs may still need to be within the usual therapeutic range for the treatment of major depression.)

The principal side effects with the TCAs—particularly the tertiary amines—are anticholinergic, orthostatic, sedative, and cardiovascular effects. Anticholinergic effects (dry mouth, constipation, urinary retention, gastric reflux, blurry vision) are especially to be avoided in cancer patients with xerostomia or stomatitis and in those recovering from gastrointestinal or genitourinary surgery (Harnett 1994; Massie and Holland 1990). (*Central* anticholinergic side effects include confusion and memory impairment and should also be avoided in patients already prone to neurotoxic drug effects.) Cancer patients (and other medically ill patients) with volume depletion and hypotension are not good candidates for trazodone or the tertiary-amine tricyclics; nortriptyline, however, at dosages of 50–75 mg/day, may be relatively free of hypotensive effects. Because of their quinidine-like properties, all TCAs can cause cardiac conduction abnormalities and generally are contraindicated in patients with preexisting cardiac arrhythmias. The SSRIs have far fewer anticholinergic, hypotensive, sedating, and cardiovascular side effects than the tertiary-amine TCAs and are far less toxic in "overdose" situations; however, they can provoke anorexia, nausea, diarrhea, weight loss, tremor, extrapyramidal effects, and hyponatremia in some patients (Harnett 1994; Massie and Holland 1990). There have also been scattered case reports of sinus node slowing with fluoxetine (Ellison et al. 1990; Feder 1991a), and this slowing might be particularly likely when SSRIs are used together with beta-blockers. Despite these potential drawbacks, fluoxetine and other SSRIs have been used successfully in cancer patients, usually by beginning with a low dose and increasing the dose slowly. Serotonin$_3$ (5-HT$_3$) receptor antagonists, such as ondansetron, may ameliorate SSRI-related nausea (Harnett 1994). Bupropion—a nontricyclic, non-SSRI—may also be safe in this population, but its use is relatively contraindicated in patients with a history of seizures. Data on newer ADs (nefazodone, fluvoxamine, venlafaxine, mirtazapine) are still incomplete vis-à-vis use in cancer patients.

Harnett (2001) has reviewed the use of psychotropics in patients with cardiovascular disease, diabetes mellitus, and respiratory disease. As a rough generalization, SSRIs appear to be the class of AD with the best overall safety and tolerability in these groups. However, in such medically ill patients, the risk of drug–drug interactions and alterations in drug metabolism (see below) must be carefully considered on a case-by-case basis; for example, fluoxetine, but not citalopram, would be expected to raise plasma levels of the antiarrhythmic agent encainide (Cozza et al. 2003).

Q. What about depressed patients with cancer and other diseases who cannot tolerate oral ADs?

A. Many medically ill patients become too weak to swallow even liquid medications; others cannot take medications orally because of stomatitis or oral, pharyngeal, or esophageal surgery (Massie and Holland 1990). In such cases, the use of intramuscular preparations or rectal suppositories may be considered. Amitriptyline, imipramine, and doxepin can be given intramuscularly, and the successful use of rectal doxepin and carbamazepine in patients with cancer has been reported (Massie and Lesko 1989; Storey and Trumble 1992). The rectal administration of amitriptyline (50 mg in cocoa butter twice daily) resulted in clinical improvement in one severely depressed cancer patient (Adams 1982). Doxepin capsules (25 mg) with no suppository base have also been used in a small number of patients, with apparent clinical benefit (Storey and Trumble 1992). Measurements of these drugs in the serum suggest that they are well absorbed via the rectum.

Q. Are the psychostimulants useful in treating depressed cancer patients and other depressed medically ill populations?

A. The psychostimulants (methylphenidate, pemoline, and D-amphetamine) may also be useful in treating depressed cancer patients, promoting a sense of well-being, decreased fatigue, and improved appetite (when used in low doses) (Massie and Holland 1990). These agents have a rapid onset of AD action and are not abused in the medically ill population; however, tolerance may sometimes develop. Psychostimulants, like ADs, also potentiate the pain-relieving effects of narcotic analgesics and help counteract their sedating effects. Some clinicians regard psychostimulants as first-line treatments of depression in the medical setting, because of their rapid therapeutic effect and low frequency of adverse reactions.

Q. What drug–drug interactions have importance in medically ill patients taking ADs?

A. Since most medically ill patients will be taking several nonpsychotropic medications, the issue of drug–drug interactions often becomes critical (Ciraulo et al. 1995a, 1995b; Gelenberg 1995). It should be borne in mind that some SSRIs (notably fluoxetine, paroxetine, and fluvoxamine) are strong inhibitors of the cytochrome P450 system, which is responsible for the metabolism of numerous "nonpsychiatric" drugs and medications. The CYP 2D6 system—which is strongly inhibited by paroxetine and fluoxetine—metabolizes many antiarrhythmics (e.g., encainide, propafenone), beta-blockers, opiates, and donepezil. CYP 3A4—which is moderately inhibited by fluvoxamine, strongly inhibited by nefazodone, and modestly inhibited by sertraline—metabolizes lidocaine, quinidine, carbamazepine, calcium channel blockers, erythromycin, steroids, protease inhibitors, cisapride, and the nonsedating antihistamine loratadine (which is also metabolized by CYP 2D6; Cozza et al. 2003). HIV patients receiving protease inhibitors (e.g., ritonavir, saquinavir) are at especially high risk for drug–drug interactions in the CYP 3A4 system, which is affected by several ADs (Cozza et al. 2003). In all patients—but especially in medically ill populations—the clinician is well advised to assume a drug–drug interaction until proved otherwise.

Q. What are the risks of AD use during pregnancy and the postpartum period? What special concerns arise when dosing ADs in the pregnant patient?

A. With respect to ADs, most data come from studies of the TCAs and fluoxetine; we have only limited information about other SSRIs or newer agents such as duloxetine and escitalopram (Altshuler et al. 1996; Newport et al. 2004; Stowe and Nemeroff 1995). The TCAs (e.g., desipramine [Norpramin], imipramine [Tofranil], nortriptyline [Pamelor]) appear to have little potential for teratogenicity. However, the more anticholinergic tricyclics (e.g., amitriptyline, doxepin) can occasionally induce fetal tachyarrhythmias, urinary retention, or intestinal obstruction. Clomipramine (Anafranil), a tricyclic used mainly in the treatment of OCD, also has substantial anticholinergic effects and would be expected to produce similar effects in the neonate. With respect to dosing, Wisner and colleagues (1993) found that the doses of TCA required to achieve remission actually increased during the second half of pregnancy, reaching 1.6 times the mean dose required when the patients were not pregnant. The necessity for a higher dose was attributed, in part, to enhanced hepatic metabolism of ADs during pregnancy and to increased volume of distribution. Neonatal irritability, tachypnea, tremor, and hypotonia may result from tricyclic toxicity or withdrawal. It is therefore prudent to monitor maternal TCA blood levels throughout pregnancy and gradually to reduce the dosage during the week before delivery.

SSRIs also appear safe during gestation. A study by Pastuszak and colleagues (1993) found no evidence of teratogenicity in 128 women taking fluoxetine during the first trimester, when compared with matched control subjects. Although there was a trend toward higher miscarriage rates in the fluoxetine group compared with the control women taking known nonteratogens, the risk was small (relative risk=1.9) and comparable to that of TCAs. (Interestingly, depression itself may also raise the risk of miscarriage.) A study by Chambers and colleagues (1996) found no significant differences between fluoxetine-treated pregnant women and control women in number of spontaneous pregnancy losses of major structural anomalies; however, the incidence of three or more minor anomalies was significantly higher in the fluoxetine cohort, and women who took fluoxetine during the third trimester were at increased risk for perinatal complications. The Chambers et al. study has been criticized on a variety of methodological grounds, including its failure to control for coexisting diseases (Nulman et al. 1997). Nulman and colleagues (1997) found that in utero exposure to either TCAs or fluoxetine does not affect global IQ, language development, or behavioral development in preschool children. Summarizing the published reports of SSRI use during gestation (*N*=2,219), including use of fluoxetine, citalopram, paroxetine, sertraline, and fluvoxamine, Newport et al. (2004) concluded that, collectively, "these data provide no evidence that prenatal SSRI exposure is associated with an increased incidence of congenital malformation" (p. 1118). In their comprehensive review, Altshuler et al. (1996) concluded that the "use of psychotropic medications during pregnancy is appropriate in many clinical situations and should include thoughtful weighing of risk of prenatal exposure versus risk of relapse following drug discontinuation" (p. 592). Finally, the clinician should keep in mind that ECT appears to be a safe and effective alternative for the pregnant patient with severe depression.

Q. Is there an AD of "first choice" during pregnancy?

A. There are insufficient data from well-designed studies to allow a confident answer. Miller (1994) concluded that the *tricyclics* of choice during pregnancy are desipramine and nortriptyline, because of the comparative wealth of data about them, the ability to monitor serum levels, and a favorable side-effect profile. Among the SSRIs, fluoxetine (Prozac) may be a reasonable choice for the pregnant patient with major depression, in light of the large database (*N*=1,241 exposures; Newport et al. 2004) and the data from Pastuszak et al. (1993) and Nulman et al. (1997)—notwithstanding the data from Chambers et al. (1996). Though very preliminary, some recent reports have implicated SSRIs in postdelivery *withdrawal symptoms* (hypotonia, reduced respiratory rate, EEG abnormalities) and *abnormal bleeding* in neonates (Rosenblatt and Rosenblatt 2004); however, such putative neonatal discontinuation syndromes appear to be rare and do not warrant drug discontinuation (Cohen 2004).

Q. How safe is breastfeeding while taking an AD?

A. Little is known about the excretion of ADs into breast milk or the effects of these agents on the nursing infant. Some studies indicate that several ADs or their metabolites can accumulate in breast milk, possibly peaking about 4–6 hours after an oral dose. It is not clear to what extent ADs accumulate in the blood of the nursing infant or whether significant adverse effects result from such accumulation; nevertheless, some clinicians believe that breastfeeding is best avoided when the mother is taking ADs postpartum. A report by Spigset and colleagues (1996), however, found no adverse effects in an infant whose mother was breastfeeding while taking paroxetine. This report noted that accumulation of paroxetine in breast milk may be lower than that seen with fluoxetine or fluvoxamine. In a recent review, Newport and colleagues (2004) concluded, first, that quantitative infant exposure to SSRIs during lactation is considerably lower than *transplacental* exposure during gestation, and second, that "although infant follow-up data are limited, only a few isolated cases of adverse effects have been reported" (p. 1120). Finally, the psychological importance of breastfeeding to the mother must also be weighed in the decision.

Vignettes/Puzzlers

Q. An elderly depressed woman is taking 75 mg of nortriptyline per day, with a plasma level of 120 ng/mL (therapeutic range: 50–150 ng/mL). Her hepatic and renal functions are normal. She presents to her primary physician with a 1-week history of fever, dysuria, and malaise. Urine culture at that time reveals evidence of infection, but BUN (blood urea nitrogen) and creatinine levels and liver functions are at baseline. The patient shows no evidence of postural hypotension, tachycardia, new-onset anticholinergic side effects, or confusion. An ECG shows no evidence of conduction abnormality. A nortriptyline level at that time comes back at 170 ng/mL. Does the patient have a "toxic" nortriptyline level, and should her dose be reduced?

A. This apparent elevation of nortriptyline level most likely reflects elevation of *total* serum nortriptyline levels (free plus protein-bound), and not increased or "toxic" levels of the free drug. Many psychotropic medications are bound to α_1 acid glycoprotein, termed an *acute phase reactant,* since levels may increase in response to myocardial infarction, shock, severe burns, or infectious processes (Friedman and Greenblatt 1986). This causes increased binding of some basic (nonacidic) drugs, without increased clinical or toxic effects. The clinician's "therapeutic range" for a given drug may therefore shift, such that—as in the present case—a plasma level of 170 ng/mL is very likely well within the therapeutic range for nortriptyline (Friedman and Greenblatt 1986). It is possible, but quite expensive, to order levels of only the free drug. In the present case, no adjustment of the patient's nortriptyline dose is necessary, particularly since there is no clinical evidence of tricyclic toxicity.

Q. A 67-year-old woman with major depression is prescribed nortriptyline 25 mg hs, with subsequent increases to 50 mg hs. Her plasma level is 74 ng/mL. After about 2 weeks, the patient complains of severe eye and face pain, nausea, vomiting, loss of visual acuity, and "colored halos" in her visual field. What is the most likely diagnosis?

A. This case strongly suggests *narrow-angle glaucoma* precipitated by the anticholinergic effects of nortriptyline. The most common adult form of glaucoma—chronic, open-angle type—is not usually worsened by anticholinergic agents. Narrow-angle (or "angle-closure") glaucoma may be worsened by psychotropics with anticholinergic properties, leading to blockage of aqueous humor flow and an acute rise in intraocular pressure. Thus, a careful medical and ophthalmological history is necessary before prescribing a TCA or similar agents (Gelenberg 1994). Although exacerbation of glaucoma is rare with SSRIs, there are scattered reports of such instances (Jimenez-Jimenez et al. 2001).

Q. **An elderly patient with recurrent depression has responded poorly to several SSRI trials but responds well to nortriptyline. This agent works well at 75 mg/day given at bedtime, but the patient notes "a funny feeling in my chest" when the total dose is given at bedtime. ECGs done in the morning show second-degree atrioventricular block. The patient's regimen is converted to a 25 mg bid and 25 mg hs schedule. Both the chest discomfort and the ECG abnormalities disappear. What is the pharmacokinetic explanation?**

A. While the average steady-state plasma drug level does not change whether the total dose is given once a day or in divided doses, the "height" of C_{max} (peak plasma drug concentration after a dose) does increase when a drug is given in a single large dose. This increase may be associated with greater direct quinidine-like effects of nortriptyline on cardiac nerve fibers and, thus, greater conduction delay and arrhythmias (see Preskorn 1993).

Q. **A 64-year-old woman with severe major depression is prescribed venlafaxine at 75 mg po bid. The patient is also taking "over-the-counter" cimetidine 200 mg bid for "heartburn" and quinidine sulfate 200 mg tid for occasional premature ventricular contractions. Because of ongoing psychotic symptoms, haloperidol 1 mg po bid is added 5 days after the venlafaxine is started. Four days later, the patient complains of severe nausea, somnolence, and dizziness. What is the likely cause?**

A. Venlafaxine is metabolized by the CYP 2D6 system (Cozza et al. 2003). All of the other medications noted—quinidine, haloperidol, and cimetidine—inhibit CYP 2D6 and probably raised plasma venlafaxine levels into the toxic range for this patient (the nausea being a clue). (**Note:** Quinidine is itself metabolized via the CYP 3A4 system but is an inhibitor of CYP 2D6.)

Q. A bipolar patient receiving maintenance carbamazepine 200 mg tid (with a plasma level of 7.0 μg/mL) is admitted to the hospital with severe depression. He is begun on a generic form of nefazodone 100 mg bid, which is increased to 150 mg bid. Four days later, the patient is ataxic, with slurred speech and nystagmus. A carbamazepine level comes back at 12 μg/mL, which is within the putative therapeutic range (5–12 μg/mL). What is a likely explanation for the patient's clinical picture?

A. Nefazodone is an inhibitor of CYP 3A4, which is the pathway involved in the metabolism of carbamazepine. The 10,11-epoxide of carbamazepine can cause neurotoxicity even when the plasma level of the parent compound is within the "therapeutic" range. Most likely, this epoxide metabolite had increased to toxic levels in this case. (This metabolite is apparently *not* formed when the keto-congener of carbamazepine, oxcarbazepine [Trileptal], is used.)

Q. A 73-year-old woman with major depression has had a partial response to a generic form of nefazodone 250 mg/day and is tolerating it without significant side effects. Since the effective dosage range is usually between 300 and 600 mg/day, the patient's psychiatrist increases the dosage of nefazodone (over a period of 5 days) to 400 mg/day. Two days after the final dosage adjustment, the patient complains of somnolence, nausea, dizziness, and confusion. What is the likely explanation for the patient's clinical picture?

A. Nefazodone exhibits nonlinear pharmacokinetics at steady state; that is, an increase in dose results in a greater-than-proportional increase in plasma levels. Thus, mean peak plasma levels following daily doses of 100, 200, and 400 mg are, respectively, 270, 730, and 2,050 ng/mL (DeVane 1995). In this case, the patient probably experienced a marked increase in plasma levels, leading to side effects, despite being well within the usual "therapeutic" dose range; her advanced age may well have been a factor (DeVane 1995).

Q. A 43-year-old man with major depression and HIV/AIDS is prescribed citalopram 40 mg/day. His other medications include ritonavir (a protease inhibitor), which was started the week before, and oral amoxicillin, initiated 3 days prior to his starting citalopram, for a recent lower respiratory infection. Within 5 days of taking the citalopram, the patient complains of muscle twitches, shivering, diarrhea, and confusion. He is disoriented to day and date and has difficulty with short-term memory. His affect is hypomanic. What is the likely syndrome, and what is the etiology?

A. This patient's symptoms probably represent a case of serotonin syndrome (see Table 2–22) due to elevated levels of citalopram. Citalopram is metabolized via CYP 2C19, 2D6, and 3A4. Ritonavir and other protease inhibitors are (at least initially) significant *inhibitors* of CYP 3A4 and 2D6 (Cozza et al. 2003). Patients taking fluoxetine and other SSRIs may develop serotonin syndrome when protease inhibitors are coadministered (DeSilva et al. 2001). However, over time, protease inhibitors may actually *induce* CYP enzymes, including 3A4, thus creating complex and puzzling effects on psychotropics (Cozza et al. 2003). Similarly, over-the-counter herbal agents, such as St. John's wort, may induce CYP 3A4 and cause significant drops in blood levels of protease inhibitors (Sandson 2003). The use of amoxicillin in this case is not likely to have affected the cytochrome system or the clinical picture.

Q. A 45-year-old man with major depression, panic attacks, and asthma is started on fluvoxamine, 50 mg qd. The dosage is increased over the next 5 days to 100 mg bid. He is also taking theophylline as Theo-dur, 200 mg bid, and alprazolam, 1.0 mg tid. Five days after beginning the fluvoxamine, the patient is tachycardic and anxious, yet also drowsy with mildly slurred speech. What is a likely explanation for the patient's clinical picture?

A. Fluvoxamine is a potent inhibitor of CYP 1A2, which metabolizes theophylline (Cozza et al. 2003). It also inhibits CYP 3A4, which metabolizes the triazolobenzodiazepines (including alprazolam). Most likely, this patient developed toxic levels of both theophylline (leading to tachycardia and anxiety) and alprazolam (leading to drowsiness and slurred speech).

Q. A 14-year-old girl with a diagnosis of "conduct disorder" and major depressive disorder (first episode) is prescribed paroxetine 10 mg qam. Past psychiatric history is negative with respect to psychosis or manic episodes, and there have been no previous AD trials. There is, however, a long history of "moodiness," "poor impulse control," and "severe temper tantrums" associated with damage to surroundings. Medical history is noncontributory. A workup for neurological disorder/epilepsy and attention-deficit/hyperactivity disorder is negative. Family history is positive for "mood swings" in the girl's maternal grandmother. Six days after beginning paroxetine, the patient begins to develop intense suicidal ideation accompanied by mild, self-injurious behavior (skin cutting). She presents in the ER with screaming, crying, and increased psychomotor activity. What is the most likely etiology?

A. It is difficult to tell, but a manic episode would be high on the list of suspects. On June 10, 2003, the British counterpart of the U.S. Food and Drug Administration (FDA) issued a "Dear Doctor" letter, announcing that the British equivalent of Paxil (Seroxat, paroxetine) should not be used to treat depression in patients younger than age 18. This recommendation was based on a putatively high risk of suicidal ideation in this group. Subsequently, the FDA also recommended against use of paroxetine in children and adolescents. Controlled studies of paroxetine and sertraline in younger populations have not yielded robustly positive results (Carlat 2003a; Keller et al. 2001; Wagner et al. 2003), and the only FDA-approved SSRI for depressed younger populations is fluoxetine (Emslie et al. 1997). Nevertheless, the claim that Paxil, Effexor (venlafaxine), or other ADs "cause" increased suicidal behavior in younger populations is difficult to substantiate on the basis of carefully controlled studies (Perlis 2003), and the concept of "suicidal behavior" may be overly broad.

A preliminary report from the American College of Neuropsychopharmacology (ACNP) also casts doubt on any link between SSRI-type ADs and suicide (Harris 2004). The situation may differ, however, in younger bipolar patients, who may not have been correctly diagnosed, as may have been the case with the patient in our vignette. These patients may sometimes develop a mixed or irritable manic state in response to ADs, which in turn may lead to suicidal ideation or self-injurious behavior (Perlis 2003). One should treat the diagnosis of "conduct disorder" or "ADHD" with some skepticism in children with histories of severe mood instability, irritability, behavioral "dyscontrol," and positive family histories of bipolar disorder (Fergus et al. 2003;

Mota-Castillo 2002). Major depressive episodes in such patients should raise the question of bipolar disorder and may require treatment with mood stabilizers (Pies 2002). Recent changes in the product information for Serzone reflects some awareness that inappropriate treatment of bipolar disorder with an AD may lead to precipitation of mixed or manic episodes (Bristol-Myers-Squibb, "Dear Physician" letter, June 18, 2004). Notwithstanding uncertainties in the data, the FDA recently required black box warnings regarding increased risk of "suicidality" for all antidepressants (FDA news release, October 15, 2004).

Q. A 27-year-old man with a history of opiate abuse, dysthymia, and OCD has been taking methadone 50 mg/day, with good behavioral control of his addiction. However, he begins to develop signs and symptoms of major depression and worsening OCD after losing his job of 7 years. He is prescribed fluvoxamine 50 mg/day, and the dosage is increased to 150 mg/day after 2 weeks. With no improvement in depression at that point, and a new complaint of sexual dysfunction, the physician adds a generic form of nefazodone, 50 mg/day, to the patient's regimen. Within 5 days, the patient appears somnolent and slightly euphoric and complains of constipation. On physical examination, the patient's pupils are slightly constricted and reflexes are diminished symmetrically. What is the cause of these changes?

A. Most likely, the patient is experiencing signs and symptoms of methadone toxicity. Methadone is metabolized mainly via CYP 3A4, and perhaps to some extent via CYP 2D6. Although fluvoxamine is only a moderate inhibitor of CYP 3A4, nefazodone is a strong inhibitor (Cozza et al. 2003). The combination of the two ADs most likely raised plasma methadone levels considerably.

References

Adams S: Amitriptyline suppositories. N Engl J Med 306:996, 1982

Agras WS: Treatment of eating disorders, in The American Psychiatric Publishing Textbook of Psychopharmacology, 3rd Edition. Edited by Schatzberg AF, Nemeroff CB. Washington, DC, American Psychiatric Publishing, 2004, pp 1031–1040

Akiskal HS: Dysthymic disorder: psychopathology of proposed chronic depressive subtypes. Am J Psychiatry 140:11–20, 1983

Albert R, Ebert D: Full efficacy of SSRI treatment in refractory dysthymia is achieved only after 16 weeks (letter). J Clin Psychiatry 57:176, 1996

Altshuler LL, Post RM, Leverich GS, et al: Antidepressant-induced mania and cycle acceleration: a controversy revisited. Am J Psychiatry 152:1130–1138, 1995

Altshuler LL, Cohen L, Szuba MP et al: Pharmacologic management of psychiatric illness during pregnancy: dilemmas and guidelines. Am J Psychiatry 153:592–606, 1996

Altshuler LL, Cohen LS, Moline ML et al: The Expert Consensus Guidelines Series. Treatment of depression in women. Postgrad Med (spec no 1), March 2001, pp 1–107

Altshuler L, Suppes T, Black D, et al: Impact of antidepressant discontinuation after acute bipolar depression remission on rates of depressive relapse at 1-year follow-up. Am J Psychiatry 160:1252–1262, 2003

American Psychiatric Association: Diagnostic and Statistical Manual of Mental Disorders, 3rd Edition, Revised. Washington, DC, American Psychiatric Association, 1987

American Psychiatric Association: Diagnostic and Statistical Manual of Mental Disorders, 4th Edition. Washington, DC, American Psychiatric Association, 1994

American Psychiatric Association: Diagnostic and Statistical Manual of Mental Disorders, 4th Edition, Text Revision. Washington, DC, American Psychiatric Association, 2000

American Psychiatric Association: Practice guideline for the treatment of patients with bipolar disorder (revision). Am J Psychiatry 159:1–50, 2002

Amsterdam JD, Garcia-Espana F, Fawcett J, et al: Efficacy and safety of fluoxetine in treating bipolar II major depressive episode. J Clin Psychopharmacol 18:435–440, 1998

Apter JT, Birkett M: Fluoxetine treatment in depressed patients who failed treatment with sertraline. Presentation at the 34th annual meeting of the American College of Neuropsychopharmacology, San Juan, Puerto Rico, December 1995

Apter JT, Kushner SF: A guide to selection of antidepressants. Primary Psychiatry 3:14–16, 1996

Arana GW, Hyman SE: Handbook of Psychiatric Drug Therapy, 2nd Edition. Boston, MA, Little, Brown, 1991

Arana GW, Rosenbaum JF: Handbook of Psychiatric Drug Therapy, 4th Edition. Philadelphia, PA, Lippincott Williams & Wilkins, 2000

Aranth J, Lindberg C: Bleeding, a side effect of fluoxetine (letter). Am J Psychiatry 149:412, 1992

Arias B, Catalan R, Gasto C, et al: 5HTTLPR polymorphism of the serotonin transporter gene predicts non-remission in major depression patients treated with citalopram in a 12-weeks follow up study. J Clin Psychopharmacol 23:563–567, 2003

Artigas F, Perez V, Alvarez E: Pindolol induces a rapid improvement of depressed patients treated with serotonin reuptake inhibitors. Arch Gen Psychiatry 51:248–251, 1994

Ayd FJ: Lexicon of Psychiatry, Neurology, and the Neurosciences. Baltimore, MD, Williams & Wilkins, 1995

Barr LC, Goodman WK, Price LH: Physical symptoms associated with paroxetine discontinuation (letter). Am J Psychiatry 151:289, 1994

Belanoff JK, Flores BH, Kalezhan M, et al: Rapid reversal of psychotic depression using mifepristone. J Clin Psychopharmacol 21:516–521, 2001

Bezchlibnyk-Butler KZ, Jeffries JJ: Clinical Handbook of Psychotropic Drugs. Seattle, WA, Hogrefe and Huber, 2000

Blier P: Cellular basis for the mechanisms of action of drugs in treating mood disorders. Current Psychiatry 2 (September supplement):26–29, 2003

Blumer D: The Dysthymic Pain Disorder: Chronic Pain as Masked Depression. New York, Biomedical Information Corporation, 1987

Bostic JQ, Prince J, Frazier J, et al: Pediatric psychopharmacology update. Psychiatric Times 20:88–94, 2003

Bowden CL, Goldberg JF: Switching and Destabilization in Bipolar Disorder. Boston, MA, Continuing Medical Education, Boston University School of Medicine, 2003

Bowden CL, Calabrese JR, Sachs G, et al: A placebo-controlled 18-month trial of lamotrigine and lithium maintenance treatment in recently manic or hypomanic patients with bipolar I disorder. Arch Gen Psychiatry 60:392–400, 2003

Boyer W, Bunt R: Selective-serotonin reuptake inhibitors and serotonin-norepinephrine reuptake inhibitors in treatment-resistant depression, in Treatment-Resistant Mood Disorders. Edited by Amsterdam JD, Hornig M, Nierenberg AA. Cambridge, England, Cambridge University Press, 2001, pp 159–179

Branconnier RJ, Cole JO, Ghazvinian S: Clinical pharmacology of bupropion and imipramine in elderly depressives. J Clin Psychiatry 44(sec 2):130–133, 1983

Brown WA, Harrison W: Are patients who are intolerant to one serotonin selective reuptake inhibitor intolerant to another? J Clin Psychiatry 56:30–34, 1995

Browne G, Steiner M, Roberts J, et al: Sertraline and/or interpersonal psychotherapy for patients with dysthymic disorder in primary care: 6-month comparison with longitudinal 2-year follow-up of effectiveness and costs. J Affect Disord 68:317–330, 2002

Bschor T, Bauer M: Is successful lithium augmentation limited to serotonergic antidepressants? J Clin Psychopharmacol 24:240–241, 2004

Burt VK, Suri R, Altshuler L, et al: The use of psychotropic medications during breast-feeding. Am J Psychiatry 158:1001–1009, 2001

Carlat D: Do antidepressants work for kids? The Carlat Report 1(11):1–2, 2003a

Carlat D: Psychostimulants: bringing order out of chaos. The Carlat Report 1(4):2–4, 2003b

Carlat D: Cymbalta: dual the reuptake, triple the hype. The Carlat Report 2(1):1–2, 2004

Castillo E, Rubin RT, Holsboer-Trachsler E: Clinical differentiation between lethal catatonia and neuroleptic malignant syndrome. Am J Psychiatry 146:324–328, 1989

Chambers CD, Johnson KA, Dick LM, et al: Birth outcomes in pregnant women taking fluoxetine. N Engl J Med 335:1010–1015, 1996

Charney DS, Miller HL, Licinio J, et al: Treatment of depression, in The American Psychiatric Press Textbook of Psychopharmacology, Edited by Schatzberg AF, Nemeroff CB. Washington, DC, American Psychiatric Press, 1995, pp 575–601

Ciraulo DA, Creelman WL, Shader RI, et al: Antidepressants, in Drug Interactions in Psychiatry, 2nd Edition. Edited by Ciraulo CA, Shader RI, Greenblatt FJ, et al. Baltimore, MD, Williams & Wilkins, 1995a, pp 29–63

Ciraulo DA, Shader RI, Greenblatt DJ: SSRI drug-drug interactions, in Drug Interactions in Psychiatry, 2nd Edition. Edited by Ciraulo CA, Shader RI, Greenblatt FJ, et al. Baltimore, MD, Williams & Wilkins, 1995b, pp 64–89

Cohen L: Treating the depressed and pregnant. Clinical Psychiatry News, November 2004, p 12

Cole SA, Woodard JL, Juncos JL et al: Depression and disability in Parkinson's disease. J Neuropsychiatry Clin Neurosci 8:20–25, 1996

Cornelius JR, Soloff PH, Perel JM, et al: Continuation pharmacotherapy of borderline personality disorder with haloperidol and phenelzine. Am J Psychiatry 150:1843–1848, 1993

Coryell W, Solomon D, Turvey C, et al: The long-term course of rapid-cycling bipolar disorder. Arch Gen Psychiatry 60:914–920, 2003

Cozza KL, Armstrong SC, Oesterheld JR: Concise Guide to Drug Interaction Principles for Medical Practice: Cytochrome P450s, UGTs, P-Glycoproteins, 2nd Edition. Washington, DC, American Psychiatric Publishing, 2003, pp 60–166, 345–369

Creelman W, Ciraulo DA: Monoamine oxidase inhibitors, in Drug Interactions in Psychiatry, 2nd Edition. Edited by Ciraulo CA, Shader RI, Greenblatt FJ, et al. Baltimore, MD, Williams and Wilkins, 1995, pp 90–128

Dalton SO, Johansen C, Mellemkjoer L, et al: Use of selective serotonin reuptake inhibitors and risk of upper gastrointestinal tract bleeding. Arch Intern Med 163:59–64, 2003

Davidson JRT: Monoamine oxidase inhibitors, in Handbook of Affective Disorders, 2nd Edition. Edited by Paykel ES. New York, Guilford, 1992, pp 345–358

de Abajo FJ, Rodriguez LAG, Montero D: Association between selective serotonin reuptake inhibitors and upper gastrointestinal bleeding: population based case-control study. BMJ 319:1106–1109, 1999

DeBattista C, Doghramji K, Menza MA, et al: Adjunct modafinil for the short-term treatment of fatigue and sleepiness in patients with major depressive disorder: a preliminary double-blind, placebo-controlled study. J Clin Psychiatry 64:1057–1064, 2003

Demitrack MA: Can monoamine-based therapies be improved? J Clin Psychiatry 63(suppl 2):14–18, 2002

Denys D, van Megen HJ, van der Wee N, et al: A double-blind switch study of paroxetine and venlafaxine in obsessive-compulsive disorder. J Clin Psychiatry 65:37–43, 2004

Depression Guideline Panel: Depression in Primary Care, Vol 2: Treatment of Major Depression (Clinical Practice Guideline No 5; AHCPR Publ No 93-0551). Rockville, MD, U.S. Dept of Health and Human Services, Public Health Service, Agency for Health Care Policy and Research, 1993

Derogatis LR, Morrow GR, Fetting J, et al. The prevalence of psychiatric disorders among cancer patients. JAMA 249:751–757, 1983

DeSilva KE, Le Flore DB, Marston BJ, et al: Serotonin syndrome in HIV-infected individuals receiving antiretroviral therapy and fluoxetine. AIDS 15:1281–1285, 2001

DeVane CL: Nefazodone—pharmacology and efficacy of a new antidepressant agent: formulary considerations. Pharmacy and Therapeutics, June 1995, pp 363–374

Dewan MJ, Pies RW (eds): The Difficult-to-Treat Psychiatric Patient. Washington, DC, American Psychiatric Publishing, 2001

Dong J, Blier P: Modification of norepinephrine and serotonin, but not dopamine, neuron firing by sustained bupropion treatment. Psychopharmacology (Berl) 155:52–57, 2001

Drug Facts and Comparisons. St Louis, MO, Facts and Comparisons, 1995, pp 1356–1505

Dubovsky SL: Geriatric neuropsychopharmacology, in The American Psychiatric Press Textbook of Geriatric Neuropsychiatry. Edited by Coffey CE, Cummings JL. Washington, DC, American Psychiatric Press, 1994, pp 596–631

Duman RS, Heninger GR, Nestler EJ: A molecular and cellular theory of depression. Arch Gen Psychiatry 54:597–606, 1997

Dunbar GC, Cohn JB, Feighner JP, et al: A comparison of paroxetine, imipramine, and placebo in depressed outpatients. Br J Psychiatry 159:394–398, 1991

Dunner DL: Treating depression in the elderly. J Clin Psychiatry 55 (12, suppl):48–58, 1994

Dunner DL, Zisook S, Billow AA: A prospective safety surveillance study for bupropion sustained-release in the treatment of depression. J Clin Psychiatry 59:366–373, 1998

Edwards JG, Long SK, Sedgwick EM, et al: Antidepressants and convulsive seizures: clinical, electroencephalographic, and pharmacologic aspects. Clin Neuropharmacol 9:329–360, 1986

Ellison JM, Milofsky JE, Ely E: Fluoxetine-induced bradycardia and syncope in two patients. J Clin Psychiatry 51:385–386, 1990

Emslie GJ, Rush AJ, Weinberg WA, et al: A double-blind, randomized, placebo-controlled trial of fluoxetine in depressed children and adolescents. Arch Gen Psychiatry 54:1031–1037, 1997

Ereshefsky L: Drug interactions of antidepressants. Psychiatr Ann 26:342–350, 1996

Ereshefsky L, Overman GP, Karp JK: Current psychotropic dosing and monitoring guidelines. Primary Psychiatry 3:21–45, 1996

Fava M: Management of nonresponse and intolerance: switching strategies. J Clin Psychiatry 61 (suppl 2):10–12, 2000

Fava M: The role of the serotonergic and noradrenergic neurotransmitter systems in the treatment of psychological and physical symptoms of depression. J Clin Psychiatry 64 (suppl 13):26–29, 2003

Fava M, Judge R, Hoog SL, et al: Fluoxetine versus sertraline and paroxetine in major depressive disorder: changes in weight with long-term treatment. J Clin Psychiatry 61:863–867, 2000

Fava M, Dunner DL, Greist JH, et al: Efficacy and safety of mirtazapine in major depressive disorder patients after SSRI treatment failure: an open-label trial. J Clin Psychiatry 62(6):413–420, 2001

Fava M, McGrath PJ, Sheu WP, and the Reboxetine Study Group: Switching to reboxetine: an efficacy and safety study in patients with major depressive disorder unresponsive to fluoxetine. J Clin Psychopharmacol 23:365–3699, 2003

Favale E, Rubino V, Mainardi P, et al: Anticonvulsant effect of fluoxetine in humans. Neurology 45:1926–1927, 1995

Fawcett J, Kravitz HM, Zajecka JM, et al: CNS stimulant potentiation of monoamine oxidase inhibitors in treatment-refractory depression. J Clin Psychopharmacol 11:127–132, 1991

Feder R: Bradycardia and syncope induced by fluoxetine. J Clin Psychiatry 52:139, 1991a

Feder R: Reversal of antidepressant activity of fluoxetine by cyproheptadine in three patients. J Clin Psychiatry 52:163–164, 1991b

Feighner JP, Herbstein J, Damlouji N: Combined MAOI, TCA, and direct stimulant therapy of treatment resistant depression. J Clin Psychiatry 46:206–209, 1985

Fergus EL, Miller RB, Luckenbaugh DA, et al: Is there a progression from irritability/dyscontrol to major depressive and manic symptoms? A retrospective community survey of parents of bipolar children. J Affect Disord 77:71–78, 2003

Fink M: Response to "Neuroleptic malignant-like syndrome due to cyclobenzoprine"? J Clin Psychopharmacol 16:97–98, 1996

Fink M: Separating psychotic depression from nonpsychotic depression is essential to effective treatment. J Affect Disord 76:1–3, 2003

Fink M, Bush G, Francis A: Catatonia: a treatable disorder, occasionally recognized. Directions in Psychiatry 13:1–7, 1993

Fogelson DL, Bystritsky A, Pasnau R: Bupropion in the treatment of bipolar disorders: the same old story? J Clin Psychiatry 53:443–446, 1992

Forest Pharmaceuticals: Lexapro (package insert). St Louis, MO, Forest Pharmaceuticals, 2003

Friedman H, Greenblatt DJ: Rational therapeutic drug monitoring. JAMA 256:2227–2233, 1986

Gadde KM, Parker CB, Maner LG, et al: Bupropion for weight loss: an investigation of efficacy and tolerability in overweight and obese women. Obes Res 9:544–551, 2001

Gammon GD: Incentive bias? (letter) J Clin Psychiatry 57:265, 1996

Gardner DM, Shulman KI, Walker SE: The making of a user friendly MAOI diet. J Clin Psychiatry 57:99–104, 1996

Gelenberg AJ: Angle-closure glaucoma and tricyclic antidepressants. Biological Therapies in Psychiatry Newsletter 17:35–36, 1994

Gelenberg AJ: The P450 family. Biological Therapies in Psychiatry Newsletter 18:29–31, 1995

Gelenberg AJ: Switching SSRIs. Biological Therapies in Psychiatry Newsletter 19:9–10, 1996

Gelenberg AJ: Can an SSRI lower cholesterol? Biological Therapies in Psychiatry Newsletter 20:6, 1997

Gelenberg AJ: SSRIs for children. Biological Therapies in Psychiatry Newsletter 26:33, 2003

Ghaemi SN: Mood Disorders: A Practical Guide. Philadelphia, PA, Lippincott Williams & Wilkins, 2003

Ghaemi SN, Boiman EE, Goodwin FK: Diagnosing bipolar disorder and the effect of antidepressants: a naturalistic study. J Clin Psychiatry 61:804–808, 2000

Giakas WJ, Davis JM: Intractable withdrawal from venlafaxine treated with fluoxetine. Psychiatr Ann 27:85–92, 1997

Giller E, Bialos D, Harkness L, et al: Assessing treatment response to the monoamine oxidase inhibitor isocarboxazid. J Clin Psychiatry 45:44–48, 1984

Glassman AH, Roose SP, Bigger JT: The safety of tricyclic antidepressants in cardiac patients: risk-benefit reconsidered. JAMA 26:2673–2675, 1993

Goff DC, Baldessarini RJ: Antipsychotics, in Drug Interactions in Psychiatry, 2nd Edition. Edited by Ciraulo CA, Shader RI, Greenblatt FJ, et al. Baltimore, MD, Williams & Wilkins, 1995, pp 129–174

Goldberg JF, Whiteside JE: The association between substance abuse and antidepressant-induced mania in bipolar disorder: a preliminary study. J Clin Psychiatry 63:791–795, 2002

Golden RN, Bebchuck JM, Leatherman ME: Trazodone and other antidepressants, in The American Psychiatric Press Textbook of Psychopharmacology, Edited by Schatzberg AF, Nemeroff CB, Washington, DC, American Psychiatric Press, 1995, pp 195–214

Golden RN, Dawkins K, Nicholas L: Trazodone and nefazodone., in The American Psychiatric Publishing Textbook of Psychopharmacology, 3rd Edition. Edited by Schatzberg AF, Nemeroff CB. Washington, DC, 2004, pp 315–325

Goldstein DJ, Mallinckrodt C, Lu Y, et al: Duloxetine in the treatment of major depressive disorder: a double-blind clinical trial. J Clin Psychiatry 63:225–231, 2002

Goldstein L, Barker M, Segall F, et al: Seizure and transient SIADH associated with sertraline (letter). Am J Psychiatry 153:732, 1996

Goodnick PJ, Henry JH, Buki VMV: Treatment of depression in patients with diabetes mellitus. J Clin Psychiatry 56:128–136, 1995

Goodwin FK, Jamison KR: Manic-Depressive Illness. New York, Oxford University Press, 1990

Gorman JM: Special considerations in switching antidepressants. Teleconference (chaired by Keller MB), Providence, RI, August 18, 1995

Greden J: Maintenance antidepressant treatment. Progress Notes (American Society of Clinical Psychopharmacology) 6(Fall–Winter):28–34, 1995–1996

Greenblatt DJ, Sellers EM, Koch-Weser J: Importance of protein binding for the interpretation of serum or plasma drug concentrations. J Clin Pharmacol 22:259–263, 1982

Grossman R, Hollander E: Treatment of obsessive-compulsive disorder with venlafaxine (letter). Am J Psychiatry 153:576–577, 1996

Hallward A, Ellison JM: Antidepressants and Sexual Function. London, Harcourt Health Communications (Mosby International), 2001

Harnett DS: Psychopharmacologic treatment of depression in the medical setting. Psychiatr Ann 24:545–551, 1994

Harnett DS: The difficult-to-treat psychiatric patient with comorbid medical illness, in The Difficult-to-Treat Psychiatric Patient. Edited by Dewan MJ, Pies RW. Washington, DC, American Psychiatric Publishing, 2001, pp 325–357

Harris G: Panels says Zoloft and cousins don't increase suicide risk. New York Times, January 22, 2004. Available at American College of Neuropsychopharmacology Web site (www.acnp.org). Accessed August 19, 2004.

Harrison WM, Stewart JW: Pharmacotherapy of dysthymic disorder, in Diagnosis and Treatment of Chronic Depression. Edited by Kocsis JH, Klein DN. New York, Guilford, 1995, pp 124–145

Herr KD, Nemeroff CB: Paroxetine, in The American Psychiatric Publishing Textbook of Psychopharmacology, 3rd Edition. Edited by Schatzberg AF, Nemeroff CB. Washington, DC, American Psychiatric Publishing, 2004, pp 259–281

Hoehn-Saric R, Harris GJ, Pearlson GD, et al: A fluoxetine-induced frontal lobe syndrome in an obsessive-compulsive patient. J Clin Psychiatry 52:131–133, 1991

Hopkins HS: Fluoxetine-bupropion interaction. Biological Therapies in Psychiatry Newsletter 19:31–32, 1996

Jacobson SA, Pies RW, Greenblatt DJ: Handbook of Geriatric Psychopharmacology. Washington, DC, American Psychiatric Publishing, 2002

Janicak PG, Davis JM, Preskorn SH, et al: Principles and Practice of Psychopharmacotherapy. Baltimore, MD, Williams & Wilkins, 1993

Jenkins SC, Tinsley JA, Van Loon JA: A Pocket Reference for Psychiatrists, 3rd Edition. Washington, DC, American Psychiatric Press, 2001

Jimenez-Jimenez FJ, Orti-Pareja M, Zurdo JM: Aggravation of glaucoma with fluvoxamine. Ann Pharmacother 35:1565–1566, 2001

Joffe RT: Thyroid augmentation, in Treatment-Resistant Mood Disorders. Edited by Amsterdam JD, Hornig M, Nierenberg AA. Cambridge, England, Cambridge University Press, 2001, pp 239–251

Joffe RT, Levitt AJ, Sokolov STH: Augmentation strategies: focus on anxiolytics. J Clin Psychiatry 57 (suppl 7):25–31, 1996a

Joffe, RT, Levitt AJ, Sokolov STH, et al: Response to an open trial of a second SSRI in major depression. J Clin Psychiatry 57:114–115, 1996b

Johnston JA, Lineberry CG, Ascher JA: A 102-center prospective study of seizure in association with bupropion. J Clin Psychiatry 52:450–456, 1991

Kaufman KR, Gerner R: Lamotrigine toxicity secondary to sertraline. Seizure 7:163–165, 1998

Kehoe WA, Schorr RB: Focus on mirtazapine. Formulary 31:455–469, 1996

Keller M: Depression in adults. Presentation at the 8th annual U.S. Psychiatric and Mental Health Congress, New York, NY, November 18, 1995

Keller MB, Ryan ND, Strober M, et al: Efficacy of paroxetine in the treatment of adolescent major depression: a randomized, controlled trial. J Am Acad Child Adolesc Psychiatry 40:762–772, 2001

Kennedy GJ: Psychopharmacology of late-life depression. Annals of Long-Term Care 9:35–40, 2001

Ketter TA, Jenkins JB, Schroeder DH, et al: Carbamazepine but not valproate induces bupropion metabolism. J Clin Psychopharmacol 15:327–333, 1995

Kline NA, Dow BM, Brown SA, et al: Sertraline efficacy in depressed combat veterans with post-traumatic stress disorder. Presentation at the 146th annual meeting of the American Psychiatric Association, San Francisco, CA, May 22–27, 1993

Kocsis JH, Thase M, Koran L, et al: Pharmacotherapy of pure dysthymia: sertraline vs imipramine and placebo. Eur Neuropsychopharmacol 4:204–206, 1994

Koran LM, Sallee FR, Pallanti S: Rapid benefit of intravenous pulse loading of clomipramine in obsessive-compulsive disorder. Am J Psychiatry 154:396–401, 1997

Krishnan KRR, Steffens DC, Doraiswamy PM: Psychotropic drug interactions. Primary Psychiatry 3:21–49, 1996

Lavretsky H, Kim M-D, Kuman A, et al: Combined treatment with methylphenidate and citalopram for accelerated response in the elderly: an open trial. J Clin Psychiatry 64:1410–1414, 2003

Leonard BE: New approaches to the treatment of depression. J Clin Psychiatry 57 (suppl 4):26–33, 1996

Lowry MR, Dunner FJ: Seizures during tricyclic therapy. Am J Psychiatry 137:1461–1462, 1980

Markovitz PJ, Wagner S: An open-label trial of modafinil augmentation in patients with partial response to antidepressant therapy. J Clin Psychopharmacol 23:207–209, 2003

Marshall RD, Liebowitz MR: Paroxetine/bupropion combination treatment for refractory depression (letter). J Clin Psychopharmacol 16:80–81, 1996

Marshall RD, Johannet CM, Collins PY, et al: Bupropion and sertraline combination treatment in refractory depression. J Clin Psychopharmacol 9:284–286, 1995

Massie MJ, Holland JC: Depression and the cancer patient. J Clin Psychiatry 51 (7, suppl):12–17, 1990

Massie MJ, Lesko L: Psychopharmacological management, in Handbook of Psychooncology: Psychological Care of the Patient With Cancer. Edited by Holland JC, Rowland JH. New York, Oxford University Press, 1989, pp 470–491

McElroy SL: Clinical management of antidepressant side effects. Presentation at the 8th annual U.S. Psychiatric and Mental Health Congress, New York, NY, November 18, 1995

Mechcatie E: Manufacturer halts shipments of nefazodone. Clinical Psychiatry News, June 2004, p 7

Menza MA, Kaufman KF, Castellanos AM: Modafinil augmentation of antidepressant treatment in depression. J Clin Psychiatry 61:378–381, 2000

Metz A, Shader RI: Combination of fluoxetine with pemoline in the treatment of major depressive disorder. Int Clin Psychopharmacol 6:93–96, 1991

Miller LJ: Psychiatric medication during pregnancy: understanding and minimizing risks. Psychiatr Ann 24:69–75, 1994

Montejo AL, Llorca G, Izquierdo JA, et al: Incidence of sexual dysfunction associated with antidepressant agents: a prospective multicenter study of 1022 outpatients. J Clin Psychiatry 62 (suppl 3):10–21, 2001

Morishita S, Arita S: The clinical use of milnacipran for depression. Eur Psychiatry 18:34–35, 2003

Mota-Castillo M: Five red flags that rule out ADHD in children. Current Psychiatry 4:56, 2002

Narendran R, Young CM, Valenti AM, et al: Is psychosis exacerbated by modafinil? Arch Gen Psychiatry 59:292–293, 2002

Nelson JC: Are the SSRIs really better tolerated than the TCAs for treatment of major depression? Psychiatr Ann 24:628–631, 1994

Nemeroff CB: Drug interactions in perspective. Progress Notes (American Society of Clinical Psychopharmacology) 6(Fall–Winter):35–37, 1995–1996

Nemeroff CB: Dr Nemeroff replies (letter). J Clin Psychiatry 57:267–268, 1996

Nemeroff CB, Devane CL, Pollack BG: Summary and review of antidepressants and the cytochrome P450 system. Progress Notes (American Society of Clinical Psychopharmacology) 6(Fall–Winter):38–40, 1995–1996

Newport DJ, Fisher A, Graybeal S, et al: Psychopharmacology during pregnancy and lactation, in The American Psychiatric Publishing Textbook of Psychopharmacology, 3rd Edition. Edited by Schatzberg AF, Nemeroff CB. Washington, DC, American Psychiatric Publishing, 2004, pp 1109–1146

Nierenberg AA: The treatment of severe depression: is there an efficacy gap between SSRI and TCA antidepressant generations? J Clin Psychiatry 55 (9, suppl A):55–59, 1994

Nierenberg AA, Papakostas GI, Peterson T, et al: Lithium augmentation of nortriptyline for subjects resistant to multiple antidepressants. J Clin Psychopharmacol 23:92–95, 2003

Nulman I, Rovet J, Stewart DE, et al: Neurodevelopment of children exposed in utero to antidepressant drugs. N Engl J Med 336:258–262, 1997

Oesterheld J, Kallepalli BR: Grapefruit juice and clomipramine: shifting metabolic ratios. J Clin Psychopharmacol 17:62–63, 1997

Oesterheld JR, Shader RI, Wender PH: Diagnosis and treatment of attention deficit hyperactivity disorder in youth and adults, in Manual of Psychiatric Therapeutics, 3rd Edition. Edited by Shader RI. Philadelphia, PA, Lippincott Williams & Wilkins, 2003, pp 346–364

O'Reardon J: On antidepressant augmentation. The Carlat Report 2(1):4–5, 2004

Ottervanger JP, Stricker BHCH, Huls J, et al: Bleeding attributed to the intake of paroxetine (letter). Am J Psychiatry 151:781–782, 1994

Pallanti S, Quercioli L, Koran LM: Citalopram intravenous infusion in resistant obsessive-compulsive disorder: an open trial. J Clin Psychiatry 63:796–801, 2002

Pastuszak A, Schick-Boschetto B, Zuber C, et al: Pregnancy outcome following first-trimester exposure to fluoxetine (Prozac). JAMA 269:2246–2248, 1993

Pearlman CA: Neuroleptic malignant syndrome: a review of the literature. J Clin Psychopharmacol 6:257–273, 1986

Peck AW, Stern WC, Watkinson C: Incidence of seizures during treatment with tricyclic antidepressant drugs and bupropion. J Clin Psychiatry 44 (5, sec 2):197–201, 1983

Perlis RH: Child proof: first, do no harm? Paroxetine and suicide. Curbside Consultant (Massachusetts General Hospital) 2(October/November):1, 2003

Peselow ED, Filippi AM, Goodnick P, et al: The short- and long-term efficacy of paroxetine HCl, B: data from a double-blind crossover study and from a year-long trial vs imipramine and placebo. Psychopharmacol Bull 25:272–276, 1989

Petersdorf RG: Hypothermia and hyperthermia, in Harrison's Principles of Internal Medicine, 12th Edition. Edited by Wilson JD, Braunwald E, Isselbacher KJ, et al. New York, McGraw-Hill, 1991, pp 2194–2200

Phillips KA: Body dysmorphic disorder: the distress of imagined ugliness. Am J Psychiatry 148:1138–1149, 1991

Phillips KA, Nierenberg AA: The assessment and treatment of refractory depression. J Clin Psychiatry 55 (2, suppl):20–26, 1994

Phillips KA, Albertini RS, Rasmussen SA: A randomized placebo-controlled trial of fluoxetine in body dysmorphic disorder. Arch Gen Psychiatry 59:381–388, 2002

Physicians' Desk Reference, 58th Edition. Montvale, NJ, Thomson PDR, 2004

Physicians' Desk Reference Concise Prescribing Guide, Montvale, NJ, Thomson PDR, Issue 4, 2004, pp. 7-12

Pies R: Atypical depression, in Handbook of Clinical Psychopharmacology, 2nd Edition. Edited by Tupin JP, Shader RI, Harnett DS. Northvale, NJ, Jason Aronson, 1988, pp 329–356

Pies R: One foot on the bandwagon? (editorial). J Clin Psychopharmacol 15:303–305, 1995

Pies R: Psychotropic medications and the oncology patient. Cancer Pract 4:1–3, 1996

Pies R: Time and the art of psychopharmacology. Harv Rev Psychiatry 5:1–4, 1997

Pies R: Mastering the cytochromes: a practical primer. J Psychiatr Pract 6:267–271, 2000

Pies R: The "softer" end of the bipolar spectrum. J Psychiatr Pract 8:189–195, 2002

Pies RW, Shader RI: Approaches to the treatment of depression, in Manual of Psychiatric Therapeutics, 3rd Edition. Edited by Shader RI. Philadelphia, PA, Lippincott Williams & Wilkins, 2003, pp 240–270

Pies R, Weinberg AD: Quick Reference Guide to Geriatric Psychopharmacology. Branford, CT, American Medical Publishing, 1990, pp 11–16

Pollock BG, Sweet RA, Kirshner M, et al: Bupropion plasma levels and CYP2D6 phenotype. Ther Drug Monit 18:581–585, 1996

Post RM: Mechanisms underlying the evolution of affective disorders: implications for long-term treatment, in Severe Depressive Disorders. Edited by Grunhaus L, Greden JF. Washington, DC, American Psychiatric Press, 1994, pp 23–65

Potter WZ, Manji HK, Rudorfer MV: Tricyclics and tetracyclics, in The American Psychiatric Press Textbook of Psychopharmacology, Edited by Schatzberg AF, Nemeroff CB. Washington, DC, American Psychiatric Press, 1995, pp 141–160

Preskorn SH: Pharmacokinetics of psychotropic agents: why and how they are relevant to treatment. J Clin Psychiatry 54 (9, suppl):3–7, 1993

Preskorn SH: Advances in Antidepressant Therapy: The Pharmacologic Basis. San Antonio, TX, Dannemiller Memorial Educational Foundation, 1994

Preskorn SH: Comparison of the tolerability of bupropion, fluoxetine, imipramine, nefazodone, paroxetine, sertraline, and venlafaxine. J Clin Psychiatry 56 (suppl 6):12–21, 1995

Preskorn SH: Clinical Pharmacology of Selective Serotonin Reuptake Inhibitors. Caddo, OK, Professional Communications, 1996

Preskorn SH: Outpatient Management of Depression: A Guide for the Primary Care Practitioner, 2nd Edition. Caddo, OK, Professional Communications, 1999

Price LH, Carpenter LL, Rasmussen SA: Drug combination strategies, in Treatment-Resistant Mood Disorders. Edited by Amsterdam JD, Hornig M, Nierenberg AA. Cambridge, England, Cambridge University Press, 2001, pp 194–222

Quitkin FM, Stewart JW, McGrath PJ: Phenelzine vs imipramine in the treatment of probable atypical depression: defining syndrome boundaries of selective MAOI responders. Am J Psychiatry 145:306–311, 1988

Quitkin FM, McGrath PJ, Stewart JW, et al: Chronological milestones to guide drug change. Arch Gen Psychiatry 53:785–792, 1996

Rauch SL, O'Sullivan RL, Jenike MA: Open treatment of obsessive-compulsive disorder with venlafaxine: a series of ten cases. J Clin Psychopharmacol 16:81–83, 1996

Ravindran AV, Bialik RJ, Lapierre YD: Therapeutic efficacy of specific serotonin reuptake inhibitors (SSRIs) in dysthymia. Can J Psychiatry 39:21–26, 1994

Richelson E: Pharmacology of antidepressants—characteristics of the ideal drug. Mayo Clin Proc 69:1069–1081, 1994

Richelson E: Interactions of antidepressants with neurotransmitter transporters and receptors and their clinical relevance. J Clin Psychiatry 64 (suppl 13):5–12, 2003

Rinne T, van den Brink W, Wouters L, et al: SSRI treatment of borderline personality disorder: a randomized, placebo-controlled clinical trial for female patients with borderline personality disorder. Am J Psychiatry 159:2048–2054, 2002

Roose SP, Glassman AH, Attia E, et al: Comparative efficacy of selective serotonin reuptake inhibitors and tricyclics in the treatment of melancholia. Am J Psychiatry 151:1735–1739, 1994

Rosenblatt JE, Rosenblatt NC (eds) Currents in Affective Illness 22:4, 2003

Rosenblatt JE, Rosenblatt NC (eds): Currents in Affective Illness 23:4, 2004

Rosenstein DL, Nelson JC, Jacobs SC: Seizures associated with antidepressants: a review. J Clin Psychiatry 54:289–299, 1993

Roth BL, Meltzer HY: The role of serotonin in schizophrenia, in Psychopharmacology: The Fourth Generation of Progress. Edited by Bloom FE, Kupfer DJ. New York, Raven, 1995, pp 1215–1227

Sachs GS, Guille C: Weight gain associated with use of psychotropic medications. J Clin Psychiatry 60 (suppl 21):16–19, 1999

Sachs GS, Lafer B, Stoll AL, et al. A double-blind trial of bupropion versus desipramine for bipolar depression. J Clin Psychiatry 55:391–393, 1994

Sandson NB: Drug Interactions Casebook. Washington, DC, American Psychiatric Publishing, 2003

Schatzberg AF: Efficacy and tolerability of duloxetine, a novel dual reuptake inhibitor, in the treatment of major depressive disorder. J Clin Psychiatry 64 (suppl 13):30–37, 2003

Schatzberg AF, Cole JO: Manual of Clinical Psychopharmacology, 2nd Edition. Washington, DC, American Psychiatric Press, 1991, pp 313–318

Segraves RT: Effects of psychotropic drugs on human erection and ejaculation. Arch Gen Psychiatry 46:275–284, 1989

Shader RI: Dissociative, somatoform, and paranoid disorders, in Manual of Psychiatric Therapeutics, 2nd Edition. Edited by Shader RI. Boston, MA, Little, Brown, 1994, pp 15–23

Shelton RC, Tollefson GD, Tohen M, et al: A novel augmentation strategy for treating resistant major depression. Am J Psychiatry 158:131–134, 2001

Sherman C: SSRIs benefit cognition in elderly who are depressed. Clinical Psychiatry News 24:19, 1996

Shim J, Yonkers KA. Sertraline, in The American Psychiatric Publishing Textbook of Psychopharmacology, 3rd Edition. Edited by Schatzberg AF, Nemeroff CB. Washington, DC, American Psychiatric Publishing, 2004, pp 247–257

Silver JM: Clinical update on the management of agitation in the elderly. Presentation at the 8th annual U.S. Psychiatric and Mental Health Congress, New York, NY, November 16, 1995

Skolnick P: Beyond monoamine-based therapies: clues to new approaches. J Clin Psychiatry 63 (suppl 2):19–23, 2002

Smith BD, Salzman C: Do benzodiazepines cause depression? Hosp Community Psychiatry 42:1101–1102, 1991

Smoller JW, Pollack MH, Systrom D, et al: Sertraline effects on dyspnea in patients with obstructive airways disease. Psychosomatics 39:24–29, 1998

Sofuoglu M, DeBattista C: Development of obsessive symptoms during nefazodone treatment (letter). Am J Psychiatry 153:577–578, 1996

Spigset O, Carleborg L, Nordstrom A, et al: Paroxetine level in breast milk (letter). J Clin Psychiatry 57:39, 1996

Stahl SM: Remeron (mirtazapine): designing specific serotonergic actions. Psychiatr Ann 27:138–139, 1997a

Stahl SM: Serotonin pathways: mediators of SSRI side effects. Psychiatr Ann 27:82–84, 1997b

Stahl SM: Basic psychopharmacology of antidepressants, Part 1: antidepressants have seven distinct mechanisms of action. J Clin Psychiatry 59 (suppl 4):5–14, 1998

Stahl SM, Grady MM: Differences in mechanism of action between current and future antidepressants. J Clin Psychiatry 64 (suppl 13):13–17, 2003

Stearns V, Johnson MD, Rae JM, et al: Active tamoxifen metabolite plasma concentrations after coadministration of tamoxifen and the selective serotonin reuptake inhibitor paroxetine. J Natl Cancer Inst 95:1758–1764, 2003

Sternbach H: The serotonin syndrome. Am J Psychiatry 148:705–713, 1991

Stoll AL, Pillay SS, Diamond L, et al: Methylphenidate augmentation of serotonin selective reuptake inhibitors: a case series. J Clin Psychiatry 57:72–76, 1996

Storey P, Trumble M: Rectal doxepin and carbamazepine therapy in patients with cancer. N Engl J Med 327:1318–1319, 1992

Stoudemire A, Moran MG, Fogel BS: Psychopharmacology in the medically ill patient, The American Psychiatric Press Textbook of Psychopharmacology. Edited by Schatzberg AF, Nemeroff CB. Washington, DC, American Psychiatric Press, 1995, pp 783–801

Stowe ZN, Nemeroff CB: Psychopharmacology during pregnancy and lactation, in The American Psychiatric Press Textbook of Psychopharmacology. Edited by Schatzberg AF, Nemeroff CB. Washington, DC, American Psychiatric Press, 1995, pp 823–837

Sutherland SM, Krishnan KR: The difficult-to-treat patient with anxiety disorder, in The Difficult-to-Treat Psychiatric Patient. Edited by Dewan MJ, Pies RW. Washington, DC, American Psychiatric Publishing, 2001, pp 115–148

Taylor CB: Treatment of anxiety disorders, in The American Psychiatric Press Textbook of Psychopharmacology. Edited by Schatzberg AF, Nemeroff CB. Washington, DC, American Psychiatric Press, 1995, pp 641–655

Teitelman E: Off-label uses of modafinil (letter). Am J Psychiatry 158:1341, 2001

Thase ME, Rush AJ: Treatment-resistant depression, in Psychopharmacology: The Fourth Generation of Progress. Edited by Bloom FE, Kupfer DJ. New York, Raven, 1995, pp 1081–1097

Thase ME, Sloan DME: Venlafaxine, in The American Psychiatric Publishing Textbook of Psychopharmacology, 3rd Edition. Edited by Schatzberg AF, Nemeroff CB. Washington, DC, American Psychiatric Publishing, 2004, pp 349–360

Theoharides TC, Harris RS, Weckstein D: Neuroleptic malignant-like syndrome due to cyclobenzaprine? J Clin Psychopharmacol 15:79–81, 1995

Thompson JW Jr, Ware MR, Blashfield RK: Psychotropic medication and priapism: a comprehensive review. J Clin Psychiatry 51:430–433, 1990

Tielens JA: Vitamin C for paroxetine- and fluvoxamine-associated bleeding. Am J Psychiatry 154:883–884, 1997

Tollefson GD: Selective serotonin reuptake inhibitors, in The American Psychiatric Press Textbook of Psychopharmacology. Edited by Schatzberg AF, Nemeroff CB. Washington, DC, American Psychiatric Press, 1995, pp 161–182

Trestman RL, deVegvar M, Siever LJ: Treatment of personality disorders, in The American Psychiatric Press Textbook of Psychopharmacology. Edited by Schatzberg AF, Nemeroff CB. Washington, DC, American Psychiatric Press, 1995, pp 753–768

Velamoor VR, Swamy GN, Parmar RS, et al: Management of suspected neuroleptic syndrome. Can J Psychiatry 40:545–550, 1995

Venlafaxine: a new dimension in antidepressant pharmacotherapy. J Clin Psychiatry 54:119–126, 1993

von Moltke LL, Greenblatt DJ, Shader RI: Clinical pharmacokinetics of antidepressants in the elderly: therapeutic implications. Clin Pharmacokinet 24:141–160, 1993

Wagner KD, Ambrosini P, Rynn M, et al: Efficacy of sertraline in the treatment of children and adolescents with major depressive disorder. JAMA 290:1033–1041, 2003

West ED, Dally PJ: Effect of iproniazid in depressive syndromes. Br Med J 1:1491–1494, 1959

Wise MG: Special considerations in switching antidepressants. Teleconference (chaired by Keller MB), Providence, RI, August 18, 1995

Wisner KL, Perel JM, Wheeler SB: Tricyclic dose requirements across pregnancy. Am J Psychiatry 150:1541–1542, 1993

Witcher JW, Long A, Smith B, et al: Atomoxetine pharmacokinetics in children and adolescents with attention deficit hyperactivity disorder. J Child Adolesc Psychopharmacol 13:53–63, 2003

Yudofsky SC, Silver JM, Hales RE: Treatment of aggressive disorders, in The American Psychiatric Press Textbook of Psychopharmacology. Edited by Schatzberg AF, Nemeroff CB. Washington, DC, American Psychiatric Press, 1995, pp 735–751

Zajecka, JM: Treatment strategies for depression complicated by anxiety disorders. Presentation at the 8th annual U.S. Psychiatric and Mental Health Congress, New York, NY, November 16, 1995

Zajecka JM, Fawcett J, Guy C: Coexisting major depression and obsessive-compulsive disorder treated with venlafaxine (letter). J Clin Psychopharmacol 10:152–153, 1990

Zanarini MC, Silk K: The difficult-to-treat patient with borderline personality disorder, in The Difficult-to-Treat Psychiatric Patient. Edited by Dewan MJ, Pies RW. Washington, DC, American Psychiatric Publishing, 2001, pp 179–208

Zarate CA, Kando JC, Tohen M, et al: Does intolerance or lack of response with fluoxetine predict the same will happen with sertraline? J Clin Psychiatry 57:67–71, 1996

CHAPTER 3

ANTIPSYCHOTICS

Overview

Drug Class

The designation *antipsychotic* is often used synonymously with *neuroleptic* or *major tranquilizer.* The last term should be avoided, because these agents do not merely "tranquilize" but have specific effects on core features of psychosis, such as auditory hallucinations. *Neuroleptic* implies something that "seizes the nervous system"—a vestige of the belief that effective antipsychotics were associated with extrapyramidal side effects (EPS). Experience with newer, atypical antipsychotics has refuted this view (Janicak et al. 1993). Thus, whereas haloperidol may be termed a *neuroleptic,* clozapine, risperidone, olanzapine, and other atypical agents are properly termed *antipsychotics* (APs). However, we will apply the term *antipsychotic* generically to all agents discussed in this chapter. The specific classes of AP agents include the *phenothiazines* (e.g., chlorpromazine); *thioxanthenes* (e.g., thiothixene); *butyrophenones* (e.g., haloperidol); *dihydroindolones* (e.g., molindone); *dibenzoxazpines* (e.g., loxapine); *diphenylbutylpiperidines* (e.g., pimozide); *dibenzodiazepines* (e.g., clozapine, loxapine); *thienobenzodiazepines* (e.g., olanzapine); *dibenzothiazepines* (e.g., quetiapine); *benzisoxazoles* (e.g., risperidone, ziprasidone); and *quinolinones* (e.g., aripiprazole).

Indications

It may seem redundant to say that the main indication for an AP is psychosis, but since these agents are often used (and misused) for other conditions (such as agitation), the point bears emphasizing. The main psychiatric disorders for which an AP is indicated are schizophrenia, schizoaffective disorder, bipolar disorder, schizophreniform disorder, and brief psychotic disorder. Currently, five of the atypical APs—olanzapine, risperidone, aripiprazole, ziprasidone, and quetiapine—have U.S. Food and Drug Administration (FDA)–approved labeling for the short-term treatment of mania. In addition, olanzapine and aripiprazole recently received FDA approval for the *maintenance* treatment of bipolar disorder. The APs also play a role in the treatment of various "secondary" psychotic states (e.g., secondary to cocaine intoxication, Alzheimer's disease, AIDS dementia) and major depression with psychotic features. There is also interest in atypical APs as augmentation agents in treating unipolar nonpsychotic depression. This list is not exhaustive, nor is it necessarily inappropriate to use an AP in treating a nonpsychotic individual; thus, APs are used to treat the tics of Tourette's syndrome; certain severe cases of obsessive-compulsive disorder (OCD) when comorbid schizotypal personality disorder or tics are present; and (in low doses) borderline personality disorder (BPD).

The evidence that APs are effective in treating nonpsychotic disorders is limited, and the risk of tardive dyskinesia (TD) (see subsection "Main Side Effects" later in this chapter) must constantly be borne in mind. The same applies to the use of APs in treating violent or aggressive developmentally disabled individuals, in whom inappropriately high doses of APs may exacerbate the unwanted behaviors. But whereas APs are intended primarily for psychotic conditions, these agents may be used acutely in various medical contexts, even when the patient does not manifest psychotic features in the strict sense. For example, the early tranquilizing effect of the APs may be useful in calming the severely agitated, delirious patient in the intensive care unit. APs are also used widely (if sometimes inappropriately) in managing the behavioral disturbances associated with dementia.

Mechanisms of Action

The precise mechanism by which APs exert their AP effects is not known; however, nearly all compounds with significant AP activity block central dopamine (DA) receptors of some kind (Janicak et al. 1993; Kapur and

Mamo 2003). The *dopamine hypothesis* of AP action was proposed in the 1960s by Carlsson and Lindquist (1963), who observed that patients treated with traditional APs exhibited symptoms of Parkinson's disease. They concluded that AP medications affect the dopaminergic system in the brain. Indeed, the DA hypothesis has been the mainstay in explaining and treating schizophrenia for almost 30 years.

DA receptors belong to two main "families": the D_1 and D_5 types, and the D_2, D_3, and D_4 types. The clinical effects of classical neuroleptics are correlated with their affinity for the D_2 receptor. Indeed, Kapur and Mamo (2003) observed that "modulation of the dopamine D_2 receptor remains both necessary and sufficient for antipsychotic drug action, with affinity to the D_2 receptor being the single most important discriminator between a typical and atypical drug profile" (p. 1081). In the 1980s, a new agent with reduced D_2 antagonism but with significant $serotonin_2$ receptor (5-HT_2) antagonism—clozapine—was introduced. Clozapine's reduced antagonism of the D_2 receptor was thought to underlie the virtual absence of EPS or TD with this agent. Clozapine and several other atypical agents also act more selectively on mesolimbic DA receptors (so-called A10 neurons) than on striatal (A9) DA receptors, perhaps contributing to these agents' low rates of EPS (see subsection "Main Side Effects" later in this chapter). Older data suggested that a ratio of 5-HT_2 to D_2 receptor blockade (or binding affinity) greater than 10:1 contributes to the "atypicality" of an AP (Meltzer et al. 1989). Moreover, the simultaneous antagonism of DA receptors and 5-HT_{2A}/5-HT_{2C} receptors was implicated in the amelioration of *negative symptoms* of schizophrenia—aspects of the disease that respond poorly to neuroleptics. However, more recent data have cast doubt on the role of simultaneous D_2/5-HT_2 blockade in conferring atypicality (Seeman 2002). Rather, a "fast-off-D_2" hypothesis seems to be emerging as the leading explanation for atypicality (see subsection "Mechanisms of Action" in "Questions and Answers" section later in this chapter). Despite these hypotheses, the actual clinical advantages of the atypicals—including their effect on negative symptoms—remain somewhat controversial (Davis et al. 2003; Rosenheck et al. 2003).

Neuroleptics and atypical APs have many effects on neurotransmitters and receptors that may be related to their therapeutic effects, such as their effects on norepinephrine (NE) release. Blockade of α_2-adrenergic autoreceptors (leading to increased NE release from the presynaptic neuron) seems to occur with clozapine and perhaps risperidone; such noradrenergic effects may be associated with improved mood or negative symptoms. These agents also have anticholinergic, antihistaminic, and antiadrenergic effects that contribute to side effects (see subsection "Main Side Effects" later in this chapter). The most recent atypical agent approved, aripiprazole, appears to be a *partial agonist* at D_2 and 5-HT_{1A} receptors and an antagonist at 5-HT_{2A} receptors (Burris et al. 2002; J.A. Lieberman 2004).

Recently, the DA hypothesis of schizophrenia has been challenged (or modified) by several lines of evidence suggesting that *glutamate dysfunction* is crucially involved in the pathophysiology of schizophrenia—a mechanism that may explain the antipsychotic effects seen with some anticonvulsants that reduce glutamatergic activity (Dursun and Deakin 2001).

Pharmacokinetics

Like the antidepressants, the APs undergo hepatic metabolism via the cytochrome P450 (CYP) system (DeVane 1994). Most APs appear to be metabolized via the CYP 2D6 system (e.g., perphenazine, thioridazine, risperidone), whereas others are at least partially metabolized through CYP 1A2 (e.g., clozapine, olanzapine) and CYP 3A4 (quetiapine). Several atypical APs are metabolized via multiple CYP pathways, as well as via glucuronidation. APs undergo extensive "first-pass" hepatic extraction with oral dosing, leading to lower initial plasma levels than with intramuscular injection. Peak plasma levels are reached in about 2–3 hours after oral dosing and about 20–30 minutes after intramuscular injection. Because the intramuscular route avoids first-pass effects, plasma levels are roughly twice as high (initially) as with oral agents; thus, the usual intramuscular dose of an AP is about one-half the oral dose of the drug. Most APs have elimination half-lives of 20–24 hours, with longer times in the elderly or individuals with hepatic dysfunction. Two exceptions are aripiprazole, which has a $t_{1/2}$ of more than 70 hours; and ziprasidone, with a $t_{1/2}$ of only 6–7 hours. Some APs (e.g., chlorpromazine) generate dozens of active metabolites; others, such as haloperidol, only two or three. Still, these metabolites may have therapeutic implications, as with the potentially neurotoxic *haloperidol pyridinium* (Tsang et al. 1994). Few laboratories report plasma levels of AP metabolites. Moreover, for most APs, there is no well-established relationship between plasma AP concentration and clinical efficacy, though modest evidence supports a "therapeutic window" (roughly 4–15 ng/mL) for haloperidol. Similarly, response to clozapine seems to be correlated with plasma levels above the "threshold" of 400 ng/mL, though higher and lower levels may be effective for any given patient. Plasma levels of olanzapine appear to be therapeutic at roughly 23 ng/mL, but as yet no "therapeutic window" has been determined for olanzapine or other atypical APs, with the exception of clozapine. However, plasma AP levels may be useful in detecting noncompliance and extremes of abnormal metabolism, or in confirming toxicity. Blood levels may also be useful when the patient is taking multiple psychotropics undergoing hepatic metabolism.

Main Side Effects

APs have a variety of side effects, arising from their actions at many different neuronal receptors. *Extrapyramidal side effects,* including acute dystonic reactions, akathisia, and "parkinsonism," are seen more commonly with high-potency neuroleptics, such as haloperidol and fluphenazine. However, EPS may occasionally be seen with atypical agents and are not uncommon with higher doses of risperidone. Lower-potency agents, such as thioridazine and chlorpromazine, are more likely to cause *anticholinergic, antihistaminic,* and *antiadrenergic* side effects. Clozapine may cause anticholinergic effects but may also provoke *sialorrhea,* perhaps due to cholinergic effects at a subtype of muscarinic receptor. Blockade of peripheral α_1-adrenergic receptors appears to mediate the *hypotensive effects* of some APs. The antihistaminic effect of low-potency APs may mediate their sedating and weight-promoting side effects.

Other side effects associated with the APs include *hepatic dysfunction* (probably mostly with aliphatic phenothiazines); rare cases of *pancreatitis* (especially with clozapine and olanzapine); *sexual dysfunction* (mainly with low-potency agents and risperidone); *prolactin elevation, menstrual irregularities,* and *gynecomastia; skin rash; photosensitivity reactions; decreased seizure threshold,* particularly with clozapine and olanzapine (Centorrino et al. 2002); *neuroleptic malignant syndrome* (NMS); and *tardive dyskinesia*. The cumulative yearly incidence of TD in patients taking classical neuroleptics is about 4%–5% and is much higher (around 20%) in elderly populations. TD rates with most atypicals are roughly one-tenth as high.

With optimal monitoring, the incidence of clozapine-induced *agranulocytosis* is about 0.3% per year and usually occurs within the first 5 months of treatment. Low-potency APs (especially thioridazine), ziprasidone, and quetiapine also have some sodium ion channel–blocking properties, which may occasionally cause *QTc prolongation.* Finally, several atypical APs have been implicated in causing or exacerbating *type 2 diabetes, weight gain, dyslipidemia,* and *glucose dysregulation.* Although the data are not conclusive, clozapine and olanzapine seem to be more likely to produce one or more of these problems than are other atypical APs.

Management of AP side effects involves dosage reduction; very slow increases in dose (especially in the elderly); adjustment of scheduling (e.g., giving the drug mainly at bedtime); change of agent class (e.g., from a low- to a high-potency or atypical agent); use of antiparkinsonian agents for EPS; use of Urecholine for peripheral anticholinergic side effects; and the use of thromboembolic disease (TED) stockings or salt tablets for AP-induced postural hypotension. Clozapine-induced sialorrhea may be effectively treated with a peripherally acting anticholinergic agent (e.g., glycopyrrolate) rather than with centrally acting agents (e.g., benztropine). Patients taking atypical APs need careful monitoring so that abnormalities in glucose or lipid regulation can be detected, and they may require ancillary drugs to control these side effects.

Drug–Drug Interactions

APs with anticholinergic side effects (dry mouth, blurry vision, urinary retention, constipation, and confusional states) may be potentiated by *other anticholinergic agents,* such as trihexyphenidyl (Artane) and benztropine (Cogentin), which are used to counteract EPS. (Thus, the combination of a low-potency AP, clozapine, or olanzapine with anticholinergic agents is often unnecessary and unwise, particularly in elderly patients and patients with dementia.) The QTc-prolonging effect of some atypical APs may be augmented by concomitant use of other medications that prolong QTc (e.g., some fluoroquinolone antibiotics, erythromycin, tricyclic antidepressants [TCAs], quinidine, sotalol, and amiodarone). APs may lead to increased EPS when used concomitantly with *lithium* or *SSRIs,* such as fluoxetine (Prozac)—most likely because of pharmacodynamic interactions in the brain. Fluoxetine and paroxetine also have the pharmacokinetic effect of inhibiting the CYP 2D6 system, thus increasing plasma levels of many APs. Agents that strongly inhibit CYP 1A2, such as fluvoxamine, mexiletine, or propafenone, may greatly elevate blood levels of clozapine or olanzapine. *Valproate* may modestly increase plasma AP levels, but this effect is of doubtful clinical significance. Conversely, *phenytoin* (Dilantin), *phenobarbital,* and *carbamazepine* (Tegretol) may significantly reduce plasma AP levels. In addition, *cigarette smoking* has been reported to induce the hepatic metabolism of clozapine and olanzapine. *Antacids* such as Maalox may impair absorption of APs from the gastrointestinal tract.

Potentiating Maneuvers

As many as 25% of all psychotic patients do not respond adequately to their first trial of a conventional AP agent (Cole et al. 1964). After issues of incorrect diagnosis, poor compliance, and inadequate dose/bioavailability (Osser 1989) have been ruled out, a variety of potentiation strategies are possible. Combining two (or more) atypical agents is practiced frequently and has some theoretical rationale, based on the varying receptor affinities of some atypical APs (e.g., clozapine and risperidone). However, controlled studies supporting this practice are rare. In some schizoaffective patients, the addition of a mood stabilizer (lithium or valproate) may reduce emotional lability or dysphoric manic symptoms. Moreover, both valproate and lamotrigine appear to potentiate some APs in schizophrenia patient populations (Casey et al. 2003; Dursun and Deakin 2001), possibly owing to their effects on glutamate and/or γ-aminobutyric acid (GABA). Beta-blockers may reduce aggressive/violent or self-injurious behaviors, and benzodiazepines may sometimes improve "negative" symptoms in schizophrenia (Janicak et al. 1993). For women with chronic schizophrenia and anxious-depressive symptoms, the addition of a TCA (desipramine) may be beneficial after 3 months of treatment (Hogarty et al. 1995). Also, limited data suggest that SSRIs may have adjunctive benefits in patients with schizophrenia.

Use in Special Populations

As with all psychotropics, use of APs in elderly patients and medically ill patients generally requires dosage reduction and careful monitoring of vital signs and side effects. Elderly patients, in general, should not be treated with the highly anticholinergic APs, such as thioridazine or chlorpromazine. (Anticholinergic side effects can include urinary retention, bowel obstruction, and confusional states.) Such low-potency agents also tend to promote postural hypotension. Clozapine may be effective in both geriatric and medically ill older patients (e.g., Parkinson's disease patients with psychosis) but produces many side effects; thus, clozapine dosage should begin extremely low (6.25 mg/day), with very gradual increases. Olanzapine appears to be safe and generally well tolerated in elderly patients, despite its strong anticholinergic properties observed in vitro. Though anticholinergic side effects are rarely problematic in elderly patients taking olanzapine, olanzapine-related constipation and urinary retention may be more frequent than observed with risperidone in some older patients or patients with dementia. However, although risperidone appears to be safe and effective in the elderly, it must be used at low dosages (0.5–1.5 mg/day) to avoid hypotension, EPS, and drug–drug interactions. Recently, the makers of risperidone and olanzapine issued a warning regarding the increased risk of cerebrovascular adverse events in elderly patients with dementia who are taking these agents. However, a direct causal relationship between risperidone, olanzapine, or other atypical agents and increased risk of stroke has not been clearly established. Nevertheless, given the risk of α_1 (noradrenergic) receptor blockade and resultant orthostatic hypotension, all APs should be used cautiously in elderly and dementia patient populations. This is especially true for patients who are at high risk for falls and who have various cardiac conditions (e.g., congestive heart failure).

The use of APs in children and adolescents is complicated by resistance to medication and both over- and undermedication (Dulcan et al. 1995). Age, weight, and severity of symptoms do not provide clear guidelines; moreover, although children metabolize APs more rapidly than adults, they may also require lower plasma levels for efficacy (Dulcan et al. 1995). The best advice is to begin with a very low dose and to increase the dose very gradually (no more than once or twice a week). On the other hand, older adolescents with schizophrenia may require AP doses comparable to those of adults. It is not yet clear which class of AP is safest and most efficacious in children and adolescents (Gelenberg 1994). Both typical and atypical agents have shown some efficacy in younger schizophrenic patients, but the studies have had small sample sizes and have been short term. However, given the reduced risk of EPS and TD with the atypicals, these are probably first-line agents in younger patients, with the exception of clozapine (Wagner 2004).

The use of APs in the pregnant patient—as with any medication—should be avoided, if clinically feasible. Unfortunately, the dangers from untreated psychosis may require aggressive treatment and often outweigh the rather remote risks of teratogenesis or neonatal toxicity from APs (Stowe and Nemeroff 1995). Ideally, one should defer treatment until after the first trimester, when organ formation is most susceptible to teratogenic effects, but this is often impractical. Despite their widespread use, atypical APs have not been well studied, prospectively, in pregnancy (Newport et al. 2004). Electroconvulsive therapy is a viable option in the acutely psychotic/manic pregnant patient but, despite its safety in such circumstances, is often restricted by the courts.

Tables

Drug Class

TABLE 3–1. Dosages and putative therapeutic levels of currently available antipsychotics

Chemical class/subclass	Generic name	Brand name	Usually effective oral dosage (adults)[a] (mg/day)	Putative therapeutic plasma level (ng/mL)
Benzisothiazolylpiperazine	ziprasidone	Geodon	60–180	—
Benzisoxazole	risperidone	Risperdal	1.0–6.5	? 25–40[b]
Butyrophenones	haloperidol	Haldol	2–25	2–12
Dibenzodiazepines	clozapine	Clozaril	100–900	350–550
Dibenzothiazepine	quetiapine	Seroquel	150–900	—
Dibenzoxazepines	loxapine	Loxitane	30–150	—
Dihydroindolones	molindone	Moban	20–225	—
Dihydroquinolinone	aripiprazole	Abilify	10–30[c]	—
Diphenylbutylpiperidines	pimozide	Orap	2–12	—
Phenothiazines				
Aliphatic	chlorpromazine	Thorazine	150–1,000	30–100
	triflupromazine	Vesprin	20–150	—
	promazine	Sparine	25–1,000	—
Piperazine	fluphenazine	Prolixin, Permitil	2–20	0.2–2
	perphenazine	Trilafon	8–40	0.8–3
	trifluoperazine	Stelazine	5–30	1–2.5
	acetophenazine	Tindal	40–80	—

TABLE 3–1. Dosages and putative therapeutic levels of currently available antipsychotics *(continued)*

Chemical class/subclass	Generic name	Brand name	Usually effective oral dosage (adults)[a] (mg/day)	Putative therapeutic plasma level (ng/mL)
Phenothiazines *(continued)*				
Piperidine	mesoridazine	Serentil	75–300	—
	thioridazine	Mellaril	100–800	—
Thienobenzodiazepine	olanzapine	Zyprexa	10–35	? 25–30
Thioxanthenes				
Aliphatic	chlorprothixene	Taractan	30–600	—
Piperazine	thiothixene	Navane	6–50	2–15

Note. —=insufficient data; ?=data are preliminary or there is no well-established correlation between plasma level and therapeutic response.

[a]Doses reflect consensus of listed references and author's clinical experience. Acute doses are generally somewhat higher than maintenance doses for many patients. Dosage recommendations vary considerably depending on the age of patient; first-episode versus multiepisode patient; diagnosis (e.g., dementia vs. schizophrenia); and plasma levels attained. Initial doses of antipsychotic that induces hypotension (e.g., mesoridazine, chlorpromazine, quetiapine, risperidone) may need to be significantly lower than the ultimately effective dose. Examples: 1) Initial and final doses of risperidone may need to be lower in elderly or medically ill patients. 2) Clozapine dose may be substantially lower in elderly Parkinson's patients with psychosis, or in patients with Lewy body dementia, than in young, healthy patients with schizophrenia. 3) For a patient who achieves a plasma haloperidol level of only 1 ng/mL at 10 mg/day, a dosage increase may be necessary.

[b]Sum of risperidone and 9-hydroxyrisperidone.

[c]*Inducers* of cytochrome P450 (CYP) 2D6 or 3A4 may substantially *decrease* aripiprazole blood levels; conversely, *inhibitors* of these CYP enzymes may substantially *increase* aripiprazole blood levels. The manufacturer suggests adjustments in dose of as much as 50%; however, the patient's clinical status should be the determining factor.

Source. P.F. Buckley and Meltzer 1995; Janicak et al. 1993; Jenkins et al. 2001; Kane et al. 2003b; Kaplan et al. 1994; Lindenmayer and Apergi 1996; Physicians' Desk Reference 1996; Shader 2003a; Van Putten et al. 1990b.

TABLE 3–2. First-generation ("typical" or "neuroleptic") antipsychotic dosage equivalents of 10 mg of haloperidol

Agent	**Tablet/capsule strengths (mg)**	**Approximate mg equivalent to 10 mg of haloperidol daily**[a]
chlorpromazine	10, 25, 50, 100, 200	500
fluphenazine	1, 2.5, 5, 10	10
perphenazine	2, 4, 8, 16	32
thioridazine	10, 15, 25, 50, 100, 150, 200	450
thiothixene	1, 2, 5, 10, 20	25
trifluoperazine	1, 2, 5, 10	25
fluphenazine decanoate (mg/2–3 weeks)	—	25
haloperidol decanoate (mg/4 weeks)	—	150

Note. Long-acting risperidone (Risperdal Consta) was recently approved by the U.S. Food and Drug Administration for treatment of schizophrenia. The likely therapeutic dose, after lead-in phase with oral antipsychotic, is 25 mg every 2 weeks (Kane et al. 2003a).

[a]Data on equivalent doses vary considerably, depending on whether in vitro or clinical data are used. Equivalent doses also vary from patient to patient.

Source. Kane et al. 2003b.

TABLE 3–3. Second-generation ("atypical") antipsychotic dosage equivalents of 10 mg of haloperidol

Agent	Tablet/capsule strengths (mg)	Approximate mg equivalent to 10 mg of haloperidol daily[a]
aripiprazole	5, 10, 15, 20, 30	20
clozapine	25, 100	425
olanzapine[b,c]	2.5, 5, 7.5, 10, 15, 20	20
quetiapine	25, 100, 200, 300	600
risperidone[b]	0.25, 0.5, 1, 2, 3, 4	5.5
ziprasidone[d]	20, 40, 60, 80	140

[a]Data on equivalent doses vary considerably, depending on whether in vitro or clinical data are used. Equivalent doses also vary from patient to patient.
[b]Both olanzapine and risperidone are now available in orally disintegrating tablet formulations. Risperidone is also available as an oral solution.
[c]Olanzapine (Zyprexa Intramuscular) recently became available for intramuscular injection, with U.S. Food and Drug Administration–approved labeling for agitation in schizophrenia and bipolar mania. The recommended dose is 10 mg, with lower doses (2.5–5 mg) in geriatric or medically ill patients. Seventy percent of patients appear to benefit from just one dose in a 24-hour period. Somnolence may be observed when benzodiazepines are coadministered.
[d]Ziprasidone (Geodon) is also available as the mesylate for intramuscular injection. Recommended dose is 10–20 mg im every 2–4 hours, up to a maximum of 40 mg/day. *Use of this intramuscular preparation for more than 3 consecutive days has not been studied.*
Source. Kane et al. 2003b; Physicians' Desk Reference 2004.

TABLE 3–4. Comparative costs of some atypical antipsychotics

Agent (dosage)	Cost per day (AWP)
clozapine (400 mg/day)	$18.25 (brand) $13.80 (generic)
risperidone (6 mg/day)	$14.36 $21.66 (M-Tab)
risperidone (long-acting[a])	
(25 mg)	$284.54[b]
(37.5 mg)	$426.83[b]
(50 mg)	$569.09[b]
olanzapine (20 mg/day)	$21.56 $24.00 (Zydis)
olanzapine (intramuscular) (10 mg)	$22.19 (per dose)
quetiapine (600 mg/day)	$16.00
ziprasidone (160 mg/day)	$11.00
ziprasidone (intramuscular) (20 mg)	$47.86 (per dose)
aripiprazole	
(15 mg/day)	$11.50
(20 mg/day)	$16.28

Note. AWP = average wholesale price
[a]Every 2 weeks.
[b]Per injection.
Source. D. P. Rogers, Pharm.D., B.C.P.S., Tewksbury State Hospital, Tewksbury, MA; prices based on wholesaler database (McKesson, December 2004).

Indications

TABLE 3–5. Indications for use of antipsychotics

Indication	Comments/Special considerations
Schizophrenia	**Large database.** Dose generally equivalent to 10 mg of haloperidol per day; dosages of haloperidol above 10–15 mg/day usually unnecessary. Plasma haloperidol levels of 2–12 ng/mL may be optimal; plasma haloperidol levels above 30 ng/mL may be associated with increased toxicity and unclear benefit; plasma levels less certain with other antipsychotics. Clozapine indicated for refractory schizophrenia, negative symptoms; probable correlation between clozapine levels >350 ng/mL and efficacy. With the exception of clozapine, no atypical antipsychotic is clearly superior for refractory schizophrenia. Atypical agents have roughly equal efficacy for schizophrenia per se.
Schizophreniform disorder Brief psychotic disorder	**Very limited database.** Patients with first onset of acute or subacute psychosis may respond rapidly to lower doses of APs than do patients with schizophrenia. Lithium may be effective in a small percentage of patients. Use of AP for 3–6 months with gradual taper-off may suffice in many cases of schizophreniform disorder. ECT may be indicated in cases in which patient has marked catatonic or depressive features. Benzodiazepines (e.g., lorazepam 2–6 mg/day) may suffice in brief psychotic episodes or "brief reactive psychosis."
Delusional disorder	**Very limited database.** Delusional disorder relatively uncommon (incidence 25 times less than that of schizophrenia). Subtypes include erotomanic, grandiose, jealous, persecutory, somatic. Large-scale studies of APs lacking in these patients; anecdotal reports indicate that some patients, including those with particularly paranoid psychoses of late life, do respond to APs. Erotomanic and jealous subtypes may be more resistant to AP treatment.

TABLE 3–5. Indications for use of antipsychotics *(continued)*

Indication	Comments/Special considerations
Paranoid personality disorder Schizoid personality disorder Schizotypal personality disorder Borderline personality disorder	**Database limited.** Low-dose AP trial may be helpful in some BPD patients, though long-term studies are not encouraging. Some recent open-label studies find atypicals (clozapine, olanzapine) useful in BPD patients. Even more limited database for paranoid, schizoid, and schizotypal personality disorders, in which low-dose APs reported useful in a few studies. Paranoid personality disorder patients often extremely resistant to medication and experience it as coercive, and the benefits are not clear.
Schizoaffective disorder	**Limited controlled database and variably defined, heterogeneous syndrome.** Probably "schizomanic" and "schizodepressed" subgroups represent different disorders, with latter group very heterogeneous. In schizomanic patients, AP plus mood stabilizer often used; clozapine seems very promising in the manic-excited phase of schizoaffective disorder, but less useful for the schizodepressive type. For patients with acute exacerbations of schizoaffective disorder, or schizophrenia with depressive symptoms, controlled studies find that APs are drugs of choice and that ADs are not usually useful. Atypical agents may have an advantage (especially clozapine in suicidal patients), but controlled studies are lacking. ECT may be useful in both types of schizoaffective illness.
Psychosis secondary to drug/toxin	**Limited database.** In psychiatric emergencies in which patients present with psychotic symptoms due to delirium or street drug abuse (hallucinogens), a response is usually achieved with haloperidol at low-moderate dosages (1–5 mg/day), sometimes in combination with lorazepam (0.5–1.5 mg po, im, or iv, q 1–2 hours). Avoid low-potency APs with anticholinergic effects, especially if PCP toxicity is suspected.

TABLE 3–5. Indications for use of antipsychotics *(continued)*

Indication	Comments/Special considerations
Psychosis and/or behavioral disturbance secondary to dementia	**Moderately large but mostly uncontrolled database.** In dementia patients with psychotic features (hallucinations, paranoia), APs more effective than placebo but probably not as effective as in younger schizophrenia patients. The closer the disruptive behaviors of the dementia patient resemble psychotic features of schizophrenia, the more effective the AP will be. Low-potency first-generation agents generally avoided because of peripheral and central anticholinergic effects (e.g., increased cognitive dysfunction in Alzheimer's disease patients). Haloperidol 0.5–1.0 mg/day may be an alternative in dementia patients with psychotic features or severe behavioral disturbance (e.g., aggression). Clozapine may be useful in psychotic Parkinson's patients (6.25–50 mg/day may suffice); olanzapine and quetiapine may perhaps be useful. Lewy body dementia patients are exquisitely sensitive to extrapyramidal effects of APs, even atypicals; keep dose extremely low. There is some concern regarding risk of cerebrovascular accident/adverse events with risperidone, olanzapine, and aripiprazole treatment of dementia patients, but a causal link has not been established with any atypical agent (e.g., most affected patients in risperidone studies had history of prior stroke, atrial fibrillation, hypertension). Buspirone, trazodone, SSRI, and an anticonvulsant may be alternatives to AP in disruptive, aggressive dementia patients without true psychotic symptoms.

TABLE 3–5. Indications for use of antipsychotics *(continued)*

Indication	Comments/Special considerations
Bipolar disorder	**Moderate but growing database.** Five well-controlled trials comparing lithium with first-generation APs in acute manic episode: overall, lithium was superior (89% vs. 54% response rate). First-generation (conventional) APs (so-called neuroleptics) have faster onset of action than lithium and may be useful as adjuncts to lithium or valproate in initial management of mania; benzodiazepines also useful acutely. Conventional APs may worsen depressive symptoms long term in bipolar patients. Ideally, AP is tapered and discontinued as the mood stabilizer gains control. *Currently olanzapine, risperidone, aripiprazole, ziprasidone, and quetiapine have FDA-approved labeling for the treatment of manic and mixed bipolar episodes.* Olanzapine, risperidone, and quetiapine also have labeling for use in combination with lithium or divalproex for treatment of acute mania in bipolar I disorder. Olanzapine also has FDA-approved labeling for maintenance treatment of bipolar disorder, based on one placebo-controlled study. The combination of fluoxetine and olanzapine (Symbyax) has been approved for treatment of bipolar depression. Aripiprazole also recently received FDA approval for the maintenance treatment of bipolar disorder. The Texas Medication Algorithm includes the addition of an atypical AP in the second tier of treating bipolar disorder.

TABLE 3–5. Indications for use of antipsychotics *(continued)*

Indication	Comments/Special considerations
Major depression with psychotic features (? and without psychotic features)	**Large database in psychotic major depression.** Combination of AP and AD works better than either AP or AD alone. (Some delusionally depressed patients may worsen on AD alone.) Amoxapine may also be effective. Limited, uncontrolled data suggest clozapine, olanzapine monotherapy may be effective in psychotic depression. Combination of AP and AD may lead to increased plasma levels of either or both agents. ECT is excellent alternative and treatment of choice in severe cases. **Nonpsychotic major depression.** One double-blind, controlled study (N=28) found that olanzapine (5–20 mg/day) plus fluoxetine produced significantly greater improvement than either olanzapine or fluoxetine alone in patients with nonbipolar, nonpsychotic, refractory major depression. Combination was generally well tolerated.
Obsessive-compulsive disorder	**Small database.** AP rarely indicated in OCD, except as augmenting agent (with serotonergic drug) in patients with comorbid tic disorder, schizotypal features, or OCD refractory to SSRI alone. Clozapine may exacerbate obsessive-compulsive symptoms in some patients.
Mental retardation with behavioral dyscontrol (no psychotic symptoms)	**Limited controlled data.** APs widely used in developmentally disabled patients, but few data are available from well-controlled trials. APs may exacerbate agitation, akathisia, and/or self-injury in some mentally retarded patients. Dopamine D_1 blockers and clozapine may have theoretical advantages in patients with self-injurious behavior. Use lowest feasible dose of AP or consider alternatives (valproate, beta-blocker, buspirone, SSRI, lithium).

TABLE 3–5. Indications for use of antipsychotics *(continued)*

Indication	Comments/Special considerations
Tourette's syndrome	**Large database.** Clonidine (or guanfacine) is usual first-line treatment. Haloperidol (0.2 mg/kg per day), pimozide (3 mg/day) are effective, but cardiac arrhythmias are associated with higher doses of pimozide, and EPS are associated with haloperidol. Atypical APs appear to be effective, with most data for risperidone, and limited data for olanzapine, quetiapine, and ziprasidone.

Note. ?=data preliminary. AD=antidepressant; AP=antipsychotic; BPD=borderline personality disorder; EPS=extrapyramidal symptoms; ECT=electroconvulsive therapy; FDA=U.S. Food and Drug Administration; OCD=obsessive-compulsive disorder; PCP=phencyclidine; SSRI=selective serotonin reuptake inhibitor.

Source. Cornelius et al. 1991, 1993; Janicak et al. 1993; Janssen Pharmaceutica, "Dear Doctor" letter, April 16, 2003; Kaplan et al. 1994; Keck et al. 1995; Keith and Schooler 1989; Levinson et al. 1999; Lindenmayer and Apergi 1996; Marder and Wirshing 2004; Peterson 1995; Pies and Popli 1995; Raskind 1995; Roth 1989; Schexnayder et al. 1995; Schulz et al. 2004; Shelton et al. 2001; Suppes et al. 2001; Tueth et al. 1995; Wagner 2004; Zanarini and Silk 2001; Zarate et al. 1995.

Mechanisms of Action

TABLE 3–6. Relative receptor affinities of haloperidol versus available atypical agents

Receptor	haloperidol	clozapine (Clozaril)	risperidone (Risperdal)	olanzapine (Zyprexa)	quetiapine (Seroquel)	ziprasidone (Geodon)	aripiprazole (Abilify)
D_2	+++	+	+++	++	+	+++	++++[a]
$5\text{-}HT_{2A}$	+	++	++++	+++	+	++++	++
α_1	++++	++++	++++	++	+++	+++	++
H_1	+/–	++++	++	++++	+++	+	++
M_1	+/–	++++	+/–	+++	+	+/–	+/–

Note. +/–=none to minimal affinity; +=slight affinity; ++=moderate affinity; +++=high affinity; ++++=strong affinity. In vitro receptor affinities do not always reflect *clinical* effects or side effects of the agent, which are often dose-dependent. The semiquantitative symbols shown here are merely approximations derived from K_i (dissociation constant) values (Miyamoto et al. 2002). A large K_i indicates a low receptor affinity.

$\alpha_1=\alpha_1$ noradrenergic receptor; D_2=dopamine$_2$ receptor; $5\text{-}HT_{2A}$=serotonin$_{2A}$ receptor; H_1=histamine$_1$ receptor; M_1=muscarinic (cholinergic) receptor.

Implications of receptor binding affinity/antagonism: Higher $5\text{-}HT_2/D_2$ ratio, in part, may confer "atypicality," though this claim has been questioned (Seeman 2002); M_1 blockade produces anticholinergic side effects, such as dry mouth; H_1 blockade is associated with sedation, weight gain; α_1 blockade is associated with orthostatic hypotension.

[a]Although aripiprazole has very high D_2 affinity, its pharmacodynamic action at this receptor appears to be that of a *partial agonist.*

Source. J.A. Lieberman 2004; Miyamoto et al. 2002.

Pharmacokinetics

TABLE 3–7. Pharmacokinetic profiles of first-generation (neuroleptic) antipsychotics

Agent	Mean half-life ($t_{1/2}$), hours	Main CYP elimination pathway[a]	Main CYP enzymes inhibited by drug
chlorpromazine	20	2D6	2D6
fluphenazine	20	2D6	2D6
haloperidol	22	2D6, 3A4	2D6
loxapine	7	?2D6, ?3A4	None known
perphenazine	15	2D6, 3A4	2D6
pimozide	55	3A4	2D6
thioridazine	20	2D6	2D6

Note. ? = metabolic route not well described. CYP = cytochrome P450.

[a]Most antipsychotics have alternate metabolic pathways.

Source. Modified and condensed from Cozza et al. 2003; Perry et al. 1997; Physicians' Desk Reference 2004.

TABLE 3–8. Pharmacokinetic profiles of second-generation (atypical) antipsychotics

Agent	Mean half-life ($t_{1/2}$), hours	Main CYP elimination pathway[a]	Main CYP enzymes inhibited by drug
aripiprazole	75 (parent compound)	2D6, 3A4	None known
	94 (active metabolite dehydroaripiprazole)	2D6, 3A4	None known
clozapine	16	1A2, 3A4, 2C19 (glucuronidation)	2D6
olanzapine	30	Glucuronidation, 1A2	None known
quetiapine	6[b]	3A4	None known
risperidone	4 (parent compound)	2D6, 3A4	2D6
	22 (active metabolite 9-hydroxyrisperidone)	2D6, 3A4	2D6
ziprasidone	6.6	Aldehyde oxidase[c], 3A4	None known

Note. ? = metabolic rate not well described. CYP = cytochrome P450.

[a]Most antipsychotics have alternate metabolic pathways.

[b]Binding to dopamine D_2 receptor is longer and may permit once-daily dosing (J.A. Lieberman 2004).

[c]A non–cytochrome P450 enzyme, responsible for about two-thirds of ziprasidone's metabolism.

Source. Modified and condensed from Cozza et al. 2003; Physicians' Desk Reference 2004.

Main Side Effects

TABLE 3–9. Comparative side effects among available first-generation (typical) antipsychotics

Agent	Sedation	EPS	Anticholinergic effects	Orthostasis
chlorpromazine	+++	+	+++	+++
fluphenazine	+	+++	+	+
haloperidol	+	+++	+	+
loxapine	++	++	+	++
mesoridazine	+++	+	++	++
molindone	+	++	+	+
perphenazine	+	++	+	++
pimozide	+	+++	+	+
thioridazine	+++	+	+++	+++
thiothixene	+	+++	+	+
trifluoperazine	+	+++	+	+

Note. +/−= minimal; += mild; ++= moderate; +++= substantial. Effects may differ in acute vs. chronic treatment, in young vs. elderly patients, and with dose and route of administration.

EPS = extrapyramidal side effects.

Source. Drug Facts and Comparisons 1995; Shader 2003a. Values also based on the author's clinical experience.

TABLE 3–10. Comparative side effects among selected second-generation (atypical) antipsychotics

Agent	Sedation/ Somnolence	EPS	Anticholinergic effects	Orthostasis	Prolactin level elevation	Weight gain
aripiprazole	0	+	+/–	0/+	0	+/–
clozapine	+++	0	+++[a]	+++	0	++++
olanzapine	++	0/+	+	+/++	0/+	+++
quetiapine	++	0	+	++	0/+	+/++
risperidone	+	+/++[b]	+	++	++/+++	++
ziprasidone	+	+	+	+	0/+	+/–

Note. 0=almost no effect; +/–=equivocal or very minor effect; ++++=strong/severe effect. The semiquantitative effects depicted here are only approximations and may differ depending on dose, early vs. later phase of treatment, and individual sensitivity. Note that clinical side effects do not always mirror in vitro receptor affinities.

EPS=extrapyramidal side effects.

[a]Clozapine has high in vitro affinity for muscarinic receptor (see Table 3–6) but has variable clinical effects; for example, some patients may experience hypersalivation and/or enuresis, but others may experience dry mouth, urinary retention, and other anticholinergic effects. There is some evidence that supposed hypersalivation from clozapine may actually reflect an impaired swallowing mechanism rather than a cholinergic effect; alternatively, it may be mediated via α-adrenergic blockade (Marder and Wirshing 2004).

[b]EPS usually at higher risperidone dosages (>2.5 mg/day).

Source. J.A. Lieberman 2004; Marder and Wirshing 2004; Schulz et al. 2004; Weiden 2003; values also based on the author's clinical experience.

TABLE 3–11. Motor and mental symptoms of neuroleptic-induced extrapyramidal side effects

Syndrome	Motor symptoms	Mental symptoms	Psychiatric differential diagnosis
Akathisia	Restlessness, pacing, fidgeting, shifting from foot to foot	Jitteriness, anxiety, irritability, anger, difficulty concentrating, suicidality	Psychotic agitation, anxiety disorder, agitated depression, mixed manic state
Dystonia	Muscle contractions, tongue protrusion, torticollis, opisthotonos	Fear, distress, paranoia	Catatonic posturing, seizure, conversion disorder
Tardive dyskinesia (TD)	Buccolingual masticatory movements of irregular (nonrhythmic) nature; choreiform or athetoid (writhing) movements of fingers, extremities, trunk; rarely, respiratory dyskinesia. Not present during sleep. Tardive dystonia related to TD and may coexist with it (late-onset of twisting movements of limbs, trunk, neck).	In mild, early cases, patient often not aware of and not distressed by TD. In more severe cases, TD interferes with chewing or causes dysphagia, which may be very distressing, as may (rare) respiratory dyskinesia.	Other choreiform disorders, such as Huntington's chorea, Sydenham's chorea; diseases/lesions affecting basal ganglia, electrolyte or other metabolic disease must be ruled out.
Parkinsonism	Tremor (resting), rigidity, bradykinesia, masklike facies	Bradyphrenia (slowed thinking), mental clouding	Negative symptoms of schizophrenia; depression; neuroleptic malignant syndrome

Source. Modified from Ayd 1995; Casey 1995.

TABLE 3–12. Selected agents for treatment of extrapyramidal side effects (EPS) of first-generation (neuroleptic) antipsychotics

Generic name	Trade name	Usual daily dosage for EPS
amantadine	Symmetrel	100–200 mg bid
benztropine	Cogentin	0.5–2 mg po bid 1–2 mg im for acute dystonic reaction
biperiden	Akineton	2–6 mg po tid 2 mg im
clonazepam	Klonopin	0.5–1 mg bid
diphenhydramine	Benadryl	25–50 mg po bid 25 mg im for acute dystonic reaction
procyclidine	Kemadrin	2.5–5 mg tid
trihexyphenidyl	Artane, Tremin, others	2–5 mg tid

Source. Kaplan et al. 1994: Stanilla and Simpson 2004.

TABLE 3–13. Neuroleptic malignant syndrome (NMS): differential diagnosis

	NMS	Serotonin syndrome	Malignant hyperthermia	Lethal (pernicious) catatonia	Central anticholinergic syndrome
Core symptoms	Hyperthermia Severe muscle rigidity (usually "lead pipe") Diaphoresis Delirium Muteness Incontinence Rhabdomyolysis Autonomic instability (fluctuating BP, pallor/ flushing) Tremulousness Tachycardia Tachypnea EPS	Variable temperature elevation (37.4°C–42.5°C) Mental status changes Hypomania Restlessness Myoclonus Hyperreflexia Diaphoresis Shivering/teeth chattering Tremor Diarrhea Incoordination	Hyperthermia (core temperature>41°C) Muscle rigidity Ischemia Hot skin Mottled cyanosis Hypotension Rhabdomyolysis	Hyperthermia Muscle rigidity Diaphoresis Delirium Extreme hyperactivity (often early in syndrome) or stupor Psychotic prodrome Mutism Posturing Stupor alternating with excitement Hypertension Tremulousness	Hyperthermia Decreased sweating Hot, dry skin Dilated, sluggish pupils Tachycardia Constipation Urinary retention Confusion Impaired memory Delirium Hallucinations

TABLE 3–13. Neuroleptic malignant syndrome (NMS): differential diagnosis *(continued)*

	NMS	Serotonin syndrome	Malignant hyperthermia	Lethal (pernicious) catatonia	Central anticholinergic syndrome
Core symptoms *(continued)*	? Most common temporal sequence: mental status change → rigidity → autonomic instability → hyperthermia				
Laboratory findings	Elevated CPK, WBC, LFTs, myoglobinuria	No specific findings	Disseminated intravascular coagulation Respiratory/metabolic acidosis Hyperkalemia Hypermagnesemia	No specific findings	No specific findings

TABLE 3–13. Neuroleptic malignant syndrome (NMS): differential diagnosis *(continued)*

	NMS	Serotonin syndrome	Malignant hyperthermia	Lethal (pernicious) catatonia	Central anticholinergic syndrome
Causes/ Mechanisms	Presumed: blockade of dopaminergic pathways in basal ganglia and hypothalamus; also may result from sudden withdrawal of dopamine agonist; lithium may precipitate NMS. Low serum iron may be associated with NMS.	Activation of 5-HT_{1A} receptors in brain stem, spinal cord; enhancement of overall serotonin neurotransmission. Most commonly due to interaction between MAOI and serotonergic agent (L-tryptophan, SSRI), but may occur with any serotonergic drug.	Inherited disorder; triggering anesthetic (halothane, methoxyflurane) causes calcium release from sarcoplasmic reticulum, leading to activation of myosin ATPase, heat production.	Manic and depressed mood states; schizophrenia (also secondary to infection, metabolic disorders, other medical disorders).	Blockade of central and peripheral muscarinic receptors (e.g., due to tricyclic phenothiazine).

TABLE 3–13. Neuroleptic malignant syndrome (NMS): differential diagnosis *(continued)*

	NMS	Serotonin syndrome	Malignant hyperthermia	Lethal (pernicious) catatonia	Central anticholinergic syndrome
Management	Use supportive measures (cooling, hydration, airway, cardiovascular support); stop neuroleptic; no well-validated "antidote" of choice, but dopamine agonists (bromocriptine 5 mg tid) or dantrolene (1–2 mg/kg q 6 hrs) have been helpful in case reports. Benzodiazepines may ↓ rigidity; ECT may be effective and appropriate in severe cases.	Discontinue suspected agent; use supportive measures (cooling blanket for hyperthermia); propranolol, methysergide, or cyproheptadine may help.	Administer dantrolene sodium 1 mg/kg via rapid intravenous infusion; 100% O_2; Na bicarb; use external cooling.	ECT recommended by some as treatment of choice (within first 5 days); lorazepam 1–2 mg po or im up to qid also useful; neuroleptics generally best withheld (may worsen catatonia).	Remove offending agent; physostigmine usually not indicated (? unless cardiac arrhythmia present).

TABLE 3–13. Neuroleptic malignant syndrome (NMS): differential diagnosis *(continued)*

	NMS	Serotonin syndrome	Malignant hyperthermia	Lethal (pernicious) catatonia	Central anticholinergic syndrome
Management *(continued)*	*Caution:* Dopamine agonists may worsen psychosis and cause hypotension, emesis.				

Note. ?=data uncertain. BP=blood pressure; CPK=creatine phosphokinase; ECT=electroconvulsive therapy; EPS=extrapyramidal side effects; 5-HT_{1A}=$serotonin_{1A}$; LFTs=liver function tests; MAOI=monoamine oxidase inhibitor; SSRI=selective serotonin reuptake inhibitor; WBC=white blood cell count.

Source. Ayd 1995; Caroff 2003; Castillo et al. 1989; Fink 1996; Fink et al. 1993; Jenkins et al. 2001; Pearlman 1986; Petersdorf 1991; Sternbach 1991; Theoharides et al. 1995; Velamoor et al. 1995.

TABLE 3–14. Management of antipsychotic (AP) side effects

Side effect	Strategy
Dry mouth, blurry vision, constipation, other anticholinergic effects; hypersalivation	Encourage fluid intake (nonsugar); use of sugarless gum; use of high-fiber diet and/or stool softener for constipation; use of bethanechol for peripheral anticholinergic side effects; switch to more potent agent, or to atypical agent with low anticholinergic effect (e.g., aripiprazole, ziprasidone) if above unsuccessful. For clozapine-related hypersalivation, consider dosage reduction if clinically feasible; benztropine (1–2 mg hs), hyoscine patch, terazosin (begin with 1 mg qhs, monitor blood pressure), possibly ipratropium spray. Behavioral modification, chewing sugarless gum to aid swallowing of secretions may help.
EPS/Akathisia	If patient is taking a neuroleptic, switch to atypical agent. If patient is taking risperidone, switch to an atypical with ↓ EPS risk (e.g., quetiapine, olanzapine). Other options: reduce dose of AP if clinically feasible; add anticholinergic (benztropine, trihexyphenidyl); for akathisia, add beta-blocker (propranolol 10 mg tid or atenolol 50 mg bid); for refractory EPS, consider amantadine 100 mg bid (may worsen psychosis in some patients). Benzodiazepines are sometimes helpful.
Dizziness, hypotension	If patient is taking agent with high risk of ↓ BP (clozapine, risperidone, quetiapine), switch to agent with lower risk (aripiprazole, ziprasidone). Instruct patient to dangle legs, rise slowly from bed; reduce dose of AP and/or divide into smaller amounts given more frequently. Increase salt intake (e.g., salt tablets); consider use of TED (compressive) stockings; in difficult cases, consider fludrocortisone (Florinef).
Daytime sedation	Reduce dose of AP if clinically feasible; try giving most at bedtime; use higher-potency agent, or atypical agent with less sedation (risperidone, ziprasidone, aripiprazole). Some preliminary evidence suggests modafinil may be useful, but there are also some reports of worsening psychosis, dizziness, and elevated AP level (via CYP 2C19 inhibition?) with this agent.

TABLE 3–14. Management of antipsychotic (AP) side effects *(continued)*

Side effect	Strategy
Prolonged QTc (>450 msec)	Avoid use of concomitant agents that can prolong QTc (e.g., quinidine, sotalol); make sure patient's potassium and magnesium levels are within normal range; avoid thioridazine; olanzapine, risperidone have less effect on QTc than ziprasidone.
Weight gain	Obtain pretreatment weight and monitor periodically. Try to increase patient's exercise level; implement dietary counseling and restrict fat, sugar, etc. Atypical agents usually cause more weight gain than typical agents, with clozapine and olanzapine the most likely to promote weight gain. (One study implicates quetiapine as major weight promoter). Consider change to ziprasidone, aripiprazole, or risperidone. Consider concomitant use of orlistat, H_2 antagonist (start nizatidine along with atypical agent), possibly topiramate.
Glucose dysregulation	Obtain pretreatment (baseline) glucose level; check at least annually during treatment; in patients with risk factors for diabetes mellitus (e.g., family history), measure glycosylated hemoglobin A_{1c} every 3 months. Clozapine, olanzapine, and perhaps quetiapine appear more likely than risperidone or ziprasidone to cause glucose dysregulation, but randomized, controlled data are lacking, and causal relationships are hard to establish.
Lipid dysregulation	Obtain baseline lipid profile; monitor lipids at least twice a year during treatment. Clozapine and olanzapine are more likely than other atypicals to cause hyperlipidemia. May require addition of lipid-lowering agent (e.g., atorvastatin).
Sexual side effects	Avoid thioridazine, most other typical APs. Reduce dose of AP if possible; switch to more potent agent; add small amount of cyproheptadine (? yohimbine in males); bethanechol, possibly sildenafil.

Note. BP=blood pressure; CYP=cytochrome P450; EPS=extrapyramidal side effects; TED=thromboembolic disease.

Source. Allison et al. 1999; Anghelescu et al. 2000; Breier et al. 2001; Freudenreich et al. 2004; Gelenberg 2003a, 2003b; Hallward and Ellison 2001; D.Z. Lieberman et al. 2002; Mathews et al. 2003; McIntyre et al. 2003; Navarro et al. 2001; Osser et al. 1999; Weiden 2003.

TABLE 3–15. Clozapine and white blood cell count (WBC): managing abnormalities

WBC (/mm^3)	Absolute neutrophil count (/mm^3)	Management
<3,500, or history of myeloproliferative disorder, or previous clozapine-induced agranulocytosis/granulocytopenia		Do not initiate clozapine treatment.
<3,500 after initiation of clozapine from normal WBC baseline; drops by 3,000 or more from baseline; or shows cumulative drop of 3,000 or more over 3 weeks		Repeat WBC and differential counts. Evaluate patient for signs of infection, fever, sore throat, malaise. (If signs and symptoms of infection present, consider holding clozapine.)
Between 3,000 and 3,500 subsequently	>1,500	Maintain clozapine but perform twice-weekly WBC and differentials.
	<1,500	Hold clozapine; get daily WBC and differential counts. Monitor for infection. Do not resume clozapine unless/until granulocyte count returns to >1,500 and patient shows no signs of infection. Continue to get twice-weekly WBC and differential until total WBC >3,500.

TABLE 3–15. Clozapine and white blood cell count (WBC): managing abnormalities *(continued)*

WBC (/mm^3)	Absolute neutrophil count (/mm^3)	Management
WBC < 3,000 or →	<1,500	Hold clozapine. Obtain daily WBC and differential counts. Monitor for infection. Do not resume clozapine unless/until granulocyte count returns to >1,500 and patient shows no signs of infection. Continue to get twice-weekly WBC and differential until total WBC >3,500.
WBC < 2,000 or →	<1,000	Continue to hold clozapine. Consider bone marrow aspiration, protective isolation if patient is granulopoiesis-deficient. If infection develops, perform cultures, start antibiotics. Obtain daily WBC and differential counts. Do not rechallenge with clozapine, because agranulocytosis is likely to reappear with shorter latency.

Source. Modified from Novartis Pharmaceutical Company product information, 2004; Physicians' Desk Reference 2004.

Drug–Drug Interactions

TABLE 3–16. Antipsychotic (AP) drug interactions

Medication/drug combined with AP	Effect/Interaction
Antacids, cimetidine, antidiarrheals	Impaired GI absorption of chlorpromazine, ? haloperidol, other APs. Cimetidine may impair metabolism of clozapine and lead to toxicity; may impair absorption of some APs. Omeprazole greatly reduces clozapine levels.
Anticholinergics	Additive anticholinergic effects (e.g., ileus, confusion) when given with low-potency APs, clozapine, and perhaps olanzapine; in theory, may worsen tardive dyskinesia, but evidence is equivocal.
Anticonvulsants	Effect depends on agent: CBZ may lead to significantly lower plasma levels of haloperidol, clozapine, aripiprazole, and other APs; valproate may inhibit metabolism of chlorpromazine and (to a modest degree) clozapine, thus raising levels of AP; valproate has little effect on haloperidol. Chlorpromazine (but not haloperidol) may inhibit metabolism of phenytoin; phenytoin may reduce levels of haloperidol, clozapine. Lamotrigine may possibly elevate clozapine levels (? via effect on glucuronidation). APs, in general, lower seizure threshold and antagonize anticonvulsants. Combination of clozapine and CBZ increases risk of bone marrow suppression.
Antidepressants	TCAs: Increased plasma levels of both AP and AD; increase in anticholinergic effects with TCA and low-potency AP. SSRIs and newer ADs: Fluoxetine, paroxetine, bupropion (strong inhibitors of CYP 2D6) may inhibit metabolism of APs, including haloperidol, risperidone, aripiprazole, with potential worsening of EPS in some cases. Nefazodone may raise blood levels of APs metabolized via CYP 3A4 (e.g., quetiapine). Venlafaxine may increase blood levels of haloperidol, risperidone, perhaps via inhibition of CYP 2D6.

TABLE 3–16. Antipsychotic (AP) drug interactions *(continued)*

Medication/drug combined with AP	Effect/Interaction
Antihypertensives	Effect depends on agent: with captopril and perhaps other ACE inhibitors, propranolol and methyldopa lead to increased hypotensive effect (with chlorpromazine, haloperidol); but coadministration of chlorpromazine and methyldopa sometimes produces hypertension; antihypertensive effect of guanethidine may be reduced by chlorpromazine and similar APs; molindone does not have this effect, and haloperidol and thiothixene have less interference.
Antiretroviral agents	Ritonavir is inhibitor of CYP 2D6 and may impair clearance of risperidone, clozapine, and other APs.
Benzodiazepines	Clozapine plus BZD may lead to respiratory suppression (probably most common with high-dose BZD). Alprazolam may increase serum levels of fluphenazine or haloperidol.
Beta-blockers (e.g., propranolol)	Increased levels of both AP and beta-blocker; ? enhanced antipsychotic effect.
CNS depressants (e.g., opiates, barbiturates)	Increased sedation, confusion, falls, hypotension. Phenobarbital may decrease chlorpromazine levels via induction of hepatic metabolism.
L-Dopa/Carbidopa	Decreased antiparkinsonian effect of L-dopa, due to dopamine receptor blockade by AP. *Note:* L-Dopa is not effective for AP-induced EPS. L-Dopa may precipitate psychosis.
Lithium	Increased EPS; rarely, cases of encephalopathy (lethargy, fever, confusion). Not clear this is more common with any one AP, though haloperidol–lithium combination is more frequently reported.
Other APs	May mutually inhibit each other's metabolism, thus raising plasma level of one or both. Combinations may have potentially dangerous effects on QTc (especially true of ziprasidone plus another AP), postural hypotension.

Note. ACE=angiotensin-converting enzyme; AD=antidepressant; BZD=benzodiazepine; CBZ=carbamazepine; CNS=central nervous system; CYP=cytochrome P450; EPS = extrapyramidal side effects; GI=gastrointestinal; SSRI=selective serotonin reuptake inhibitor; TCA = tricyclic antidepressants.

Source. Adapted from data in Cozza et al. 2003; Frick et al. 2003; Kossen et al. 2001; Venkatakrishnan et al. 2003.

TABLE 3–17. Second-generation (atypical) antipsychotics (APs): potential drug–drug interactions

Antipsychotic	Major (and minor) cytochrome system involved in AP metabolism	Potential drug–drug interactions
aripiprazole	2D6, 3A4	Enzyme inhibition by fluoxetine, paroxetine, erythromycin, fluconazole, itraconazole, ketoconazole would raise blood levels. Enzyme induction by carbamazepine would reduce blood levels.
clozapine	1A2 (3A4, 2D6)	Enzyme inhibition by cimetidine, erythromycin, clarithromycin, fluoxetine, paroxetine, fluvoxamine, ciprofloxacin, quinidine may raise blood levels. Enzyme induction by cigarette smoking, carbamazepine, phenytoin, omeprazole.
olanzapine	1A2 (3A4, 2D6)	Enzyme inhibition by fluvoxamine, ciprofloxacin; probably some effect from CYP 3A4 inhibitors. Enzyme induction by cigarette smoking.
quetiapine	3A4 (2D6)	Enzyme inhibition by cimetidine, erythromycin, clarithromycin, fluconazole, itraconazole, ketoconazole, nefazodone, grapefruit juice. Enzyme induction by carbamazepine, phenytoin.
risperidone	2D6	Enzyme inhibition by fluoxetine, paroxetine, quinidine.
ziprasidone	Aldehyde oxidase (3A4, 1A2)	Since most metabolism is via aldehyde oxidase, cytochrome P450 (CYP) effects should be small; however, potent CYP 3A4 inhibitors may increase blood levels, potentially affecting QTc. Enzyme induction by carbamazepine may slightly reduce ziprasidone levels.

Source. Cozza et al. 2003; D. Z. Lieberman et al. 2002; Venkatakrishnan et al. 2003.

Potentiating Maneuvers

TABLE 3–18. Potentiation of antipsychotics (APs)

Agent added to AP	Potential benefits	Potential risks/side effects
Antidepressants	Some open and controlled data suggest improvement in depressive and negative symptoms with addition of either TCA or SSRI.	Added cardiovascular side effects; occasional reports of worsening psychosis. SSRIs may elevate AP drug levels (e.g., fluvoxamine and olanzapine). Some cases of worsening of EPS with addition of SSRIs to APs.
Benzodiazepines	May improve comorbid anxiety; perhaps improve negative features (?alprazolam), some core symptoms of psychosis (reduced auditory hallucinations). Lorazepam (also clonazepam, diazepam) transiently improves "functional catatonic" symptoms (may or may not be due to schizophrenia). BZDs may permit use of lower doses of APs for acute psychosis.	BZD-related side effects, such as memory impairment, sedation, risk of dependency; high BZD doses may cause respiratory suppression in patients taking clozapine. Some reports of behavioral disinhibition, exacerbation of psychosis, anxiety, depression; several controlled studies found tolerance developed by fourth week of BZD treatment.
Beta-blockers	May reduce aggression, perhaps self-injurious behavior in some psychotic patients. May reduce some core features of psychosis.	May alter hepatic metabolism of APs (?increase plasma levels). Side effects include hypotension, bradycardia, worsening of COPD, masking of hypoglycemia in diabetic patients; some patients may become depressed. Not all studies show efficacy.

TABLE 3–18. Potentiation of antipsychotics (APs) *(continued)*

Agent added to AP	Potential benefits	Potential risks/side effects
Carbamazepine	May improve affective lability, aggression in some patients with schizoaffective disorder. Mania complicated by psychotic features responds to anticonvulsants.	May reduce plasma levels of some APs (e.g., haloperidol). Increased risk of neurotoxicity. Increased risk of hepatotoxicity when CBZ combined with phenothiazines. Increased risk of bone marrow suppression when CBZ is combined with clozapine. Side effects include sedation, GI upset, ataxia, SIADH.
Lamotrigine	Limited, naturalistic evidence of adjunctive benefit when added to clozapine in treatment-resistant schizophrenia patients; this benefit not seen when combined with risperidone, haloperidol, olanzapine.	Combination treatment with APs seems to be well tolerated, but systematic data on side effects are lacking.
Lithium	May improve mood stability, depressive–anxious features in some patients with chronic schizophrenia. May be useful in patients with schizophreniform disorder (?especially those with family history of mood disorders).	Increased EPS, cerebellar symptoms. Increased risk of neurotoxicity. Lithium-related side effects (e.g., polyuria, loose stools, tremor).

TABLE 3–18. Potentiation of antipsychotics (APs) *(continued)*

Agent added to AP	Potential benefits	Potential risks/side effects
Other APs	Anecdotal observations and case series reports suggest combining two APs (e.g., adding risperidone or haloperidol to clozapine or olanzapine) may augment partial response to original agent. Some theoretical rationale for adding potent dopamine D_2 blocker (e.g., risperidone) to atypical agent with little D_2 blockade (e.g., olanzapine).	Virtually no controlled studies have evaluated efficacy, safety, or cost-effectiveness of this practice. Clinician may misinterpret "late" response to combination as indicating that *both* agents are necessary; in fact, it may be that the second agent alone was effective, or that the original agent would have been effective, given enough time. APs may mutually raise each other's blood levels; possibly worsen side effects or increase risk of agranulocytosis. Risk of increased EPS, additive cardiovascular effects (including prolonged QTc, hypotension). (Monitoring ECG is prudent.) Additive side effects of second agent may undermine favorable side-effect profile of first agent. (For example, risperidone's high rate of EPS may nullify lack of EPS with olanzapine or quetiapine.) Some question of whether aripiprazole's AP effect is undermined by an added D_2 blocker.

TABLE 3–18. Potentiation of antipsychotics (APs) *(continued)*

Agent added to AP	Potential benefits	Potential risks/side effects
Valproate (divalproex)	May improve mood lability in some patients with schizoaffective disorder. Some evidence of adjunctive benefit (when combined with olanzapine or risperidone) in schizophrenia. May provide antiseizure prophylaxis in some patients taking high-dose clozapine, though controlled data are lacking.	May alter hepatic metabolism of some APs, but there is probably not a strong effect (e.g., 6% increase in clozapine levels). Divalproex side effects include increased tremor, GI upset, sedation, and transient alopecia. Thrombocytopenia, weight gain may occur in combination with AP.

Note. BZD = benzodiazepine; CBZ = carbamazepine; COPD = chronic obstructive pulmonary disease; ECG = electrocardiogram; EPS = extrapyramidal side effects; GI = gastrointestinal; SIADH = syndrome of inappropriate antidiuretic hormone; SSRI = selective serotonin reuptake inhibitor; TCA = tricyclic antidepressant.

Source. Casey et al. 2003; Csernansky and Newcomer 1995; Dursun and Deakin 2001; Henderson and Goff 1996; Hogarty et al. 1995; Janicak et al. 1993; Pies 2001; Raskin et al. 2000; Sussman 1997.

Use in Special Populations

TABLE 3–19. Antipsychotics (APs) in special populations

Special population	Concerns/Recommendations
Children and young adolescents	*First-generation (conventional or neuroleptic) APs:* Few controlled studies of APs in prepubertal children; haloperidol and loxapine appear superior to placebo in adolescent schizophrenia patients. Disorders in children and adolescents seem more refractory than those in adults; children and adolescents are more likely to develop sedation, perhaps earlier TD; acute dystonias may be more common in younger males; laryngeal dystonias are especially dangerous. Reduction of dose more effective than anticholinergics for EPS in children. Children may develop greater hypotensive effects than adults before becoming clinically symptomatic; monitor BP closely during initial titration. Children metabolize APs more rapidly than do adults (lower plasma level at same dose) but also require lower plasma levels for efficacy; age, weight, and severity of symptoms do not provide clear dosage guidelines. Recommended dosage for haloperidol in children is 0.5–16 mg/day, but initial dose should be very low, with no more than twice-weekly increments; divided doses are useful initially, with eventual conversion to mostly at bedtime. Monitor closely for signs of "behavioral toxicity" (apathy, cognitive dulling, sedation). Older adolescents may require a dosage similar to that in adults. *Second-generation (atypical) APs:* Few randomized, controlled studies; most data from open studies, case reports. Clozapine (mean total daily dose = 176 mg) appears superior to placebo and to haloperidol in children and adolescents with schizophrenia, but has significant side effects (e.g., seizure, neutropenia, weight gain). Olanzapine (5–20 mg/day) and risperidone (1–6 mg/day) are equal or superior in efficacy to haloperidol in children and adolescents with schizophrenia spectrum disorders but have numerous side effects, including EPS and weight gain. Open studies of quetiapine (dosage range = 300–800 mg/day) show efficacy in adolescents with psychotic disorders.

TABLE 3–19. Antipsychotics (APs) in special populations *(continued)*

Special population	Concerns/Recommendations
Elderly patients	*General points:* Concomitant medical problems, numerous psychiatric and nonpsychiatric drugs increase risk for adverse reactions and drug–drug interactions; elderly patients have increased sensitivity to anticholinergic properties of APs; they may develop confusion, memory impairment, and hallucinations; postural hypotension may be a problem with low-potency APs, also the quinidine-like properties of low-potency agents may exacerbate conduction abnormalities; some older patients may develop higher plasma AP levels than do younger patients. TD may develop more rapidly and at lower AP doses than in younger patients. "Start low, go slow" with dosage (one-half to one-third young adult dose initially); use hs or divided dosing; monitor BP and vital signs closely; watch for signs of confusion, dizziness, fever, and rigidity (risk of NMS). Attempt non-AP treatment of "agitation" (e.g., trazodone, buspirone) if possible. *First-generation (conventional or neuroleptic) APs:* Low-potency APs are generally not as well tolerated overall as higher-potency APs (haloperidol, fluphenazine), but high-potency agents have higher risk of EPS. Haloperidol in range of 0.25–1.5 mg qd to qid is usual regimen for psychosis in elderly patients, though some patients will require higher doses (dementia patients with psychosis usually respond at lower doses than do patients with schizophrenia). Haloperidol (e.g., 1–2 mg po or iv up to qid) is drug of choice for agitation in delirium; monitor cardiac status. *Second-generation (atypical) APs:* Drugs of choice for long-term treatment of psychotic illness in the elderly. Use very low initial doses of atypicals in elderly patients, dementia patients (e.g., clozapine 6.25 mg qd; risperidone 0.25–0.5 mg qd; olanzapine 2.5 mg; quetiapine 25 mg at bedtime initially). In elderly schizophrenia patients, median total daily doses of risperidone and olanzapine are approximately 2 mg and 10 mg, respectively. Recent concern about increased risk of cerebrovascular adverse events with risperidone use in agitated dementia patients; however, causal link is unclear, and other APs with α_1 antagonism (i.e., olanzapine, quetiapine, ziprasidone) may also pose risk, perhaps due to orthostatic hypotension.

TABLE 3–19. Antipsychotics (APs) in special populations *(continued)*

Special population	Concerns/Recommendations
Developmentally disabled (mentally retarded) and autistic patients	Autism differs from mental retardation (MR) in showing qualitative developmental deviations, not just delays and decreased IQ. Several studies have shown that haloperidol, trifluoperazine, and pimozide lead to improved behavior in autistic children (e.g., reduced stereotypy, withdrawal, hyperactivity) without cognitive impairment. Haloperidol may improve language acquisition when combined with behavioral interventions. Avoid highly sedating APs in this population; reassess periodically to see if AP is necessary or is causing TD. For patients with MR and schizophrenia, APs are just as effective as among non-MR patients. Use of APs for self-injurious behavior and stereotypies in MR populations has not been well validated, although some studies suggest use of mixed D_1/D_2 receptor antagonists is useful (? clozapine). Better results may be obtained for self-injurious behaviors with serotonergic agents, especially given the risks of akathisia, TD, and cognitive impairment with APs. Recent, mainly open studies with risperidone and olanzapine showed global and behavioral benefits in autistic populations but not much evidence of improvement in “core” autistic symptoms.
Pregnant patients	*First-generation (conventional or neuroleptic) APs:* Risks of untreated psychosis (e.g., command auditory hallucinations to “stab the baby”) must be weighed against the relatively rare teratogenic effects of these medications. Several studies have shown no increase in fetal malformations after first-trimester exposure to neuroleptics, though some have found increases in nonspecific congenital defects after exposure to phenothiazines. Some data suggest that haloperidol or piperazine-type agents are less teratogenic than aliphatic phenothiazines. Very little evidence of “behavioral toxicity” or impaired IQ in infants born to mothers taking neuroleptics during pregnancy. Neuroleptics can cause anticholinergic side effects in the fetus (constipation, intestinal obstruction, urinary retention) and may increase the risk of jaundice in premature infants.

TABLE 3–19. Antipsychotics (APs) in special populations *(continued)*

Special population	Concerns/Recommendations
Pregnant patients *(continued)*	*First-generation (conventional or neuroleptic) APs* (continued): Mild, transient syndrome of neonatal hypertonia, tremor, and poor motor maturity can be seen after neuroleptic use in late pregnancy. Fetal tachyarrhythmias may be more likely with maternal use of low-potency (hence, more anticholinergic) neuroleptics. To prevent fetal sedation and muscle spasms/tremor, consider tapering and then discontinuing the drug a week or two in advance of expected delivery date. Since neuroleptics are variably excreted in breast milk, breastfeeding is best avoided if the mother continues to take the drug. *Second-generation (atypical) APs:* Despite widespread use, atypical APs have not been well studied, prospectively, in pregnancy. Case reports and anecdotal data suggest that clozapine is relatively safe in pregnancy (i.e., no major congenital malformations), but reports of minor anomalies, "floppy infant syndrome," exist. Olanzapine data thus far suggest relative safety, with no evidence of teratogenesis or obstetrical complications. Data too limited with quetiapine, ziprasidone, and aripiprazole.

Note. BP = blood pressure; EPS = extrapyramidal side effects; NMS = neuroleptic malignant syndrome; TD = tardive dyskinesia.

Source. Dulcan et al. 1995; Jacobson et al. 2002; Janicak et al. 1993; Jeste et al. 2003; Martin et al. 2003; McElhatton 1992; Newport et al. 2004; Pies and Popli 1995; Salzman et al. 1995; Stowe and Nemeroff 1995; Wagner 2004.

Questions and Answers

Drug Class

Q. When is it appropriate to use intravenous antipsychotics (APs)?

A. Intravenous haloperidol has been used safely and effectively in the management of agitated, delirious patients in critical care settings (Janicak et al. 1993). For example, a delirious patient in the coronary care unit is tearing out his intravenous lines, says he is "in the wrong hotel room," and appears to be hallucinating. For many such patients, higher-than-usual doses of intravenous haloperidol may be necessary, with hourly doses of 10 mg iv necessary in severe cases (Adams 1988). Supplemental use of intravenous lorazepam (in combination with haloperidol) may be effective and may result in lower doses of haloperidol. A typical regimen might begin with 5 mg of haloperidol, followed immediately by 0.5 mg of lorazepam. If there is no response to the first injection, an additional 10 mg of haloperidol and 4 mg of lorazepam may be given every 30–60 minutes, until the patient is adequately sedated. In most cases, a dosage of less than 100 mg/day of haloperidol is required. A related compound, *droperidol,* has also been used in the treatment of agitated, delirious patients but has produced troublesome hypotension in doses of 10–20 mg given as a bolus (Adams 1988). Keep in mind that delirium is a medical emergency that requires diagnosis and treatment of the underlying condition.

Q. What are the conversion formulas for switching a patient from oral to depot neuroleptics?

A. There are no fool-proof "formulas" for such conversions, since the clinical goal is always to use the lowest effective maintenance dose for the specific patient. The required dose may vary with the patient's tolerance of the medication, hepatic metabolism, and pharmacodynamic response at the level of the neuron. However, there are some "rules of thumb" and rough conversion guides for use of fluphenazine and haloperidol decanoate. For most patients with chronic schizophrenia maintained with a total daily dose of oral fluphenazine 10–15 mg, an appropriate dose of the decanoate would be roughly 25 mg every 2–3 weeks (Kaplan et al. 1994).The custom of biweekly injections is probably unnecessary in many cases, given the long $t_{1/2}$ of fluphenazine decanoate. Some data suggest that a plasma level of 1.0–2.8 ng/mL is optimal for patients maintained on fluphenazine decanoate (Janicak et al. 1993); however, many commercial laboratories do not use assays with sufficient sensitivity to measure fluphenazine levels < 2 ng/mL.

For conversion from oral haloperidol to the *monthly* decanoate dose, the general rule is to multiply the daily oral dose by a factor of 10–20. For example, a patient receiving 10 mg of oral haloperidol daily may require around 150 mg monthly of the decanoate. Elderly patients and patients prone to significant extrapyramidal side effects (EPS) may do better when receiving lower doses (Freudenreich and McEvoy 1995), but some severely ill patients may require up to 300 mg/month. The package insert for haloperidol decanoate cites data showing that 200 mg/month provides the most consistent relapse prevention, but the relapse rates for a maintenance dose of 200 mg/month vs. 50 or 100 mg/month differ by only 8%–10%. Although this difference is quite important from an epidemiological perspective, it still suggests that the lower dose range for haloperidol decanoate may be more appropriate, at least initially, for some patients (Freudenreich and McEvoy 1995). The rate of EPS actually seems to be less with the decanoate form of haloperidol than with the oral form (Janicak et al. 1993), though this difference may reflect the lower dose required with the decanoate form compared with the equivalent oral dose (D. Osser, M.D., personal communication, December 1996).

Recently, the U.S. Food and Drug Administration (FDA) approved the use of a long-acting formulation of risperidone (Risperdal Consta). There is, as yet, no "conversion" formula provided by the manufacturer, for patients taking other agents. In general, however, the recommendation is that patients receive 25 mg of long-acting risperidone intramuscularly every 2 weeks. During the first 3 weeks of treatment, use of an oral AP is strongly recommended, since there is a 3-week delay in release of long-acting risperidone from the microsphere delivery system. In transitioning patients from a depot neuroleptic to long-acting risperidone, it is feasible simply to administer the long-acting risperidone at the next scheduled dose of the conventional neuroleptic (Ayd 2003; Kane et al. 2003a). Although experience with depot risperidone is limited, anecdotal reports from Robert R. Conley, M.D. (reported in Sherman 2004) suggest that 2–3 weeks after the first injection, the oral AP dose may be cut in half if the patient is doing well, or by a third if the patient is showing signs of instability. By 3 months, the oral drug should be discontinued. Transition to depot risperidone from multiple oral APs requires gradual and sequential tapering from each agent.

Q. What atypical APs are available for acute intramuscular injection, and how are they best administered?

A. At this time, ziprasidone and olanzapine are the only atypical APs available for acute intramuscular use. Intramuscular ziprasidone is generally given as an initial 10-mg injection, followed by a 5- to 20-mg injection every 4–6 hours, up to a dosage of 40–80 mg/day (Gelenberg 2003a). Peak plasma levels are reached in about 30 minutes, rapidly reducing psychomotor agitation and psychotic symptoms. Side effects include nausea, vomiting, and sedation; in theory, baseline and follow-up electrocardiograms (ECGs) are indicated, given ziprasidone's tendency to increase QTc (Gelenberg 2003a). A short-acting formulation of olanzapine is also available. It achieves a peak plasma concentration two to five times higher than that of oral olanzapine in about 30 minutes (vs. 4 hours with oral olanzapine). Intramuscular olanzapine (5–10 mg/injection) may also be useful in reducing agitation in mania, with intramuscular doses of 2.5–10 mg corresponding to oral olanzapine doses of about 5–20 mg (Meehan et al. 2001). Somnolence and dizziness may be reported with intramuscular olanzapine.

Indications

Q. What is the role of conventional neuroleptics in the management of acute mania?

A. Neuroleptics, historically, have often been used as an adjunct to lithium in the early stages of acute mania, prior to achievement of therapeutic blood levels of lithium. Some clinicians continue the neuroleptic even after lithium has reached therapeutic levels, in order to reduce psychomotor agitation and grandiose delusions. Results of five controlled studies comparing lithium with neuroleptics in treating acute mania suggest that lithium is superior (response rate: 89% vs. 54%), though other studies do show some benefit for neuroleptics (Janicak et al. 1993). Neuroleptics may be preferable to lithium in treating schizoaffective disorder, given their faster onset and broader spectrum of activity, though this condition is undoubtedly quite heterogeneous. Conventional APs have a relatively greater risk of inducing tardive dyskinesia (TD) in patients with affective disorders and should be used with caution in the long-term management of bipolar disorders. Moreover, neuroleptics may worsen the depressive component of bipolar disorder over the long term (Kukopulos et al. 1980). It appears that low to moderate doses of APs are sufficient to control acutely manic patients with psychotic features and that adverse effects may be minimized with this strategy (Janicak et al. 1993). In rare cases, manic or hypomanic reactions may be seen with atypical APs (Brieger 2004), though placebo-controlled studies have not confirmed this phenomenon in bipolar patients.

Q. Since clozapine was first marketed, have the indications been broadened? In what situations would clozapine be the AP of *first choice*?

A. The 2004 edition of the Physicians' Desk Reference (PDR) states that Clozaril is indicated "for the management of severely ill schizophrenic patients who fail to respond adequately to standard antipsychotic drug treatment…either because of insufficient effectiveness or the inability to achieve an effective dose due to intolerable adverse effects from those drugs." The product labeling information notes that clozapine should be used "only in patients who have failed to respond adequately to treatment with appropriate courses of standard antipsychotic drugs…" (Physicians' Desk Reference 2004). The term *courses* is generally interpreted to mean "two or more." While clinicians are not prohibited by law from going outside FDA-approved labeling information, the clinician who does so assumes the burden of medicolegal justification. Thus, on the basis of the PDR criteria, clozapine would *never* be the *first* AP prescribed for a psychotic patient, and this position is upheld in a recent review by Marder and Wirshing (2004). Similarly, on the basis of the most recent Expert Consensus Guideline (Kane et al. 2003b), use of clozapine would be withheld until, for example, the patient has either failed to respond to adequate trials of one or more conventional APs and two atypical APs or failed to respond to two or three atypical agents. However, the authors of this same document opine that "when it is appropriate to switch to clozapine remains an area of controversy and there are few data to inform clinical practice. We may in fact be doing our patients a disservice by trying multiple drugs before going to clozapine…" (Kane et al. 2003b, p. 12). In addition to using clozapine in treating schizophrenia and schizoaffective disorder, Marder and Wirshing (2004) note its utility in refractory mania, depression with psychotic features, and psychosis in Parkinson's disease. Clozapine has also proved effective in the management of dysphoric mania (Suppes et al. 1992), though the risk of agranulocytosis renders clozapine a second- or third-line agent in the treatment of mania. In addition, several studies have found a corrective effect of clozapine on polydipsia and intermittent hyponatremia (e.g., in patients who intoxicate themselves through excessive water drinking) (Lee et al. 1991; Spears et al. 1996).

One recent, 18-week, randomized, double-blind study of treatment-resistant or treatment-intolerant schizophrenic patients found that olanzapine was as effective as clozapine on all efficacy measures (Bitter et al. 2004). However, clozapine is the only agent in all of psychiatry with FDA-approved labeling for "reduction in the risk of recurrent suicidal behavior in schizophrenia or schizoaffective disorder" (Physicians' Desk Reference 2004, p. 2229). Indeed, clozapine appears to be superior even to olanzapine in reducing the risk of suicide in schizophrenia (Marder and Wirshing 2004; Meltzer 2002).

Q. What is the role of newer atypical APs in the management of bipolar disorder and schizoaffective disorder?

A. The role of newer atypical APs in treating patients with bipolar and schizoaffective disorder is an area of intense interest. We may consider this question in terms of 1) acute treatment of bipolar mania or depression and 2) maintenance or prophylactic treatment. One recent review (Brambilla et al. 2003) concluded that olanzapine was the most "appropriate atypical antipsychotic agent" for treating bipolar patients in the manic phase, but randomized, controlled, "head-to-head" studies are lacking. Olanzapine monotherapy has demonstrated antimanic effects in two placebo-controlled, double-blind trials (Tohen et al. 1999, 2000) lasting 3 and 4 weeks, respectively. Olanzapine now has FDA-approved labeling for use as monotherapy in mania and for use in combination with lithium or valproate for the treatment of acute manic episodes. Olanzapine's antimanic effect does not appear to depend on the presence of psychotic features and is also observed in patients with mixed features (Tohen et al. 2000). Recently, risperidone and quetiapine also received FDA-approved labeling for short-term treatment of mania or mixed episodes, as monotherapy or in combination with lithium or valproate. There is also controlled evidence demonstrating the efficacy of ziprasidone and aripiprazole in treating mania, and these agents have FDA-approved labeling for this use.

Ziprasidone has been proven effective in the acute treatment of schizophrenia and schizoaffective disorder, at dosages ranging from 40 to 200 mg/day (Daniel et al. 2004). Moreover, in a 3-week, placebo-controlled, randomized trial, ziprasidone monotherapy was superior to placebo in reducing symptoms of acute mania, at a dosage of approximately 135 mg/day (Keck et al. 2003c). Similarly, aripiprazole demonstrated significantly greater efficacy than placebo in the treatment of acute manic or mixed episodes and was well tolerated in a randomized, placebo-controlled trial (Keck et al. 2003b). With respect to bipolar depression, the combination of olanzapine and fluoxetine (Symbyax) was recently approved by the FDA for this indication.

Olanzapine has also received FDA approval for use in the *maintenance* treatment of bipolar disorder, based on the results of one double-blind, placebo-controlled study (Eli Lilly, data on file, 2004). This study found that the time to relapse of either mania or depression was significantly longer for olanzapine-treated patients than for patients treated with placebo. There are now four randomized, controlled trials of olanzapine in the prevention of mood episodes in bipolar disorder. Overall, given the methodological limitations of these four studies (e.g., use of "enriched" design), Ghaemi and Hsu (2004) concluded that olanzapine shows evidence of *relapse prevention* in bipolar patients *who have responded acutely* to this agent; however, confident conclusions about actual *prophylaxis* in patients with bipolar disorder may be premature. Concerns about long-term weight gain, glycemic dyscontrol, and triglyceride level elevation with olanzapine also need further evaluation when the clinician is considering long-term use. Some data suggest that risperidone may also have antidepressant (AD) and/or mood-stabilizing properties in patients with bipolar disorder. In an open, multicenter, 6-month study of 541 bipolar and schizoaffective patients (Vieta et al. 2001), adjunctive risperidone showed both antimanic and antidepressant effects. In a randomized, double-blind study of risperidone versus haloperidol in schizoaffective disorder, both drugs were equally effective in reducing psychotic and manic symptoms, but risperidone showed a trend toward greater decreases in depression scores on the Hamilton Rating Scale for Depression (Janicak et al. 2001).

Taken in toto, the available data suggest that most atypical APs may play a useful role in both the acute and maintenance treatment phases in bipolar disorder, as well as in schizoaffective disorder.

Q. Are there any significant risks in bipolar patients continuing to use neuroleptics (along with a mood stabilizer) for *maintenance therapy* if they have shown psychotic features in previous manic or depressive episodes?

A. Conventional APs have roughly double the risk of inducing TD in patients with affective disorders (vs. nonaffective populations) and should be used with caution in the long-term management of bipolar disorders. Moreover, some data suggest that whereas a patient taking a neuroleptic along with lithium has a much smaller chance of having a manic episode, there appears to be a much *greater* chance that the patient will become depressed (Gelenberg 1995a; Kukopulos et al. 1980). The risks of developing TD and depression are almost certainly reduced with use of atypical APs, but there are few studies examining these issues over the course of a year or more in bipolar populations.

Q. Is it helpful to use APs in the treatment of personality disorders?

A. In general, the pharmacological approach to personality disorders should focus on specific target symptoms and comorbid Axis I disorders (Cowdry 1987; Pies 1994). Thus, some patients with borderline personality disorder (BPD) who show mild thought process disorder or paranoid thinking may benefit from a trial on a low-dose AP medication (e.g., 2 mg/day of thiothixene [Navane]). Early work by Soloff and colleagues (1986) suggested that BPD patients show a "broad spectrum" response to haloperidol—that is, they experience positive effects on anxiety, hostility, depression, and schizotypal symptoms. However, long-term (16-week) placebo-controlled data on BPD suggest little benefit from haloperidol at dosages up to 6 mg/day, except on measures of irritability (Cornelius et al. 1993). Preliminary data suggest, on the basis of a study of 15 BPD patients with atypical psychotic symptoms (as assessed with the Brief Psychiatric Rating Scale [BPRS] and the Global Assessment Scale [GAS]), that clozapine may improve some aspects of functioning in patients with BPD (Frankenburg and Zanarini 1993). Given the risk of agranulocytosis with clozapine, use of this agent in treating BPD patients would clearly require a careful risk-benefit discussion. In a double-blind study, Zanarini and Frankenburg (2001) found that olanzapine was more effective than placebo in reducing symptoms in all four core areas (affect, cognition, impulsivity, interpersonal relationships) of borderline psychopathology. With respect to other personality disorders, there is modest (and mainly anecdotal) evidence that

APs may be helpful in some patients with paranoid and schizotypal personality disorders (Ellison and Adler 1990; Goldberg et al. 1986). Keep in mind that some patients with paranoid personality order may become more distressed when they feel they are being "experimented on" with medication—particularly if they feel heavily sedated.

Q. Is it appropriate to treat dementia patients with APs, and if so, what is the appropriate agent and dosage?

A. In general, APs should be used very sparingly and conservatively in dementia patients, particularly when psychosis per se is not the "target symptom." APs may have a modest beneficial effect in reducing "agitation" (a term in need of differential diagnosis), insomnia, irritability, and hostility in dementia patients, but consequent confusion and motoric side effects (e.g., akathisia, parkinsonism, TD [occurring at a high incidence]) frequently outweigh their marginal benefits (Dubovsky and Buzan 2000). On the other hand, *APs should not be withheld in cases of dementia complicated by secondary hallucinations and delusions* (e.g., in Alzheimer's disease or vascular dementia). High-potency APs, such as haloperidol 0.25–2.0 mg/day, may be effective in such cases. Highly anticholinergic APs (thioridazine, chlorpromazine) may exacerbate Alzheimer's disease symptoms, since this disorder already entails decreased levels of brain acetylcholine. The use of risperidone, olanzapine, aripiprazole, and perhaps other atypical APs in psychotic dementia patients has stirred controversy recently, owing to reports of increased cerebrovascular adverse events (CAEs) and, in some cases, mortality with these agents. Although the basis for this association is unclear at this time (see discussion under subsection "Use in Special Populations" in the "Overview" section of this chapter), risperidone (and *most* atypical APs) may provoke hypotension in the elderly and should be started at lower-than-recommended doses—for example, risperidone 0.25–0.5 mg/day, with slow titration up to 1.5–2.0 mg/day. Olanzapine may also cause falls in dementia patients (Martin et al. 2003), and conservative dosing is indicated.

Despite these concerns, uncontrolled and controlled data (Jeanblanc and Davis 1995; Katz et al. 1999) suggest that risperidone at a dosage of 1.5–2.5 mg/day can be helpful in managing aggression in dementia patients with psychotic features. One study found that low-dose, once-a-day olanzapine and risperidone are equally safe and effective in the treatment of dementia-related behavioral disturbances in residents of extended care facilities (Fontaine et al. 2003). Clozapine appears to be generally safe and effective—when used in very low doses—in psychotic Parkinson's disease patients with levodopa-induced hallucinations; doses in the range of 12.5 to 50 mg at bedtime are often used (Troster et al. 2000). Patients with Lewy body dementia are notoriously sensitive to APs (e.g., developing severe EPS), though clozapine is sometimes tolerated (Jacobson et al. 2002). In some cases, agitation and aggression in dementia patients are better treated with trazodone, a selective serotonin reuptake inhibitor (SSRI), a beta-blocker, buspirone, or divalproex than with an AP (Dubovsky and Buzan 2000). The underlying cause of the patient's "agitation" should always be sought, and behavioral strategies should be tried whenever feasible.

Q. What is the role of APs in the treatment of obsessive-compulsive disorder (OCD)?

A. The addition of a low-dose dopamine receptor antagonist, such as haloperidol or pimozide, has been found useful in up to 65% of SSRI-resistant OCD patients, particularly those with chronic tic disorder or schizotypal features (McDougle et al. 1990). With respect to atypical APs, the situation is somewhat complicated, and randomized, controlled data are scant. Risperidone at a dosage of 1 mg/day was added to ongoing fluvoxamine therapy (250–300 mg/day) in three patients whose OCD symptoms had been refractory to the SSRI after 12 weeks. All three patients showed significant improvement in their OCD symptoms (McDougle et al. 1995). Another study found that the addition of risperidone to ongoing fluoxetine treatment led to improvement in a patient with sexual obsessions (Bourgeois and Klein 1996). A small, 8-week, open-label study ($N = 10$) of olanzapine augmentation (Koran et al. 2000) found some evidence of benefit when olanzapine (at a dosage of up to 10 mg/day) was added to ongoing fluoxetine; however, a "dramatic response" was seen in only one subject, while four others experienced partial improvement. Response to olanzapine augmentation appears to be independent of comorbid mood disorder response. There is at least one report of clozapine's being useful in a patient with extremely refractory OCD, after failure of SSRIs and capsulotomy (Young et al. 1994). However, other studies have suggested that clozapine and other atypicals—possibly via antagonism of the serotonin$_2$ (5-HT$_2$) receptor—may *worsen* obsessive-compulsive symptoms in some schizophrenic patients (Baker et al. 1992), though this phenomenon seems to be rare. Finally, the risk of TD and drug–drug interactions must be borne in mind if classical APs are used in the treatment of OCD. Although TD is much less common with atypical agents, drug–drug interactions may be significant (e.g., when fluvoxamine is combined with olanzapine) (Cozza et al. 2003).

Q. Are APs effective in the treatment of patients with delusional disorder?

A. Delusional disorder, in which a "nonbizarre" delusion has been present for at least 1 month and is not the product of schizophrenia, has not been systematically studied with respect to AP use. Anecdotal data suggest that APs are useful in treating this disorder, though perhaps not as effective as in the treatment of schizophrenia (Shader 1994). The AP pimozide seems to be especially useful in treating the "somatic type" of delusional disorder, which has affinities with both body dysmorphic disorder and so-called monosymptomatic hypochondriasis (Shader 1994; Phillips 1991); however, randomized controlled studies are lacking. Anecdotal reports also suggest that SSRIs may be beneficial in treating delusional disorder, raising the question of whether some of these patients' conditions may fall along the "obsessive-compulsive spectrum." Low doses of risperidone and clozapine have also been found useful in treating patients with delusional disorder, but again, these results were based on anecdotal information (Manschreck 1996).

Mechanisms of Action

Q. What is the expected "lag time" for onset of therapeutic effect, in light of the mechanism of action of APs?

A. Several studies suggest that conventional neuroleptics usually require 2–4 weeks for significant effects on "core" positive and negative features of schizophrenia. Negative symptoms (e.g., apathy, anhedonia, alogia, social withdrawal) may lag behind positive symptoms in response to conventional APs such as fluphenazine (Breier et al. 1987). Earlier attempts at using high "loading" doses of APs (e.g., >40 mg of haloperidol per day or equivalent) to manage acute exacerbations of schizophrenia—so-called rapid neuroleptization—have failed to show superiority to lower-dose strategies of haloperidol

10–20 mg/day, often in combination with a benzodiazepine (BZD) (Tueth et al. 1995). It is not clear that such acute AP/BZD effects are mediated through the same mechanism of action as is long-term amelioration of core psychotic symptoms. While acute blockade of nigrostriatal dopamine (DA) D_2 receptors by neuroleptics may account for acute dystonic reactions, it is not clear that the sedative effect of acutely administered conventional APs represents much more than a nonspecific action common to other sedative agents.

With respect to orally administered atypical APs in the treatment of schizophrenia, the time to clinical effect may vary from agent to agent. Studies of clozapine suggest that benefits increase rapidly over a 29-week course and that longer exposure tends to produce further improvement. Thus, in a study of refractory schizophrenia, Kane and colleagues (2001) found that at 4 weeks, 39% of subjects met the criteria for 20% improvement; however, by 11 weeks and 29 weeks, these figures were 54% and 57%, respectively. (It could be inferred that most patients will approach maximal benefit from clozapine after about 3–4 months of treatment, but there are exceptional cases in which improvement occurs even later in treatment.) There is some evidence that risperidone may have a more rapid onset of action than clozapine, though there is no consistent evidence that risperidone is more effective in the long term (Bondolfi et al. 1998). Some data suggest that when olanzapine is begun at a daily dose of 15 mg, rather than 5 or 10 mg, it has more rapid clinical effects (Osser and Sigadel 2001). For most newer atypical APs, the author's clinical impression is that although some schizophrenia patients will show modest to moderate improvement during the first 2 weeks of treatment, a robust response may not be seen until 4–8 weeks of treatment at adequate doses. What accounts for this lag phase? Presumably, blockade of mesolimbic DA receptors is merely the first step in a chain of intracellular events resulting in altered gene expression, such as increased messenger RNA coding for various DA receptors (Chin et al. 1995). Such long-term alterations correspond more closely to the time course of AP clinical efficacy than does acute D_2 receptor blockade per se.

Q. How do the receptor profiles for classical neuroleptics differ from the new, "atypical" agents, such as clozapine and olanzapine?

A. Since most APs affect numerous receptors (see Table 3–6), only a general response to this question is possible. Classical neuroleptics (e.g., haloperidol) seem to exert their antipsychotic effects primarily via antagonism of the D_2

receptor. Newer agents, such as clozapine, are more effective in blocking the 5-HT_2 receptor than the D_2 receptor, and this high 5-HT_2-to-D_2 ratio may confer atypical properties on these agents. Thus, atypical agents seem to be more effective in treating "negative" symptoms in schizophrenia (see below), produce fewer EPS, raise serum prolactin levels only minimally, and may be less likely to promote TD (Jibson and Tandon 1996). If we consider olanzapine's receptor profile, it is clear that multiple receptor effects result in complicated pharmacodynamic effects, as well as some side effects (see Tables 3–6 and 3–10). Thus, olanzapine binds to varying degrees to dopamine D_2, D_3, D_4, and D_5 receptors; 5-HT_2 receptors; and muscarinic, histaminic, and α_1-adrenergic receptors (Schulz et al. 2004). Recent findings using positron emission tomography (PET) (Kapur et al. 2000) suggest that several atypical agents—notably, quetiapine and olanzapine—have a "fast off" property with respect to DA receptor (especially D_2) blockade. By acting on and then quickly "leaving" these receptors, atypical agents may reduce psychosis without producing significant EPS (Kapur et al. 2000; Schulz et al. 2004). Finally, nondopaminergic mechanisms of action are now under intense scrutiny with respect to atypical APs. Thus, some atypical agents appear to have complex effects on the glutamatergic system via their action at *N*-methyl-D-aspartate (NMDA) receptors (Goff et al. 2002; Schulz et al. 2004).

Q. How effective are atypical agents in treating patients with schizophrenia compared with typical neuroleptics, particularly with respect to "negative" symptoms?

A. There continues to be controversy over the question of whether atypical agents are more effective than neuroleptics in treating schizophrenia. Some psychiatrists remain convinced that the atypicals represent a "quantum leap" beyond older agents; others are equally convinced that the atypicals have only marginal superiority compared with older agents, largely due to reduced EPS. One difficulty is in the identification and classification of "negative" symptoms of schizophrenia (e.g., apathy, anhedonia, alogia, social withdrawal). Carpenter et al. (1988) distinguished between primary negative symptoms due to the disease itself and secondary negative symptoms due either to drug effects or to the presence of positive symptoms (e.g., a patient appears to be "asocial" but is really responding to a command auditory hallucination warning him against socializing). Some studies appearing to show that atypical APs produce greater effects on negative symptoms may not have distinguished primary from secondary negative symptoms—for example, they failed to distinguish improved socialization due to reduced EPS from "true" improvement in social skills. However, some researchers (e.g., Moller 2000) have concluded that the atypicals as a group have *direct* effects on primary negative symptoms that are superior to those of older neuroleptics. With respect to the overall efficacy of atypicals, Davis and colleagues (2003) caution against lumping all the atypicals together. In their meta-analysis of 10 "second-generation" APs, they found varying degrees of superiority to conventional agents. Clozapine showed the most robust "effect size" (a measure of efficacy used in meta-analyses), with risperidone and olanzapine showing more modest advantages over first-generation neuroleptics. Notably, risperidone and olanzapine were "slightly superior" to older agents for *positive* symptoms but "moderately superior" for *negative,* cognitive, and behavioral symptoms (such as impulsivity). In contrast, quetiapine, ziprasidone, and aripiprazole were found to have "about the same efficacy" as older agents. Another meta-analysis by Leucht et al. (2003) found that of the atypical agents, only clozapine was associated with greater efficacy (and significantly fewer EPS) than conventional agents. Finally, preliminary, unpublished data from the Schizophrenia Outpatient Health Outcomes (SOHO) study are of great interest (Sylvester 2004). In a naturalistic study involving more than 17,000 patients in 37 countries, the SOHO researchers found that olanzapine produced greater improvement in positive and negative symptoms than did risperidone or "other" APs (including older neuroleptics). No significant difference in efficacy was found between olanzapine and clozapine. Other studies, as one might expect, have reached different conclusions. For example, one small study (N=42) found risperidone superior to olanzapine (Ho et al. 1999). In short, although the jury is still out, some atypical agents do appear to have advantages over conventional neuroleptics beyond merely reducing EPS. The magnitude and clinical importance of these advantages remain a matter of debate.

Q. How does the mechanism of action of aripiprazole differ from that of other atypicals? What are the clinical implications of these differences?

A. Aripiprazole appears to have a unique mechanism of action among the atypicals, in that it acts as either a D_2 *antagonist* or a D_2 *agonist,* depending on the ambient DA concentration. Thus, it is classified as a *partial agonist* at

D_2 receptors. In addition, aripiprazole has 5-HT_{2A} antagonist activity and partial agonist activity at 5-HT_{1A} receptors (Burris et al. 2002; J.A. Lieberman 2004). Its effect at the 5-HT_{1A} receptor may be associated with improvement in negative, cognitive, depressive, and anxious features (Burris et al. 2002; J.A. Lieberman 2004; Millan 2000). Aripiprazole's efficacy and relatively low side-effect profile in premarketing studies have prompted some to speak of the "Goldilocks" hypothesis of AP action: not too much, not too little, but just the "right" amount of DA receptor blockade (in the "right" brain regions) is required for optimum effects. At least one meta-analysis (Davis et al. 2003) and some recent experience with aripiprazole have raised questions as to how well its putative pharmacodynamic "advantages" translate into clinical efficacy and reduced side effects (D. Osser, M.D., personal communication, February 7, 2004; see subsection "Main Side Effects" later in this "Questions and Answers" section). However, Davis et al.'s (2003) meta-analysis included only three studies of aripiprazole. One recent 4-week, randomized, placebo-controlled, double-blind study (Potkin et al. 2003) compared aripiprazole (20 and 30 mg/day) with risperidone (6 mg/day) in patients with schizophrenia/schizoaffective disorder. Both agents were significantly superior to placebo on all efficacy measures, including improvement on the PANSS (Positive and Negative Syndrome Scale) negative symptom score. Other data (Kujawa et al. 2002) suggest that aripiprazole (30 mg/day) produces greater improvement in negative and depressive symptoms than does haloperidol (10 mg/day).

In theory, using aripiprazole concomitantly with a potent D_2 antagonist (e.g., haloperidol) could cause DA receptor agonism at the D_2 receptor in some patients—*if* the patient's D_2 receptors have become "up-regulated" in the presence of chronic D_2 blockade. This mechanism has been suggested to explain the apparent paradoxical worsening of psychosis with aripiprazole in a few patients (DeQuardo 2004). However, more clinical experience with such combinations is needed to validate this hypothesis. Some anecdotally reported side effects with aripiprazole at standard dosages (15–30 mg/day) (Rosenblatt and Rosenblatt 2003) seem at odds with its putative in vitro receptor profile and premarketing data (see subsection "Main Side Effects" later in this "Questions and Answers" section). Some have suggested that lower initial total daily doses of aripiprazole (e.g., 5 mg) than currently recommended may be appropriate (DeQuardo 2004).

Pharmacokinetics

Q. Since many APs have elimination half-lives of approximately 24 hours, is *once-daily* oral dosing optimal? What about APs with shorter or longer half-lives?

A. For APs with elimination half-lives of about 24 hours, once-daily dosing (e.g., all at bedtime) should provide sustained therapeutic blood levels (e.g., 4–15 ng/mL of haloperidol) for most patients once steady state has been reached. However, it is not clear that there is a close correlation between AP blood levels *on a given day* and AP therapeutic effects. Indeed, blood levels of typical (and perhaps atypical) APs may not reflect their enduring action at D_2 brain receptor sites (Campbell and Baldessarini 1985; J.A. Lieberman 2004) or their effects at the level of the gene. This probably means that *transiently* low plasma levels (e.g., over the course of 1–2 days) do not necessarily lead to worsening of psychotic symptoms for the average patient. Thus, pharmacodynamically, it is difficult to rationalize multiple dosing (bid or tid) of an AP on the basis of the drug's $t_{1/2}\beta$. However, the *acute* side effects of APs in some patients may be correlated with once-daily dosing and/or transient increases in peak plasma levels. Thus, an elderly patient with a tendency to postural hypotension might develop dizziness (due to peripheral α_1 blockade) if given, say, 400 mg of quetiapine or 4 mg of risperidone as *a single dose.* Similarly, a young male patient might develop an acute dystonic reaction if, on the first day of treatment, he were given haloperidol 10 mg in a single dose vs. 5 mg bid. (In this case, prophylactic anticholinergic medication, or a less potent agent, would probably be indicated.) These acute effects probably relate to the higher peak plasma levels obtained when dosing is less frequent, even though, at steady state, the *average* plasma concentration over a 24-hour period is the same, whether the medication is given once, twice, or three times daily (Friedman and Greenblatt 1986). In short, most APs with half-lives of around 24 hours may be given once daily, but individual differences in side effects may sometimes favor multiple dosing. This rule of thumb may also apply to newer atypical APs with very short elimination half-lives; for example, although quetiapine has a $t_{1/2}$ of about 6 hours, recent clinical experience suggests it may be given on a once-daily basis to some patients (Chengappa et al. 2003) The new atypical AP aripiprazole, with its $t_{1/2}$ of more than 75 hours, raises an interesting question: could it be effective even if given, say, every other day? Thus far, this has not been investigated clinically, but theory suggests it might be a viable strategy in some patients.

Q. What is the relationship between clozapine plasma levels and therapeutic response? Is there any way to calculate the likely plasma level from the dose given?

A. There is great variability in the ratio of plasma level to dose of orally administered clozapine; indeed, clozapine levels may vary more than 45-fold with the same oral dose. Factors underlying such variability may include dosing schedule, timing of blood drawing, and individual differences in absorption and metabolism of clozapine (Lindenmayer and Apergi 1996). There is reasonably good evidence for a "threshold" effect, such that clozapine plasma levels >350 ng/mL lead to better therapeutic response than do lower levels; however, higher levels (such as >600 ng/mL) are not clearly associated with greater likelihood of improvement than more moderate levels (Marder and Wirshing 2004). Moreover, higher levels may be associated with more side effects, such as sleepiness, and perhaps a greater risk of seizures (McEvoy et al. 1996; VanderZwaag et al. 1996). One rule of thumb is that clozapine plasma levels average about 45 ng/mL for every mg/kg of drug given (Marder and Wirshing 2004). So, if a 70-kg patient is given 5 mg/kg per day (i.e., 350 mg/day), the plasma clozapine level should be roughly 45 × 5 = 225 ng/mL. In fact, however, patients vary considerably in the AP blood levels they achieve, so that the actual range would be more like 200–400 ng/mL in the example given. In effect, the rule of thumb can be restated as follows: expect a little less than 1 ng/mL for every milligram of clozapine given in most patients.

Main Side Effects

Q. Should anticholinergic agents be given prophylactically with certain APs in order to prevent EPS?

A. The answer depends on the type of AP, the characteristics of the patient, the risks of using such anticholinergic agents, and the time course of treatment. In general, the prophylactic use of anticholinergic agents for patients taking *low-potency* APs (thioridazine, chlorpromazine) or *most* atypical APs is of dubious value. Most such patients will not develop acute EPS, and the addition of benztropine or similar agents will add to the total "anticholinergic burden" carried by the patient, sometimes leading to severe side effects (e.g., dry mouth, dental caries, blurry vision, constipation/bowel obstruction, and confusional states). This is especially true in elderly patients, who are often given several anticholinergic agents along with a low-potency AP. However, a young male patient starting to take haloperidol—or high doses of risperidone—may well benefit from a prophylactic anticholinergic agent; indeed, an acute dystonic reaction in such a case may lead to refusal of further medication, for fear of "being poisoned." (Some clinicians, however, prefer to have such patients begin by taking a relatively low dose of haloperidol—say, 2–4 mg/day—and monitor closely for the earliest signs of EPS, often avoiding use of anticholinergic agents; see, e.g., Osser and Patterson 1996). While the data from various studies are fraught with methodological difficulties, roughly 40% (10%–70%) of patients whose anticholinergic agents are discontinued will subsequently exhibit EPS, suggesting that these agents do have prophylactic effects (Janicak et al. 1993). Nevertheless, since most acute dystonias occur within the first few days or weeks of treatment, many patients who have been chronically maintained on APs may be weaned from their anticholinergic agents after a few months (Janicak et al. 1993). A certain percentage of these patients may redevelop dystonic symptoms; show "low grade" but uncomfortable parkinsonian symptoms, such as mild cogwheeling or rigidity; or develop akathisia. These patients should have their anticholinergic agents resumed or be considered for a trial of an atypical or low-potency AP. (Akathisia may best be treated with a beta-blocker, such as propranolol—see below). Risk factors for the development of acute EPS (e.g., male gender, age under 35, history of previous dystonic reaction) also enter into the issue of maintenance on anticholinergic agents (Stanilla and Simpson 2004).

The atypical APs have greatly reduced, but not eliminated, the need for anticholinergic medication. Clozapine, olanzapine, and quetiapine are rarely associated with EPS (see Table 3–10); hence, concomitant "prophylactic" anticholinergic agents are rarely appropriate with these agents. Acute or delayed EPS are not uncommon with risperidone at dosages >4 mg/day and may occasionally be seen with ziprasidone (Daniel et al. 2004) and aripiprazole (Rosenblatt and Rosenblatt 2003), notwithstanding premarketing data showing low rates of EPS with these newer agents. Akathisia associated with aripiprazole may be ameliorated with dosage reduction; in the author's experience, some cases appear to be associated with concomitant use of serotonergic antidepressants (R. Pies, T. Cohen, D. Rulf, unpublished data).

Q. Do anticholinergic agents interfere with the therapeutic effects of APs?

A. Some studies have found that anticholinergic agents may reduce plasma AP levels, whereas others have not confirmed this effect (Leipzig and Mendelowitz 1992). Other data indicate that for some patients, anticholinergic agents may exacerbate some positive symptoms of schizophrenia (e.g., hallucinations) or produce other behavioral toxicity (Janicak et al. 1993). In contrast, anticholinergic agents have been reported to improve some "negative" features of schizophrenia. It is often difficult to distinguish such negative or "deficit" symptoms from parkinsonian side effects and/or depression. The best strategy is to *prevent* the occurrence of EPS and negative features in the first place, by using low doses of classical APs whenever feasible or by using atypical APs.

Q. Is akathisia an EPS in the sense that acute dystonic reactions and parkinsonian symptoms are considered EPS? What is the best treatment for akathisia?

A. Akathisia is usually defined as motor restlessness accompanied by an urge to move, not explained solely by anxiety, psychosis, or mood disorder (Ovsiew 1992). Typically, the patient demonstrates a "marching in place" phenomenon or, if seated, shuffles or taps his or her feet. Neuroleptic-induced akathisia, which may occur in about 20% of neuroleptic-treated patients, has been linked with higher levels of anxiety, depression, violence, and suicide in schizophrenia patients (Csernansky and Newcomer 1995). One study found that the presence of akathisia appears to predict poor response to fluphenazine (Levinson et al. 1990). However, another study found no correlation between akathisia and higher levels of psychotic symptoms during acute haloperidol treatment of inpatients with schizophrenia (Van Putten et al. 1990a). It is possible that common central neurotransmitter mechanisms underlie both akathisia and poor treatment response to APs (Levinson et al. 1990). A failure to distinguish akathisia from worsening psychosis often leads to inappropriate increases in AP medication and worsening akathisia.

Marsden and Jenner (1980) have suggested that akathisia, unlike "ordinary" EPS, may be due to *mesocortical* rather than *nigrostriatal* DA receptor blockade. Several PET studies taken together suggest that akathisia occurs at around 60%–65% D_2 receptor blockade, AP action at 65%–75% D_2 blockade, and extrapyramidal parkinsonian signs at about 90% D_2 blockade (Farde et al. 1988; Seeman 1995). This would suggest merely a quantitative difference in the pathophysiology of "ordinary EPS" (e.g., tremor) and akathisia. (It also implies that akathisia may appear at lower AP doses than are needed to produce classical parkinsonian side effects.) However, the pathophysiology of akathisia is not well understood. The apparent effectiveness of beta-blockers in treating akathisia (Shader 2003a) suggests that *noradrenergic* mechanisms are involved. However, some studies have not shown beta-blockers to be superior to anticholinergics (e.g., Sachdev and Loneragan 1993), and the agent of choice for akathisia remains somewhat controversial. If a beta-blocker is elected, propranolol 20–80 mg/day in divided doses may be more effective than less lipophilic agents such as nadolol or atenolol, but well-designed, double-blind studies are lacking. Anticholinergic agents or BZDs (e.g., lorazepam 0.5–20 mg/day) may be effective in some patients (Shader 2003a). The problem of akathisia is best avoided by using atypical APs with low rates of EPS (e.g., quetiapine or olanzapine).

Q. What are the common sexual side effects seen with APs, and which agents are most likely to cause these?

A. Drug-induced sexual dysfunction—commonly associated with ADs but also seen with APs—can include decreased libido; impaired erectile capacity; delayed, painful, retrograde, or "anhedonic" ejaculation (without orgasm); partial or complete anorgasmia; priapism (painful, prolonged erection); and various neuroendocrine side effects that affect sexuality indirectly (Hallward and Ellison 2001; Segraves 1992). For example, all "classical" APs (neuroleptics) substantially elevate prolactin levels, which may lead to amenorrhea, galactorrhea, or gynecomastia and impotence in males. Among the older neuroleptics, thioridazine (Mellaril) is probably the most common offending agent, usually causing impaired or retrograde ejaculation in one-third or more of male patients. Decreased libido has also been reported with thioridazine and fluphenazine. Medications causing α-adrenergic blockade are most often implicated in priapism, which must be considered a urological emergency; failure to treat this problem promptly may result in permanent penile damage (Thompson et al. 1990). Among the phenothiazines, chlorpromazine and thioridazine seem to account for most of the reported cases, while haloperidol, molindone, and other high-potency agents (with relatively less α-adrenergic blockade) are less frequently implicated.

Atypical APs are not free of sexual side effects, though such side effects appear to be relatively uncommon with olanzapine, quetiapine, ziprasidone, and aripiprazole (Daniel et al. 2004; J.A. Lieberman 2004; Physicians' Desk Reference 2004). A recent randomized, open study using a semistructured interview found that 16% of quetiapine-treated patients experienced sexual dysfunction, compared with 50% of risperidone-treated patients (Knegtering et al. 2004). Sexual side effects occur in a dose-related fashion with risperidone (Goff 2004), and priapism has been reported with both risperidone and clozapine (Emes and Millson 1994). Historically, sexual side effects from psychotropics have been underreported, with estimates based on inadequate premarketing assessment tools (Hallward and Ellison 2001); thus, it would not be surprising if the newer atypicals cause more sexual dysfunction than is reported in pharmaceutical company labeling information. It is important to establish baseline (premorbid and pretreatment) sexual function whenever possible and to inquire tactfully about treatment-related sexual dysfunction in patients taking APs. Few patients—particularly psychotic patients—are prone to report such problems spontaneously.

Q. What are the most common side effects with clozapine, and how are they best managed? What about clozapine-induced enuresis and hypersalivation?

A. Clozapine, while very effective in carefully selected patients, is not a "user-friendly" medication. It produces a rather high incidence of (usually) manageable side effects, including sedation (40% incidence), hypersalivation (31%), tachycardia (>25%), dizziness (20%), constipation (14%), hypotension (9%), and hypertension (9%). Seizures occur in a dose-related fashion with clozapine, with a rate of about 3% at 300 mg/day and 6% at 600 mg/day (Meltzer 1995). Less common side effects include transient benign temperature elevations, nausea, weight gain, enuresis, and leukocytosis. Neuroleptic malignant syndrome (NMS) has been reported but appears to be less common than with conventional neuroleptics. The elderly and individuals with underlying brain damage may be more sensitive to clozapine and experience side effects (and perhaps also clinical efficacy) at significantly lower doses. Hypersalivation is occasionally responsive to anticholinergic medication (e.g., atropine, benztropine, transdermal scopolamine, glycopyrrolate), clonidine, α_1-adrenergic blockers (e.g., terazosin), and beta-blockers (Mathews et al. 2003), though controlled evidence supporting these remedies is sorely lacking. There is a possibility, however, that apparent "hypersalivation" is actually a result of clozapine-impaired swallowing (esophageal dysfunction) rather than true, cholinergically mediated hypersalivation. If so, anticholinergic agents would not be expected to help. Indeed, centrally acting anticholinergic agents could impair the gag reflex, thus exacerbating impaired swallowing (Freudenreich et al. 2004). One recent uncontrolled case series reported that sublingual ipratropium spray was helpful in a small number of patients (*N*=9) taking clozapine. This muscarinic anticholinergic agent has no central nervous system (CNS) penetration; however, its benefits last only a few hours, and contact with the eyes can trigger a glaucoma attack (Freudenreich et al. 2004). Reduction of clozapine dosage, when feasible, and behavioral modification (e.g., instruction in swallowing, chewing a sugarless gum) may also reduce complaints of hypersalivation (Mathews et al. 2003; McCarthy and Terkelsen 1994; Pearlman 1994). Enuresis may be managed by reducing the dosage, if possible; dividing the daily dose and giving the nighttime dose early in the evening, so that maximum sedation is over before maximum likelihood of enuresis (C.A. Pearlman, M.D., personal communication, February 1997); and using oxybutynin (Ditropan) or nasal vasopressin (F. Frankenburg, M.D., personal communication, February 1997).

Q. What is the risk of agranulocytosis with clozapine, and are there factors that help predict whether it will occur?

A. It is difficult to find a single, definitive figure for agranulocytosis, owing to differences in pre- and postmarketing surveillance. Thus, according to early Sandoz Pharmaceuticals information (Sandoz Pharmaceuticals, personal communication, December 1995; Physicians' Desk Reference 1995), clozapine had an associated incidence of agranulocytosis of approximately 0.65%, reflecting the average of rates for women (0.9%) and men (0.4%). However, product labeling information from the current manufacturer, Novartis, continues to cite a cumulative 1-year incidence of around 1.3%, based on premarketing studies (Physicians' Desk Reference 2004). Data from the Clozaril National Registry suggest an incidence of between 0.3% and 0.4%, when agranulocytosis was defined as an absolute neutrophil count $< 500/\text{mm}^3$, probably reflecting earlier deficiencies in monitoring (Marder and Wirshing 2004). Because the risk of agranulocytosis is greatest during the first 4–6 months, monitoring frequency drops from weekly to every 2 weeks after 6 months of treatment. Agranulocytosis may occur more frequently in older patients, females, and, possibly, individuals of Eastern European Jewish extraction, but these claims are not based on firm or consistent data; thus, unfortunately, there are no well-validated clinical predictors as to which patients are most likely to develop agranulocytosis (Marder and Wirshing 2004; Meltzer 1995). A pattern of *steadily decreasing neutrophil count,* however, may herald agranulocytosis and calls for extra monitoring (Meltzer 1995). With very few exceptions, a patient who has developed clozapine-induced agranulocytosis should not be rechallenged with this agent, as recurrence is almost inevitable (Marder and Wirshing 2004).

Q. What is the risk of "withdrawal syndromes" associated with stopping AP medication?

A. All APs can produce withdrawal symptoms (e.g., insomnia, headache, nausea, vomiting, withdrawal-emergent dyskinesia) if they are suddenly or rapidly discontinued. Specific symptoms are related to the potency of the agent, its dopaminergic blockade, and its anticholinergic effects (Hegarty 1996). Low-potency APs, such as chlorpromazine, are strongly anticholinergic, and sudden withdrawal of these agents can provoke diarrhea, drooling, and insomnia ("cholinergic rebound"). Recent case reports specifically point to clozapine withdrawal as leading to rapid psychotic decompensations, evolving over a few days. These decompensations appear to be much more rapid than syndromes seen after stopping conventional APs, perhaps as a result of the rapid clearance of clozapine from plasma and/or CNS (Hegarty 1996). Alternatively, decompensation may be due to overactivity of (previously antagonized) limbic D_4 receptors when clozapine is discontinued and replaced by an AP that is less selective for D_4 receptor antagonism (i.e., most classical neuroleptics). Serotonergic effects may also be involved in clozapine-related withdrawal. There is a nearly twofold difference in relapse risk between abrupt and gradual withdrawal of APs (Viguera et al. 1997).

Q. In general, how do the side-effect profiles of the atypical APs compare?

A. We can consider this question from the standpoint of six main categories (see Table 3–10). Clozapine, olanzapine, and quetiapine are generally more *sedating* than other atypicals. Risperidone, and, to a lesser degree, ziprasidone and aripiprazole, are associated with higher rates of *EPS.* However, there are anecdotal reports of *akathisia* associated with standard doses of aripiprazole (Rosenblatt and Rosenblatt 2003). Clozapine generally has the highest risk of *anticholinergic* side effects, though high doses of olanzapine may provoke these in some patients. *Orthostasis,* though seen with all the atypical APs, may be most likely with clozapine and somewhat likely with quetiapine and risperidone. Significant *elevation in prolactin levels* appears to be largely restricted to risperidone; however, one study found no clear relationship between prolactin elevation and *menstrual dysfunction* in schizophrenic females treated with typical neuroleptics, risperidone, olanzapine, and clozapine (Canuso et al. 2002). Most data suggest that *weight gain* is most commonly seen with clozapine and olanzapine, and less so with other atypical agents, especially ziprasidone; however, one large, observational study (McIntyre et al. 2003) found that quetiapine was associated with more weight gain than either olanzapine or risperidone, and that risperidone and olanzapine had similar weight gain liability. All these rough generalizations are subject to factors such as dose effects, age of patient, concomitant medications, and medical illness.

Q. What are the comparative risks of glucose and lipid abnormalities among the atypical APs? How do they compare with the risks associated with older agents, and what are the standards for clinical and laboratory monitoring?

A. The effects of atypical APs on glucose and lipid metabolism remain a controversial area. This is partly because there are few, if any, randomized, controlled, prospective, "head-to-head" trials of atypicals aimed at answering these questions. Most data are retrospective epidemiological findings or are poorly controlled with respect to exercise, dietary restrictions, and so forth. Furthermore, there appears to be a positive association between both obesity and diabetes, on the one hand, and severe mental illness, including bipolar disorder and schizophrenia, on the other, compared with rates in the general population (see Keck et al. 2003a for review). With these caveats in mind, a few generalizations may be made:

Many patients taking atypical APs will develop the *metabolic syndrome.* Although proposed criteria differ (Rogers 2003), the syndrome is usually characterized by obesity, insulin resistance, hypertension, high triglyceride levels, and low "good cholesterol" (high-density lipoprotein, or HDL).

Olanzapine and clozapine are associated with the most case reports of de novo diabetes (mainly type 2) or exacerbation of existing diabetes, with African Americans at relatively higher risk.

Increases in serum lipid—especially triglyceride—levels are disproportionately associated with clozapine and olanzapine; the effects of risperidone, ziprasidone, and aripiprazole are less pronounced, and quetiapine has only modest effects on lipid levels. One small (N= 10) controlled, prospective study of olanzapine demonstrated significant increases in fasting glucose and fasting serum insulin over a period of 8 weeks, pointing toward the development of peripheral insulin resistance (Ebenbichler et al. 2003). Typical neuroleptics, such as haloperidol and fluphenazine, certainly may cause glucose dysregulation, but they probably cause less pronounced lipid dysregulation than do clozapine and olanzapine.

All these generalizations (Keck et al. 2003a) must be considered provisional. In the meantime, for patients taking atypical APs, the author recommends baseline and periodic checks (e.g., after 2 months and 8 months of AP treatment) of weight/body mass index (BMI), glucose, and lipid functions. More frequent monitoring may be necessary in patients at high risk or in those who develop signs of the metabolic syndrome early in treatment. Recently, the American Diabetes Association and other organizations issued a consensus statement (American Diabetes Association et al. 2004) calling for *baseline assessment* of personal and family history of obesity, diabetes, dyslipidemia, and hypertension or cardiovascular disease; weight and height (for BMI calculation); waist circumference; blood pressure; fasting glucose level; and fasting lipid profile. Weight should be rechecked at 4, 8, and 12 weeks posttreatment, with a recheck of blood pressure, fasting glucose level, and fasting lipid profile at week 12.

Q. What are the signs and symptoms of NMS, and how is it managed?

A. NMS is probably not a single, homogeneous disease entity; rather, it may represent a continuum of dysfunction related to DA receptor blockade and other poorly characterized physiological mechanisms. NMS is typically characterized by the development of fever, muscular rigidity, autonomic instability, altered level of consciousness, elevated creatine kinase (CK, or CPK [creatine phosphokinase]), and elevated white blood cell (WBC) count, in the absence of another medical explanation (Buckley and Meltzer 1995). One or more of these features may be absent, however, in the presence of serious NMS-like syndromes. While some data indicate that mental alterations may be the earliest indicator of NMS (Velamoor et al. 1995), this feature may be too nonspecific to permit reliable diagnosis (C. Pearlman, M.D., personal communication, February 1997). Although typically associated with the use of neuroleptics or other DA receptor blockers, NMS may also occur after sudden discontinuation of dopaminergic agents, such as bromocriptine. NMS has now been reported in association with both risperidone (Webster and Wijeratne 1994) and clozapine (Sachdev et al. 1995). Clozapine-induced NMS may be somewhat atypical, in that fewer EPS and lower levels of CK may be seen. Clozapine-induced NMS must be distinguished from benign, transient clozapine-related fever, often seen in the second week of treatment. Whenever NMS is suspected, the putative offending agent should be held until a workup is completed. The workup should include ruling out *infection superimposed on drug-induced EPS* as the cause of apparent NMS. Supportive measures designed to reduce hyperthermia and stabilize vital signs—especially aggressive intravenous hydration—are critical and usually require transfer of the patient to a medical unit or ICU. Although the evidence supporting specific therapeutic agents is only modest, some clinicians will use bromocriptine (30 mg/day) or dantrolene (300 mg/day) (Buckley and Meltzer 1995). Anticholinergic agents may worsen hyperthermia (because of impaired sweating). BZDs produce inconsistent effects (Pearlman 1986) but may reduce muscular rigidity. Refractory cases of NMS may respond to electroconvulsive therapy (ECT) (Fink 1996). Although one recent review recommends that "bromocriptine...should be started as soon as possible..." (Shader 2003b), evidence-based studies of NMS management strategies have not been performed, owing to its infrequent occurrence.

Q. What are the risks of "rechallenging" a patient with a neuroleptic after an episode of NMS? Is rechallenging with an atypical AP appropriate?

A. Around 30% of patients will have a recurrence of NMS after neuroleptic rechallenge. The risk may be reduced by waiting at least 2 weeks post-NMS before the rechallenge and by using a low-potency neuroleptic (e.g., thioridazine) (Rosebush and Stuart 1989). There are insufficient data to establish the safety of rechallenge with an atypical AP agent, regardless of whether the patient developed NMS while taking a neuroleptic or a different atypical AP; indeed, NMS has been reported with sequential use of atypical agents in the same patient (Bottender et al. 2002). Some preliminary data suggest that mortality rates may be lower when NMS occurs with atypical agents, but this may simply reflect earlier detection and treatment (Ananth et al. 2004). ECT may be a viable alternative to rechallenge.

Q. How cardiotoxic are the APs, and are there differences among the various agents?

A. The APs as a group are not highly cardiotoxic agents, especially in comparison to the tricyclic antidepressants (TCAs) (Gelenberg 1996). In one study, an abnormally long QTc was found in 23% of 143 patients treated with APs, vs. 2% in unmedicated control subjects. Neuroleptic doses greater than 2,000 mg chlorpromazine equivalents per day were more than four times as likely as lower doses to prolong QTc (Gelenberg 1996; Warner et al. 1996). Thioridazine's effects on the heart resemble those of the TCAs, probably due to both anticholinergic and quinidine-like effects. A study of AP overdoses showed that thioridazine is three to five times more likely than other APs to prolong cardiac conduction (Buckley et al. 1995). In general, high-potency neuroleptics, such as haloperidol and thiothixene, are safer than low-potency alternatives for patients with cardiac illness.

With respect to newer, atypical APs, the principal cardiac concern (aside from orthostatic hypotension) is the tendency of these agents to *prolong QT*—essentially the time required for depolarization and then repolarization of cardiac tissue. The QTc is usually computed as follows (Goldberger 1998):

$$QT_c = \frac{QT}{\sqrt{R-R}}$$

When the QT interval increases beyond about 450–475 milliseconds (msec), the risk of cardiac arrhythmia, such as torsade de pointes and ventricular fibrillation, increases considerably. In comparative terms, a recent randomized investigation (Harrigan et al. 2004) examined QTc prolongation in patients receiving haloperidol (15 mg/day), thioridazine (300 mg/day), ziprasidone (160 mg/day), quetiapine (750 mg/day), olanzapine (20 mg/day), or risperidone (6–16 mg/day). Mean QTc intervals did not exceed 500 msec in any patient taking any of the APs studied, either in the absence or in the presence of metabolic inhibitors. However, the agents showed a range of effects on mean QTc prolongation, as follows: thioridazine, 30.1 msec; ziprasidone, 15.9 msec; haloperidol, 7.1 msec; quetiapine, 5.7 msec; risperidone, 3.8 msec; and olanzapine, 1.7 msec (all values reflect absence of inhibitors). Thus, olanzapine had the least effect on QTc in this study. However, the upper dosage range of risperidone used in the study (8 mg bid) was much higher than the dosage generally used in clinical practice (about 4–5 mg/day). Finally, the use of *any* AP along with another agent that prolongs cardiac conduction time (e.g., quinidine, TCAs) must be monitored carefully.

Q. Is there a substantial risk of cataracts with quetiapine, and what precautions should be taken to avoid them?

A. Lenticular changes, including cataracts, were observed in animal studies of very high-dose quetiapine, but a causal relationship in humans has not been convincingly established. Postmarketing surveillance (1997–2002) suggests that lens abnormalities in patients exposed to quetiapine are very rare (i.e., fewer than 1 in 10,000 patients) (J.A. Lieberman 2004). Nevertheless, the manufacturer continues to recommend examination of the lens (e.g., via slit lamp) at initiation of treatment or shortly thereafter and every 6 months during chronic treatment.

Drug–Drug Interactions

Q. Is it safe to combine APs with TCAs and/or SSRIs?

A. AP/AD combinations are often safe and effective for the treatment of psychotic depression and some cases of schizophrenia (see subsection "Potentiating Maneuvers" in the "Overview" section of this chapter); however, pharmacokinetic and pharmacodynamic interactions may pose problems for some patients. In general, TCAs and APs tend to compete for metabolism in one or more cytochrome systems and may mutually raise each other's plasma levels. This can lead to, for example, increased anticholinergic effects (in the case, say, of combining amitriptyline and thioridazine), hypotensive effects, or EPS. Fluoxetine and paroxetine are powerful inhibitors of the CYP 2D6 system and may elevate plasma levels of many AP agents, including risperidone and, to a lesser extent, clozapine. Clozapine and olanzapine levels can also be elevated substantially by concomitant use of fluvoxamine, probably via the latter's inhibition of CYP 1A2 (Cozza et al. 2003; Hiemke et al. 1994). AP/AD combinations may have several pharmacodynamic interactions; for example, SSRIs may decrease dopaminergic activity in some brain regions, leading to exacerbation of EPS induced by an AP alone (Leo 1996). (This effect of SSRIs may also be responsible for the "flattening" of affective or hedonic capacity in some patients.) However, some serotonergic agents may enhance overall function in chronically psychotic patients, possibly by relieving comorbid depressive or obsessive features.

Q. Given the potential pharmacokinetic interactions between carbamazepine (CBZ) and some APs, what is the best way to manage coprescription of these agents?

A. CBZ may substantially reduce plasma haloperidol levels (and probably those of other APs), presumably via stimulation of hepatic metabolism; however, the clinical outcome of this interaction shows considerable variability (Ciraulo et al. 1989, 1994). In one study (Arana et al. 1986), seven patients who had not responded to either haloperidol alone or haloperidol plus lithium were treated with haloperidol plus CBZ. Prior to the addition of CBZ, haloperidol plasma levels were around 8.3 ng/mL; after the addition of CBZ, haloperidol levels dropped to around 3.4 ng/mL, with clinical deterioration seen in at least two of the patients. On the other hand, patients with initial haloperidol levels of 12–14 ng/mL might be expected to tolerate a drop to, say, 7 ng/mL. In any case, raising the haloperidol dose should overcome this pharmacokinetic problem, but plasma levels should be followed closely. (Remember that CBZ also induces its own metabolism over time, leading to lower CBZ levels at a fixed dose.) Pharmacodynamic interactions (e.g., lethargy and confusion) may also be seen when CBZ is combined with neuroleptics (Ciraulo et al. 1989). The use of the keto-congener of CBZ, oxcarbazepine (Trileptal), may reduce some of these drug–drug interactions, though this question has not been investigated systematically.

Q. What concerns should the clinician have in combining risperidone, quetiapine, ziprasidone, and aripiprazole with other psychotropics and nonpsychotropics?

A. Both pharmacokinetic and pharmacodynamic concerns should arise. First, most of these APs (risperidone, quetiapine, ziprasidone, aripiprazole) are metabolized to varying degrees via CYP 2D6 and/or 3A4. (As noted in Table 3–8, olanzapine is metabolized partly via CYP 1A2.) Ziprasidone is somewhat exceptional, in that most of its metabolism is via the non-CYP enzyme aldehyde oxidase. Any powerful inhibitor of CYP 2D6 (fluoxetine, paroxetine, bupropion, quinidine, and even diphenhydramine) or of 3A4 (nefazodone; fluoxetine's metabolite, norfluoxetine; ciprofloxacin; clarithromycin; ketoconazole; ritonavir; and even grapefruit juice) is of potential concern when combined with these APs (Cozza et al. 2003). *Inducers* of CYP 2D6 and/or 3A4, of course, run the risk of reducing plasma levels of these APs. In theory, inhibitors of aldehyde oxidase (cimetidine, hydralazine, methadone) could raise ziprasidone blood levels and thus prolong QTc, but this has not yet been demonstrated clinically (Cozza et al. 2003). However, pharmacodynamic interactions should be kept in mind whenever atypicals are combined with other agents that can prolong QTc or increase the risk of orthostatic hypotension.

Potentiating Maneuvers

Q. Is it useful to add a conventional neuroleptic with strong D_2 receptor blockade to clozapine in patients who do not respond to clozapine alone?

A. In theory, the addition of a "classic" D_2 receptor blocker might interfere with the relatively benign EPS profile of clozapine (which has a high ratio of 5-HT_2 to D_2 receptor blockade). However, given clozapine's limited D_2 receptor antagonism, there is some rationale for combining it with an agent producing greater D_2 blockade (e.g., haloperidol). There appear to be no published studies of clozapine and haloperidol combination treatment. On the other hand, the principle of "D_2 antagonist + clozapine" was supported in a double-blind, placebo-controlled study of sulpiride, a selective D_2 blocker, which was added to ongoing clozapine treatment (Shiloh et al. 1997). Some clinical experience suggests that the addition of a conventional neuroleptic (such as haloperidol) to ongoing clozapine therapy may enhance efficacy, particularly in patients who cannot tolerate high doses of clozapine (Goff and Baldessarini 1995). Thus, a patient maintained on, say, 250 mg/day of clozapine might benefit from the addition of 1–2 mg of haloperidol or thiothixene without developing significant EPS. Theoretically, concomitant use of two APs could increase the risk of agranulocytosis, but the increment above that associated with clozapine alone is probably small.

Q. What about combining clozapine or risperidone with other atypical APs in patients with disorders refractory to one or the other agent alone?

A. Anecdotal observations and case series reports suggest that combining two atypical APs may augment partial response to the original agent; however, controlled studies are lacking, and neither the safety nor the cost-effectiveness of this practice has been convincingly demonstrated. Furthermore, the addition of a second AP may be "credited" with clinical improvement via synergism with the first agent, when, in fact, it was the second agent alone that effected the improvement. This misattribution may lead to unnecessary, expensive, long-term polypharmacy for some patients (Stahl 1999). Nevertheless, the combination of atypical APs may be warranted in some carefully selected and monitored patients (Oepen 2002; Pies 2001). Henderson and Goff (1996) studied the addition of risperidone 2–6 mg/day to clozapine in 12 patients with treatment-resistant schizophrenia ($n=10$) and schizoaffective disorder ($n=2$). This regimen led to a reduction of over 20% in total 18-item BPRS scores in 10 of the subjects, 4 weeks after addition of the risperidone. Seven patients also showed a reduction of at least 20% in negative symptom scores. There was no evidence that risperidone increased clozapine blood levels, though this may occur. Thus, clozapine plasma level in one patient with schizoaffective illness, treated with a combination of clozapine 300 mg bid and risperidone 1 mg bid, increased from 344 ng/mL to 598 ng/mL. However, this increase was not associated with any adverse events; in fact, it led to an improvement in the patient's illness (Tyson et al. 1995). Similarly, Raskin et al. (2000) found that three patients with refractory schizophrenia who had not responded adequately to either clozapine or risperidone alone showed clinical improvement with clozapine–risperidone co-treatment. In two cases, patients were able to be maintained on reduced clozapine doses, and no significant adverse effects were observed. However, Chong et al. (1997) reported a case in which the clozapine–risperidone combination resulted in an atrial ectopic arrhythmia, despite no change in clozapine blood levels. Thus, it is evident that *cardiac monitoring, including monitoring for orthostatic hypotension, is advisable when APs are combined.* In addition, there is one report in which the combination of risperidone and clozapine was associated with subsequent agranulocytosis (Godleski and Sernyak 1996), suggesting that monitoring blood count may also be indicated with this combination. Finally—though the theoretical rationale is far from clear—the combination of clozapine and olanzapine apparently led to improvement in two cases reported by Gupta et al. (1998) and in one case reported by Rhoads (2000). In summary, we need much better study of combined AP treatment. In the meantime, the most "rational" polypharmacy may involve combination of a substantial D_2 blocker with either olanzapine or clozapine (Pies 2001).

Q. How useful are anticonvulsants as potentiators of APs in patients with schizophrenia?

A. While anticonvulsants alone rarely benefit schizophrenia patients, they may be of use in persistently psychotic patients who show prominent positive symptoms; aggressive and impulsive behaviors ("episodic dyscontrol"); or electroencephalogram (EEG) abnormalities (Buckley and Meltzer 1995). Okuma et al. (1989) found that CBZ was more effective than placebo (48% vs. 30% response) when added to ongoing neuroleptic treatment of schizophrenic and schizoaffective patients, particularly for symptoms of excitement, suspiciousness, and poor cooperation. However, some patients with psychosis may worsen with the addition of CBZ to neuroleptic, possibly owing to CBZ's reduction of plasma neuroleptic levels (Arana et al. 1986). Valproate appears more promising. In a retrospective study, Hayes (1989) found that 11 of 14 schizoaffective patients improved with valproate; however, some of these patients had also received lithium. Recently, Casey et al. (2003) carried out a double-blind, randomized, placebo-controlled study of divalproex (up to 30 mg/kg per day) combined with olanzapine or risperidone in patients with an acute exacerbation of schizophrenia. With respect to early improvement, divalproex was superior to placebo over a range of psychotic symptoms. There is also interest in lamotrigine as a possible adjunctive treatment in schizophrenia, perhaps related to its effects at NMDA receptors. In one naturalistic study, Dursun and Deakin (2001) found lamotrigine beneficial when added to clozapine in patients with treatment-resistant schizophrenia; somewhat surprisingly, this benefit was *not* seen when lamotrigine was combined with the closely related atypical agent olanzapine or with risperidone and haloperidol. Controlled studies are required before lamotrigine may be recommended confidently in the treatment of refractory schizophrenia.

Q. Are agents that act directly at NMDA receptors useful as adjuncts in schizophrenia?

A. Some evidence suggests that high-dose glycine, when added to either olanzapine or risperidone, may improve outcome in schizophrenia patients (Heresco-Levy et al. 2004). Glycine is an "obligatory co-agonist" at NMDA receptors and might be particularly useful for negative symptoms of schizophrenia.

Q. How useful are BZDs in the treatment of schizophrenia?

A. The effects of the use of BZDs as either sole or adjunctive agents in psychotic patients, as noted by Janicak et al. (1993), range "from deterioration, to no change in most patients, to striking improvement in a rare patient" (pp. 152–153). BZDs may ameliorate superimposed anxiety, auditory hallucinations, and perhaps negative symptoms in a few schizophrenia patients; however, sedation, ataxia, cognitive impairment, and behavioral disinhibition may occur (Janicak et al. 1993). A number of BZDs (i.e., lorazepam, clonazepam, diazepam) have proved useful in "catatonic" patients, including some with catatonic schizophrenia (Martenyi et al. 1989). Generally, these results have been obtained using intramuscular or intravenous BZDs, though some studies point to continued benefit when the patient is maintained on oral BZDs (Martenyi et al. 1989). (Keep in mind that "catatonia" is a symptom, not a diagnosis, and that treatment must be directed at the underlying pathology.) BZDs may also be helpful in the management of acute psychotic states and may reduce the need for higher doses of neuroleptics in agitated psychotic patients (Tueth et al. 1995).

Q. Can psychotic patients with obsessive-compulsive features be treated with adjunctive medication? What about the role of atypical AP in exacerbating OCD symptoms?

A. Obsessive-compulsive symptoms may be seen in as many as 25% of schizophrenia patients, and may respond to adjunctive clomipramine (Berman et al. 1995). It appears that clomipramine at dosages up to 250 mg/day may safely be combined with *high-potency* neuroleptics (e.g., haloperidol, fluphenazine) without exacerbation of psychotic symptoms and with improvement in obsessive-compulsive symptoms. (Combining this agent with low-potency neuroleptics increases the risk of hypotension and anticholinergic effects.) However, citing evidence that clomipramine may exacerbate psychotic symptoms in some patients, Berman et al. (1995) advised caution using this strategy in acutely decompensated or manic psychotic patients. Another anti-obsessional agent—fluoxetine—has been shown to improve global function in some chronic schizophrenia patients (Goldmann and Janecek 1990), but experience in adding SSRIs to newer, atypical APs is quite limited in this population. Koran (1999) noted that atypical APs may induce or exacerbate OCD symptoms in some psychotic patients, and that these symptoms may remit spontaneously within 3 weeks. If they do not remit, some case reports suggest that reducing the AP dose or adding an SSRI may be helpful. Fluvoxamine and other SSRIs can interfere with metabolism of several neuroleptics and atypical agents; moreover, adding an SSRI carries a small risk of exacerbating symptoms of schizophrenia (Koran 1999).

Q. What is the role of psychotherapy as a potentiating strategy in the treatment of schizophrenia? Does the evidence suggest an additive effect when psychotherapy is combined with medication?

A. A review by Csernansky and Newcomer (1995) noted relatively few studies where the interaction of psychosocial treatments and drug treatments has been specifically studied in schizophrenia. Nevertheless, McGlashan (1986) noted earlier that "the individual clinician remains central to any treatment effort [of the schizophrenia patient], if only to coordinate other treatment modalities and provide ongoing evaluation" (p. 108). The fostering of trust and a sense of "safety" in the patient is, in the author's experience, critical in the successful pharmacological treatment of patients with schizophrenia and other psychotic disorders. With respect to "additive effects," Harnett (1988), after reviewing the available data, cited several studies suggesting that AP medication may act synergistically with psychosocial therapies. Thus, Falloon et al. (1985) demonstrated that for schizophrenic patients on optimal AP medication regimens, "family management" not only was superior to individual therapy in reducing psychotic relapse but also was associated with reduced neuroleptic dosage and fewer deficit symptoms of schizophrenia. This approach emphasized the enhancement of problem-solving and communication skills in both the patient and his or her family/caregivers; "family management" is *not* a psychodynamically based, "exploratory" form of psychotherapy. Keeping in mind that studies of psychotherapy for schizophrenia have many methodological shortcomings, Harnett (1988) concluded that there is little evidence supporting the utility of individual psychodynamically oriented therapy in schizophrenia. On the other hand, Liberman et al. (1986) showed that *social skills training* improves social adjustment and decreases relapse rates in schizophrenia. Cognitive-behavioral approaches may also help mitigate refractory schizophrenia symptoms (Sensky et al. 2000), as may other psychosocial interventions (Bustillo et al. 2001; Pies and Dewan 2001).

Use in Special Populations

Q. What are the AP agents and doses of choice in treating patients with seizure disorders?

A. Probably all APs decrease seizure threshold (i.e., make seizures more probable) to some degree, with low-potency agents, loxapine, and clozapine having greater effects than high-potency agents such as haloperidol and molindone (Centorrino et al. 2002; Dubovsky and Buzan 2000). With clozapine, major motor seizures are induced in 1%–2% of patients at dosages <300 mg/day; 2%–4% at dosages >300 mg/day, and 4%–6% at dosages >600 mg/day (Meltzer 1995); these prevalences are in contrast to a prevalence of about 0.1% with conventional neuroleptics and risperidone. A history of epilepsy or "organic brain impairment" is a risk factor for AP-induced seizures (Buckley and Meltzer 1995). Decreasing the clozapine dose and/or adding valproate are usually sufficient to manage seizures in these patients. (It is also important that the patient avoid epileptogenic agents such as caffeine or theophylline in high doses.) With other APs, using the lowest effective dose, and perhaps checking a plasma level, may help reduce the likelihood of seizures. Thus, with haloperidol, one might begin treatment at a dosage of 4 mg/day and aim for a plasma level of about 5 ng/mL—parameters that are probably applicable to most patients being treated with haloperidol. In a study of EEG abnormalities associated with typical and atypical APs, Centorrino et al. (2002) found high risk associated with clozapine and olanzapine (47% and 39% of patients, respectively); moderate risk with risperidone and typical neuroleptics (28% and 15%, respectively); and low risk with quetiapine (0.0%). Somewhat surprisingly, they did not find a relationship between risk of EEG abnormality and AP dose. Despite the high percentages of EEG abnormalities, reported risk of actual seizures is still quite low with atypical agents other than clozapine (e.g., 0.75%–0.88%) (Centorrino et al. 2002).

Q. How dangerous are APs in pregnancy, and what are the APs of choice in this situation?

A. In general, all psychotropic medications should be avoided during at least the first trimester of pregnancy, if clinically feasible. However, the risks of untreated psychosis—for example, command auditory hallucinations to "stab the baby"—must be weighed against the relatively rare teratogenic effects of these medications (Stowe and Nemeroff 1995). A number of studies have shown no increase in malformations after first-trimester exposure to conventional neuroleptics, though a few have found an increase in nonspecific congenital anomalies after exposure to phenothiazines. APs can also cause anticholinergic side effects in the fetus (constipation, urinary retention), and may increase the risk of jaundice in premature infants. A mild, transient syndrome of neonatal hypertonia, tremor, and poor motor maturity can be seen after neuroleptic use in late pregnancy. There is very little evidence of "behavioral toxicity" or impaired IQ in infants born to mothers taking APs during pregnancy (Stowe and Nemeroff 1995). Some data suggest that haloperidol or piperazine-type phenothiazines are less teratogenic than aliphatic phenothiazines, whereas other data do not point to such an advantage. Fetal tachyarrhythmias may be more likely with maternal use of low-potency (hence, more anticholinergic) APs. To prevent fetal sedation and muscle spasms/tremor, some clinicians recommend tapering off the AP a week or two in advance of the expected delivery date. Since APs are variably excreted in breast milk, breastfeeding is best avoided if the mother continues to take an AP (McElhatton

1992). There are few systematic studies of atypical AP safety during pregnancy (Altshuler et al. 1996; Patton et al. 2002); however, Waldman and Safferman (1993) noted at least 15 cases of normal births following maternal exposure to clozapine, and a recent review found no specific risks for the mother and fetus attributable to the use of clozapine during pregnancy (Nguyen and Lalonde 2003). Olanzapine data thus far suggest relative safety in pregnancy, with no evidence of teratogenesis or obstetrical complications (Newport et al. 2004). Studies of newer atypical agents, unfortunately, are lacking. Finally, keep in mind that women with schizophrenia are at increased risk for poor obstetrical outcomes, including preterm delivery, low birth weight, and neonates who are small for their gestational age (Patton et al. 2002).

Q. How do pharmacokinetic and pharmacodynamic factors interact when conventional neuroleptics are used in the elderly?

A. In general, the volume of distribution of APs is increased—and their metabolism slowed—in the elderly. This factor would be expected to result in a longer time to reach steady state; longer time for drug elimination ("washout"); and prolongation of both therapeutic and toxic effects (Dubovsky and Buzan 2000). In a study of haloperidol pharmacokinetics, Kelly et al. (1993) found no statistically significant differences in younger versus older patients; however, the older subjects (mean age=72) showed significantly greater decreases in *cognitive function* following intravenous haloperidol administration. This finding suggests important *pharmacodynamic* mechanisms in aging, perhaps involving increased neuronal sensitivity or decreased dopaminergic transmission in the elderly (Dubovsky and Buzan 2000). On the other hand, a study of serum haloperidol levels in older psychotic patients found that the *ratio of haloperidol level to dose* was higher in elderly patients with Alzheimer's disease than in younger subjects with schizophrenia, suggesting a reduction in haloperidol clearance with age (Lacro et al. 1996). This interpretation would be consistent with studies of perphenazine, thiothixene, and other neuroleptics (Lacro et al. 1996).

Pharmacodynamically, the elderly are also more sensitive to a plethora of AP side effects, including peripheral and central anticholinergic effects (e.g., dry mouth, urinary retention, confusion, delirium); cardiac effects (tachycardia, orthostatic hypotension); autonomic instability; NMS; TD; seizure risk; and metabolic disturbance associated with weight gain (Jacobson et al. 2002;

Roose et al. 2004). All these factors make "start low, go slow" the best policy in geriatric psychopharmacology.

Q. What concerns are paramount when prescribing clozapine in the elderly?

A. Special problems may arise when atypical APs are used in the elderly (Alexopoulos et al. 2004; Jacobson et al. 2002; Naimark et al. 1995; Roose et al. 2004). Weekly and biweekly blood drawings with clozapine may lead to bruising or cellulitis from an infected phlebotomy site. Clozapine's anticholinergic side effects may cause urinary retention, fecal impaction, exacerbation of narrow-angle glaucoma, and confusional states in the elderly. Respiratory arrest when clozapine is combined with BZDs may be more likely in elderly patients, though data are lacking on this question; nevertheless, BZDs should be avoided until titration of clozapine is complete (Jacobson et al. 2002). Clozapine dosage should start at around 6.25 mg/day in the elderly, with increases in increments of 6.25 mg as tolerated every 3–4 days. Divided doses are recommended.

Q. What about the risks and benefits of using newer atypical APs in elderly and dementia patient populations?

A. In general, both risperidone and olanzapine appear to be safe and well tolerated in elderly schizophrenia patient populations, as well as in patients with dementia, provided low doses are used and careful monitoring occurs (Jacobson et al. 2002; Jeste et al. 2003; Martin et al. 2003). The recent Expert Consensus Guideline (Alexopoulos et al. 2004) found that about 93% of experts rated risperidone as a first-line treatment for geriatric schizophrenia, compared with 67% for quetiapine or olanzapine, and 60% for aripiprazole. One study (Madhusoodanan et al. 1995) of risperidone in 11 elderly patients (ages 61–79) with various types of psychoses showed this agent to be useful. At dosages of 0.5–3.0 mg/day, risperidone reduced both positive and negative symptoms of psychoses and was associated with reduced EPS and TD in four patients. However, two patients with preexisting heart disease had severe dizziness and hypotension. Special care should be taken when elderly patients are coprescribed agents or drugs that inhibit the CYP 2D6 and 3A4 systems, which metabolize risperidone (e.g., fluoxetine, paroxetine, erythromycin, and nefazodone) (Cozza et al. 2003). The dosage of risperidone in the elderly should begin at no higher than 0.5 mg/day (in divided doses) and should be slowly increased as tolerated to around 2–3 mg/day. Olanzapine also appears safe and well tolerated in elderly schizophrenic populations, as well as in patients with dementia, although its side-effect profile may differ from that of risperidone. In a comparative double-blind trial of risperidone and olanzapine in 175 elderly patients with chronic schizophrenia (Jeste et al. 2003), both agents had similar efficacy and tolerability. However, according to a 5-point anticholinergic symptom scale, urinary function worsened more in the olanzapine group. Weight gain and (surprisingly) EPS were also numerically more common in the olanzapine group. In a study of low-dose risperidone and olanzapine in patients with dementia (Martin et al. 2003), adverse events were infrequent with both agents; however, laxative use and falls were more common in the olanzapine group.

Quetiapine appears to be well tolerated in elderly patients (Tariot et al. 2000) at dosages of 50–400 mg/day (Jacobson et al. 2002); however, sedation, orthostatic hypotension, and dizziness may be seen, especially with overly zealous titration. Lens opacities and/or cataracts may be associated with chronic quetiapine use, as noted in premarketing animal studies, but it is unclear how much impact quetiapine has on these problems in elderly populations. Experience with ziprasidone and aripiprazole is still limited in the elderly; however, elderly patients with cardiac disease may not be ideal candidates for ziprasidone, given its effects on QTc.

Q. How serious are recent concerns about risperidone and risk of stroke in dementia patients? What about other atypicals?

A. On April 16, 2003, Janssen Pharmaceutica Products, in a "Dear Doctor" letter, warned U.S. physicians of CAEs (e.g., stroke, transient ischemic attack), including fatalities, in elderly patients with dementia-related psychosis (mean age 85 years). More recently, a similar letter was sent out by the manufacturer of olanzapine (Eli Lilly, January 15, 2004), citing increased cerebrovascular risks in dementia-related psychosis patients, compared with placebo. The most recent product labeling information for aripiprazole (Abilify) also includes data showing increased mortality among aripiprazole-treated Alzheimer's disease patients compared with placebo-treated patients (3.8% vs. 0%); however, there is no indication that stroke played a role in the 4 (of 105) patients who died (Physicians' Desk Reference 2004). It remains to be seen whether in the case of any atypical AP, there is a *causal* relationship between atypical use and CAEs. For example, in the risperidone trials (N=1,230), there was a significantly higher incidence of CAEs in patients treated with risperidone compared with patients treated with placebo. However, many of the patients studied had preexisting risk factors for CAEs, such as atrial fibrillation. Hence, the causal role of risperidone in these CAEs remains unclear. In a follow-up letter (September 9, 2003), Janssen Pharmaceutica, in consultation with the FDA, advised physicians that "Risperdal is not approved for the treatment of patients with dementia-related psychosis," adding that this also is true of other APs marketed in the United States. However, several studies have found that risperidone is an effective therapy for psychosis and behavioral disturbances associated with dementia (Katz et al. 1999). Another study found that low-dose, once-a-day olanzapine and risperidone both appear to be equally safe and effective in the treatment of dementia-related behavioral disturbances in residents of extended care facilities (Fontaine et al. 2003). The initial dosages were 2.5 mg/day of olanzapine and 0.5 mg/day of risperidone. Titration was allowed to maximum doses of olanzapine (10 mg/day) and risperidone (2.0 mg/day). A recent analysis of placebo-controlled studies (Greenspan et al. 2003) found the risk of stroke-related mortality to be about 12.4 per 1,000 patient-years in risperidone-treated dementia patients, versus 11.5 per 1,000 patient-years with placebo—not an impressive difference. Further large-scale, controlled studies—ideally, by independently funded researchers—are needed to ascertain the comparative risk of CAEs due to atypical APs in dementia patient populations. In the meantime, a careful risk–benefit assessment should be carried out prior to use of these agents in patients with cerebrovascular risk factors, including the informed consent of the patient and/or guardian. Doses of atypical APs should be kept low in elderly and dementia patient populations, to avoid pronounced α_1 receptor blockade and resultant hypotension, which might increase the risk of stroke.

Q. Can risperidone or other atypical agents besides clozapine be used in the treatment of psychosis in patients with Parkinson's disease or Lewy body dementia (LBD)?

A. Parkinson's disease itself may give rise to psychotic symptoms, as may use of dopamine agonists such as L-dopa. Of the atypical agents, clozapine is probably most useful in Parkinson's disease, followed by quetiapine; mixed results have been obtained with olanzapine and risperidone. Most Parkinson's disease patients may be treated effectively with about 50 mg of clozapine per day; quetiapine doses are in the range of 12.5 to 150 mg daily (Jacobson et al. 2002). In LBD, visual hallucinations and a fluctuating level of consciousness are common. Patients with LBD are notoriously sensitive to the parkinsonian side effects of virtually all APs, even atypical agents. Clozapine is the only AP that has consistently ameliorated LBD symptoms without worsening motor function in most cases (Jacobson et al. 2002); however, one study (Cummings et al. 2002) found that olanzapine (5 or 10 mg) reduced psychosis in patients with LBD without worsening parkinsonism. Quetiapine may also be well tolerated, though motor worsening may be seen in about a third of Parkinson's disease patients and in about one-quarter of those with LBD (Fernandez et al. 2002). There are conflicting data as to the benefits of risperidone in psychotic patients with Parkinson's disease or LBD (Gelenberg 1995b). If risperidone is used at all, the dosage should be kept below 1 mg/day, if possible.

Q. How do APs compare with buspirone in the treatment of agitated dementia patients?

A. One double-blind study (Cantillon et al. 1996) compared buspirone 15 mg/day with haloperidol 1.5 mg/day in a population of 26 nursing home residents with Alzheimer's disease and "agitation." Physical tension and motor activity decreased to a greater extent in the buspirone-treated patients. Although the findings from this study must be considered preliminary—for example, no placebo group was included—the results certainly suggest that in nonpsychotic dementia patients with motor agitation, buspirone is worth trying before initiating an AP trial. (Patients with psychotic features were excluded from the Cantillon et al. study.) In some cases, combined use of an AP and buspirone may be warranted in agitated dementia patients. Thus far, atypical APs have not been compared with buspirone in a head-to-head study of agitated dementia patients.

Q. What special considerations exist when prescribing APs for children and adolescents?

A. The main indication for use of APs in children is childhood schizophrenia. This disorder is now regarded as essentially the same disorder as that which occurs in adults, but with more severe symptoms and a more chronic course (Nakane and Rapoport 1995). Unfortunately, there are very few well-designed studies of AP use in this younger population. The use of APs in children and adolescents is further complicated by resistance to medication and both over- and undermedication (Dulcan et al. 1995). Children metabolize APs more rapidly than adults, but they may also require lower plasma levels for efficacy (Dulcan et al. 1995). The usual dose range of haloperidol in children is about 0.5 to 16 mg/day (0.02–0.2 mg/kg per day). Loxapine at dosages of 10–200 mg/day has also been found effective in one study of adolescents with schizophrenia (Pool et al. 1976). Notwithstanding these dosage guidelines, the best advice is to begin with a very low dose and to increase it gradually—generally no more than once or twice a week (Janicak et al. 1993). Older adolescents with schizophrenia may require neuroleptic doses comparable to those of adults; doses in younger adolescents may fall between those of children and adults. Some data suggest that adolescent boys are more susceptible to acute dystonic reactions than are older patients and are less responsive to anticholinergics, such as benztropine (Campbell et al. 1985); thus, neuroleptic dosage reduction or use of an atypical agent is the preferred strategy.

It is not yet clear which class of AP is safest and most efficacious in children and adolescents. Open studies suggest that both clozapine and risperidone may be effective (Frazier et al. 1994; Grcevich et al. 1995; Nakane and Rapoport 1995), but randomized, controlled trials are lacking. One recent open-label study of risperidone in adolescents with schizophrenia (Zalsman et al. 2003) found it effective at dosages of about 3 mg/day, but not for the *negative* symptoms of schizophrenia. The average dosage of clozapine used in an open-label study of 11 adolescents with severe, chronic schizophrenia was 370.5 mg/day (by the end of 6 weeks) (Frazier et al. 1994). By week 6 of treatment, there was an overall 58% improvement in the Clinical Global Impression scale. Tachycardia and sedation were the main limiting side effects. However, other data (Freedman et al. 1994; Rapoport 1994; Remschmidt et al. 1994) have raised concerns about potential toxicity in adolescents treated with clozapine manifested as, for example, leukopenia without agranulocytosis, ECG abnormalities, weight gain, and a high incidence of EEG abnormalities (Wagner 2004). More recent controlled and open data suggest that risperidone, olanzapine, and quetiapine may be effective in children and/or adolescents at dosage ranges comparable to those used in adults; however, EPS, weight gain, agitation, drowsiness, and other side effects may be associated with these agents (see Wagner 2004 for review). Wagner concluded that "it would be reasonable to initiate treatment with an atypical antipsychotic for a child with schizophrenia" but noted that "clozapine…should not be initiated unless there has been nonresponse to trials of at least two other antipsychotics" (Wagner 2004, p. 978). At this time, it is not possible to speak of an "atypical antipsychotic of first choice" in this population.

Vignettes/Puzzlers

Q. A 34-year-old woman presents with the complaint that "I hear this voice telling me I ran someone over in my car." The patient experiences this "voice" as "probably my own thoughts." She does not perceive two or more voices discussing her in derogatory terms; command auditory hallucinations; ideas of people "reading" her mind; ideas of influence/reference; or paranoid ideation. There is no history of psychological or physical trauma and no history of olfactory hallucinations, amnesic periods, déjà vu, or altered level of consciousness. However, the patient does stop her car periodically along the highway "just to make sure that I haven't killed anybody." She remarks, "I probably didn't run over anybody, but if I don't stop to check, I just feel like I'm going crazy." The patient has no history of psychiatric hospitalizations. However, she has been in individual psychotherapy for several years because of "strange experiences" she has had most of her life (e.g., "feeling like my soul sometimes leaves my body," or "feeling like there's somebody in the room with me when I'm alone at night"). She also expresses the view that "I think I may have ESP…I can usually tell what people are thinking before they even know what it is." Are APs indicated in this case?

A. There is no simple answer to this question, but the initial approach in this case probably does not include the use of APs (Pies 1984). Most of the clinical symptoms in this case suggest an obsessional disorder with at least partially intact "reality testing," though there are certainly some schizotypal personality features that complicate this assessment. That the patient experiences the "voices" as probably her *own thoughts* rather than as an external voice being "broadcast" to her, argues against a psychotic process. Furthermore, there is no delusional elaboration surrounding the voice (e.g., "I think someone must have put a radio transmitter into my car"). Probably, treatment should begin with an

SSRI (Goodman et al. 1992). If the patient does not respond to two or more SSRI trials (especially after attempts to potentiate with clomipramine), a small amount of risperidone (0.5–1.0 mg/day) could be added (McDougle et al. 1995). Potential pharmacokinetic interactions with the SSRI should be considered, and the risk of TD must be carefully discussed when APs are used in the treatment of OCD.

Q. A 50-year-old man with a long-standing history of schizophrenia has been maintained with partial success on oral risperidone 5 mg/day for the last 6 months. Because of numerous bouts of noncompliance, the treating psychiatrist tapers and discontinues the oral regimen, then begins Risperdal Consta 25 mg im. (The manufacturer's information recommends an initial dose of 25 mg every 2 weeks.) By the time of the second administration, nursing staff has complained that the patient is "worse than he was" while taking the oral preparation; for example, the patient notes that his baseline auditory hallucinations are "louder." The clinician reasons that the initial 25 mg was too low and increases the dose to the next available strength of 37.5 mg. How sound is the clinician's management strategy?

A. Risperdal Consta is the long-acting preparation of oral risperidone. It is available in 25-mg, 37.5-mg, and 50-mg strengths. The manufacturer recommends that all patients begin with 25 mg initially, regardless of prior oral AP dose (Janssen Pharmaceutica, package insert, 2004). In addition, increases in dose are not to occur at any less than *4-week intervals,* because of the pharmacokinetics of the long-acting microsphere preparation. It is mandatory, when starting a patient on Risperdal Consta, that *oral AP therapy be continued for the first 3 weeks.* In the case cited, the long-acting preparation had not achieved its steady-state level, and residual risperidone blood and/or brain levels had probably dropped to the subtherapeutic range for this patient. The patient should have been maintained on 5 mg/day of oral risperidone for 21 days after the first injection. On day 21 (3 weeks after the initial injection), most patients will probably have high enough plasma risperidone levels to permit discontinuation of the oral AP; however, the time needed may vary from patient to patient.

Q. A 45-year-old HIV-positive woman with a history of psychological trauma is taking Combivir (lamivudine/zidovudine) 1 tablet bid and efavirenz 600 mg hs. Three weeks after testing positive and beginning her "triple cocktail," the patient starts complaining of frightening sensory experiences, such as "flashbacks" of traumatic events. Viral load and CD4+ counts are at acceptable levels. Since the patient refuses any medication that will "make her fat," a psychiatrist decides to prescribe aripiprazole 15 mg qd. After 3 days of treatment, the patient reports headache, nausea, and feeling "real antsy" and tremulous. Pronounced akathisia is observed on evaluation. What is the most likely explanation for this sequence of events?

A. HIV medications are notorious for confounding psychiatric conditions and treatment. This patient began a standard three-drug regimen containing only three pills a day. However, efavirenz, a non-nucleoside reverse transcriptase inhibitor, is known to cause psychiatric side effects, including vivid dreams and flashbacks (Vazquez 1999). These experiences may remit after a few weeks or persist for several months. Though the initial recommendation for this medication was for "hs" dosing, some clinicians now prescribe it earlier in the evening to avoid such side effects. In addition, efavirenz and other HIV medications may have complex effects on various CYP enzymes, including CYP 3A4. Initially, efavirenz may potently *inhibit* CYP 3A4, thus increasing blood levels of 3A4 substrates; however, over time, efavirenz may *induce* this enzyme (Cozza et al. 2003; Mouly et al. 2002). CYP 3A4 is an important metabolic pathway for aripiprazole, and the side effects noted after a few days of taking aripiprazole probably reflect excessive blood and/or CNS levels of the drug. Collaboration between the psychiatrist and physician responsible for this patient's HIV medications is essential; for example, adjusting psychotropic doses in order to "keep up" with metabolic changes due to the efavirenz.

Q. **A 24-year-old man with schizophrenia currently maintained on olanzapine 15 mg hs is discharged from an inpatient unit to a group home. He has been taking his current olanzapine dose for 1 month with no adverse events. After 3 weeks at a group home, he is sent back to the inpatient facility with complaints of auditory hallucinations. Staff is concerned that he might hurt himself or others. They report that the patient keeps busy by working in the wood shop with other clients. They also report that the patient likes to spend his off time "smoking and telling jokes" with other group home residents in a nearby park. Assuming that the patient is compliant with his medication regimen, what may explain his decompensation?**

A. The patient's decompensation might simply represent the "natural course" of his illness. However, cigarette smoking has been shown to decrease olanzapine and clozapine levels by as much as 40%. This effect probably occurs through hepatic induction of CYP 1A2, thereby increasing the clearance of these drugs (Gex-Fabry et al. 2003; Physicians' Desk Reference 2004; Skogh et al. 2002). Many hospitalized patients are prohibited from smoking or are allowed only limited "smoking times." Upon discharge, however, smoking may increase substantially, causing reduction in blood levels of CYP 1A2 substrates. Monitoring AP blood levels and adjusting dose accordingly may be indicated for patients whose smoking habits change with a change in residence.

Q. **A 25-year-old man with chronic schizophrenia is having his medication converted from oral haloperidol 10 mg/day to haloperidol decanoate. The patient is also taking benztropine 1 mg/day. Using the formula of "monthly im depot dose = 10–15 times daily oral dose," the patient's haloperidol is tapered down to 5 mg/day, after which the patient is given an injection of haloperidol decanoate 100 mg im. The oral haloperidol and benztropine are then discontinued. Four days later, the patient is seen in clinic and is noted to be significantly more psychotic. Reasoning that the initial intramuscular dose may not have been sufficient, the resident in the emergency room administers an additional 50 mg haloperidol decanoate im. Two days later, the patient returns to the emergency room with severe torticollis and tongue protrusion. What is the *pharmacokinetic* explanation for this adverse event, and what should have been the initial corrective action?**

A. The concentration of haloperidol decanoate in the plasma reaches a peak at around day 6, then slowly declines (McNeil Pharmaceutical, package insert, 1987). This agent has an apparent $t_{1/2}$ of around 3 weeks and reaches steady state in about 3 months (roughly 4–5 half-lives). In this case, the second intramuscular injection was producing *rising plasma levels* just as the initial injection was "peaking," probably accounting for the severe EPS. (Discontinuation of the benztropine probably created a pharmacodynamic factor predisposing to EPS—namely, increased central cholinergic activity. There seems to be no appreciable pharmacokinetic interaction between benztropine and haloperidol [Goff et al. 1991]). It would have been wiser to add a small amount of daily oral haloperidol to the patient's regimen (e.g., 2–4 mg po qd) to "tide him over" until the haloperidol decanoate reached higher plasma levels and produced its pharmacodynamic effect on DA receptors in the brain. A significant drop from baseline in total BPRS score—a change that is correlated with clinical improvement—is clearly detectable by week 4 of haloperidol decanoate treatment (Simpson 1988). Another intervention in this case would have been continuation of an anticholinergic agent on a prophylactic basis, particularly in a young male patient.

Q. A 63-year-old man who is receiving clozapine 300 mg bid undergoes a right hemicolectomy for adenocarcinoma. His clozapine is held on the day before the surgery and on the day of the operation, then restarted at 100 mg/day, with increases up to 300 mg/day by day 4. On postoperative day 5, the patient has normal bowel sounds on auscultation and is able to tolerate a regular diet. By day 6, he complains of "gas pains" and some abdominal tenderness. He shows some abdominal distension and has one bout of vomiting. No bowel sounds are heard on auscultation. He is also noted to have significant orthostatic hypotension and dizziness on standing. What is the diagnosis and etiology?

A. Any drug with significant anticholinergic effects can cause constipation, fecal impaction, and even functional bowel obstruction ("paralytic ileus"), as in the present case. Abdominal surgery itself may also be associated with ileus, but in this case, the relatively delayed onset suggests that clozapine's strong anticholinergic effects were a contributing factor (Erickson and Morris 1995). It is important, in such cases, to avoid premature restoration of full-dose regimens of highly anticholinergic medications. Furthermore, the patient's orthostatic hypotension and dizziness were probably related to the rapid dosage escalation of clozapine *after a 48-hour hiatus.* Although sensitivity to "restart" effects of clozapine is quite variable, orthostasis and even respiratory arrest have been attributed to high restart doses of clozapine; thus, if there is a hiatus of 2 days or more, clozapine should be restarted at 12.5 mg once or twice daily.

Q. A 23-year-old woman with schizophrenia is being maintained on a stable regimen of clozapine 450 mg/day when she suffers a grand mal seizure. Her psychosis was under good control for over 5 months, and two attempts to reduce the clozapine dose led to worsening of psychosis. Owing to a previous allergic reaction to valproate, the patient is started on phenytoin 100 mg tid. Her plasma phenytoin level after 1 week is 12 μg/mL (therapeutic range = 10–20 μg/mL). Two weeks later, the patient begins to complain of "the Devil's voice rocketing through my brain" and starts to isolate herself in her room. She is oriented to day and date and shows no gross neurological impairment. What is the most likely explanation of this deterioration?

A. Phenytoin may significantly decrease clozapine levels, resulting in decreased clinical efficacy (Ciraulo et al. 1994). Phenytoin toxicity is another possibility, and a follow-up phenytoin level would be indicated; however, in the absence of mental confusion, ataxia, slurred speech, and other signs of toxicity, phenytoin toxicity seems unlikely.

Q. A 25-year-old woman with schizophrenia and apparent comorbid OCD is being treated with olanzapine 20 mg/day. Although this has ameliorated her psychotic symptoms and has been well tolerated, the patient continues to show extreme obsessive-compulsive behavior, such as counting backward from 100 every time she needs to leave her bed, and arranging her food in a highly idiosyncratic manner before eating it. There does not appear to be specific delusional content behind these behaviors. Since fluvoxamine (Luvox) has been FDA-labeled for the treatment of OCD, the patient's psychiatrist begins treatment with fluvoxamine 50 mg bid. The dosage is increased over the subsequent week to 100 mg bid. The patient complains of extreme lethargy, dizziness, dry mouth, lightheadedness, and confusion. What is the likely explanation?

A. Case reports of markedly elevated olanzapine (and clozapine) levels during fluvoxamine therapy have now been reported. This effect may be mediated through fluvoxamine's strong inhibition of the CYP 1A2 system, which is at least partly involved in olanzapine's and clozapine's metabolism (Cozza et al. 2003). (CYP 3A4, CYP 2D6, and glucuronidation are also involved in the metabolism of both drugs.) Fluvoxamine should be used with great caution in combination with olanzapine or clozapine, and clinical status should be monitored carefully. Obtaining clozapine (or olanzapine) blood levels—before and after fluvoxamine—may also help guide treatment (Nemeroff et al. 1996). However, it is usually safer and simpler to use an SSRI that lacks substantial CYP 1A2–inhibiting effects, such as citalopram or sertraline.

Q. A 43-year-old man with chronic undifferentiated schizophrenia complains of a "creepy feeling" in his legs and appears to shift from foot to foot. He also describes feeling "all wound up inside." In the 1980s, he had only minimal response to adequate doses and trials of conventional neuroleptics (fluphenazine, haloperidol, thioridazine, loxapine, trifluoperazine) and experienced the same uncomfortable feelings in his legs. In the early 1990s, a trial of clozapine led to some improvement and fewer complaints, but the patient developed severe granulocytopenia, requiring discontinuation of the clozapine. More recently, olanzapine (20 mg/day) led to significant improvement in his psychosis, but the patient gained 30 pounds and developed elevated serum glucose and triglycerides. A trial of quetiapine was not associated with the "creepy feelings" in his legs, but the patient had suboptimal AP response and felt lightheaded while taking 700 mg/day of quetiapine. His current regimen is risperidone 5 mg/day, benztropine 1 mg bid, and lorazepam 1 mg bid. Although his psychosis is under relatively good control (given his long psychiatric history), the patient is aggressive, threatening, and irritable on the inpatient unit and has required seclusion or restraints three times in the past 2 weeks. What is the most parsimonious *augmentation* strategy at this point, bearing in mind the patient's discomfort in his legs?

A. The addition of a beta-blocker may be the most efficient means of treating the patient's evident akathisia, though well-designed, controlled studies are lacking (Stanilla and Simpson 2004). A beta-blocker may also ameliorate his aggressiveness and possibly his refractory psychosis. Wirshing et al. (1995) noted that most, but not all, controlled studies found improvement in acute schizophrenia when *propranolol* was used as an adjunctive agent. Dosages have been quite high, ranging from 400 to 2,000 mg/day. Propranolol can elevate levels of some APs (e.g., thioridazine), and some clinicians have suggested that beta-blockers ameliorate psychosis through this pharmacokinetic mechanism. However, it is possible that both peripheral and centrally acting beta-blockers have *primary* effects on aggression (Yudofsky et al. 1987) and psychosis, perhaps via pharmacodynamic effects of some kind. Beta-blockers are relatively contraindicated in patients with obstructive lung disease, diabetes mellitus, or hyperthyroidism. Care must also be exercised when beta-blockers are used with other agents that may slow cardiac conduction or induce hypotension (Ratey and MacNaughton 1995). Since risperidone has significant α_1-adrenergic receptor blockade (thus increasing the risk of orthostatic hypotension), the addition of propranolol could be problematic in this case. Another parsimonious option in this case would be an increase in the patient's lorazepam dose (e.g., to 1.5 mg bid), since BZDs may ameliorate akathisia (Stanilla and Simpson 2004) and may occasionally have adjunctive AP effects. Aripiprazole could be considered as the primary AP in this case; however, despite the very benign premarketing data for this agent, there have been anecdotal reports of akathisia associated with aripiprazole (Rosenblatt and Rosenblatt, 2003).

Q. A 92-year-old woman with a history of "dementia with psychosis" is admitted to the inpatient psychiatric unit from a local nursing home. The patient was observed to be "confused" and "belligerent" over the past 2 weeks, beyond her usual baseline. Owing to significant EPS, her medications were changed recently from haloperidol 1 mg bid and benztropine 1 mg qd to thioridazine 150 mg qd and the same amount of benztropine. The patient is reportedly "intolerant" of several atypical APs, having experienced severe EPS with low-dose risperidone, and severe orthostatic hypotension while taking quetiapine and olanzapine. The patient is also taking dicyclomine (Bentyl) 40 mg qid for "irritable bowel syndrome." What is the most likely cause of the patient's recent change in mental status?

A. This is probably a case of central anticholinergic toxicity (Pies 1994). Cholinergic projections from the nucleus basalis of Meynert to the cerebral cortex have been linked to the pathophysiology of Alzheimer's disease, in which acetylcholine is generally deficient. Cholinergic dysfunction may also be important in many instances of delirium. Thus, this patient may have been at risk for central anticholinergic toxicity even at baseline. The change from 2 mg/day of haloperidol to 150 mg/day of thioridazine was not a change to an equivalent dose. The correct conversion would have been to approximately *90* mg/day of thioridazine (Kane et al. 2003b). Since thioridazine is substantially more anticholinergic than haloperidol even at equivalent doses, the change in AP markedly increased the patient's "anticholinergic burden." The benztropine and dicyclomine also have substantial anticholinergic properties and probably contributed to the patient's confusional state. In addition, given thioridazine's cardiotoxic effects, it is not an AP well suited to use in geriatric psychiatry.

Q. A 47-year-old man with chronic schizophrenia and hypertension has been refractory to monotherapy with several atypical APs, including clozapine, risperidone, olanzapine, and quetiapine. His only regular nonpsychiatric medication is nicardipine 20 mg bid for hypertension. Since he showed "partial improvement" with both risperidone and olanzapine, his doctor decides to try the two medications in combination. The patient is tapered off quetiapine and started on a combination of olanzapine 5 mg/day and risperidone 2.5 mg/day. The patient appears to improve on this combination after a period of 1 week. However, he complains of lightheadedness, dizziness, and "palpitations." In addition, he feels "sick to my stomach," experiences abdominal pain, and vomits several times. Urine output is increased, and a blood sample shows markedly elevated glucose and abnormal pH. An ECG shows a new conduction abnormality. What two pathophysiological processes may explain these findings?

A. This patient has probably developed two problems associated with atypical APs in susceptible individuals: prolonged QTc, and hyperglycemia associated with ketoacidosis. The prolonged QTc was most likely due to the combination of two atypical APs in the presence of a calcium channel blocker (nicardipine), a class of drugs known to prolong QTc (see, e.g., Physicians' Desk Reference 2004; Cardene, ESP Pharma, 2004). (Orthostatic hypotension due to α-adrenergic receptor blockade would also be a concern with atypical AP polypharmacy.) Ketoacidosis may present as acute gastrointestinal symptoms in the context of ketones in the urine, polyuria, metabolic acidosis, and an anion gap (Foster 1998). Although risperidone appears to be associated with hyperglycemia and ketoacidosis less frequently than olanzapine (Keck et al. 2003a), the FDA has recently requested that all manufacturers of atypical APs include a warning regarding hyperglycemia and diabetes mellitus in their product labeling. In the case above, one might speculate that the combination of two atypical APs increased the risk for glucose dysregulation, though controlled study of this issue is lacking.

References

Adams F: Emergency intravenous sedation of the delirious, medically ill patient. J Clin Psychiatry 49 (12, suppl):22–27, 1988

Alexopoulos GS, Streim JE, Carpenter D: Expert consensus guidelines for using antipsychotic agents in older patients. J Clin Psychiatry 65 (suppl 2):100–102, 2004

Allison DB, Mentore JL, Heo M, et al: Antipsychotic-induced weight gain: a comprehensive research synthesis. Am J Psychiatry 156:1686–1696, 1999

Altshuler LL, Cohen L, Szuba MP, et al: Pharmacologic management of psychiatric illness during pregnancy: dilemmas and guidelines. Am J Psychiatry 153:592–606, 1996

American Diabetes Association, et al: Consensus development conference on antipsychotic drugs and obesity and diabetes. J Clin Psychiatry 65:267–272, 2004

Ananth J, Parameswaran S, Gunatilake S, et al: Neuroleptic malignant syndrome and atypical antipsychotic drugs. J Clin Psychiatry 65:464–470, 2004

Anghelescu I, Klawe C, Benkert O: Orlistat in the treatment of psychopharmacologically induced weight gain. J Clin Psychopharmacol 20:716–717, 2000

Arana GW, Goff DC, Friedman H, et al: Does carbamazepine-induced reduction of plasma haloperidol levels worsen psychotic symptoms? Am J Psychiatry 143:650–651, 1986

Ayd FJ: Lexicon of Psychiatry, Neurology, and the Neurosciences. Baltimore, MD, Williams & Wilkins, 1995

Ayd F: Long-acting risperidone: first long-acting atypical antipsychotic. International Drug Therapy Newsletter 38:89–95, 2003

Baker RW, Chengappa KN, Baird JW, et al: Emergence of obsessive-compulsive symptoms during treatment with clozapine. J Clin Psychiatry 53:439–442, 1992

Berman I, Sapers BL, Chang HHJ, et al: Treatment of obsessive-compulsive symptoms in schizophrenic patients with clomipramine. J Clin Psychopharmacol 15:206–210, 1995

Bitter I, Dossenbach MR, Brook S, et al: Olanzapine versus clozapine in treatment-resistant or treatment-intolerant schizophrenia. Prog Neuropsychopharmacol Biol Psychiatry 28:173–180, 2004

Bondolfi G, Dufour H, Patris M, et al: Risperidone versus clozapine in treatment-resistant chronic schizophrenia: a randomized double-blind study. The Risperidone Study Group. Am J Psychiatry 155:499–504, 1998

Bottender R, Jager M, Hofschuster E, et al: Neuroleptic malignant syndrome due to atypical neuroleptics: three episodes in one patient. Pharmacopsychiatry 35:119–121, 2002

Bourgeois JA, Klein M: Risperidone and fluoxetine in the treatment of pedophilia with comorbid dysthymia (letter). J Clin Psychopharmacol 16:257–258, 1996

Brambilla P, Barale F, Soares JC: Atypical antipsychotics and mood stabilization in bipolar disorder. Psychopharmacology (Berl) 166:315–332, 2003

Breier A, Wolkowitz OM, Doran AR, et al: Neuroleptic responsivity of negative and positive symptoms in schizophrenia. Am J Psychiatry 144:1549–1555, 1987

Breier A, Tanaka Y, Roychowdhury S, et al: Nizatidine for the prevention of olanzapine-associated weight gain in schizophrenia and related disorders: a randomized, controlled, double-blind study. Presentation at the 41st annual meeting of the New Clinical Drug Evaluation Unit, Phoenix, AZ, May 28–31, 2001

Brieger P: Hypomanic episodes after receiving ziprasidone: an unintended "on-off-on" course of treatment. J Clin Psychiatry 65:132–135, 2004

Buckley NA, Whyte IM, Dawson AH: Cardiotoxicity more common in thioridazine overdose than with other neuroleptics. Clin Toxicol 33:199–204, 1995

Buckley PF, Meltzer HY: Treatment of schizophrenia, in The American Psychiatric Press Textbook of Psychopharmacology, 2nd Edition. Edited by Schatzberg AF, Nemeroff CB. Washington, DC, American Psychiatric Press, 1995, pp 615–639

Burris KD, Molski TF, Xu C, et al: Aripiprazole, a novel antipsychotic, is a high-affinity partial agonist at human dopamine D_2 receptors. J Pharmacol Exp Ther 302:381–389, 2002

Bustillo J, Lauriello J, Horan W, et al: The psychosocial treatment of schizophrenia: an update. Am J Psychiatry 158:163–175, 2001

Campbell A, Baldessarini RJ: Prolonged pharmacologic activity of neuroleptics (letter). Arch Gen Psychiatry 42:637, 1985

Campbell M, Green WH, Deutsch SI (eds): Child and Adolescent Psychopharmacology. Beverly Hills, CA, Sage, 1985

Cantillon M, Brunswick R, Molina D, et al: A double-blind trial for agitation in a nursing home population with Alzheimer's disease. Am J Geriatr Psychiatry 4:263–267, 1996

Canuso CM, Goldstein JM, Wojcik J, et al: Antipsychotic medication, prolactin elevation, and ovarian function in women with schizophrenia and schizoaffective disorder. Psychiatry Res 111:11–20, 2002

Carlsson A, Lindquist M: Effect of chlorpromazine or haloperidol on the formation of 3-methoxytyramine and normetanephrine in mouse brain. Acta Pharmacol Toxicol 20:140-144, 1963

Caroff SN: Neuroleptic malignant syndrome. Current Psychiatry 2:36–42, 2003

Carpenter WT, Heinrichs DW, Wagman AMI: Deficit and nondeficit forms of schizophrenia: the concept. Am J Psychiatry 145:578–583, 1988

Casey DE: Antipsychotic drug therapy and extrapyramidal symptoms: past, present, and future. Syllabus material for Progress in Psychoses, U.S. Psychiatric and Mental Health Congress, New York, NY (CME Inc., and Janssen Pharmaceutica Inc.), November 17, 1995

Casey DE, Daniel DG, Wassef AA, et al: Effect of divalproex combined with olanzapine or risperidone in patients with an acute exacerbation of schizophrenia. Neuropsychopharmacology 28:182–192, 2003

Castillo E, Rubin RT, Holsboer-Trachsler E: Clinical differentiation between lethal catatonia and neuroleptic malignant syndrome. Am J Psychiatry 146:324–328, 1989

Centorrino F, Price BH, Tuttle M, et al: EEG abnormalities during treatment with typical and atypical antipsychotics. Am J Psychiatry 159:109–115, 2002

Chengappa KN, Parepally H, Brar JS, et al: A random-assignment, double-blind, clinical trial of once- vs twice-daily administration of quetiapine fumarate in patients with schizophrenia or schizoaffective disorder: a pilot study. Can J Psychiatry 48:187–194, 2003

Chin AC, Shaw KA, Ciaranello RD: Molecular neurobiology, in The American Psychiatric Press Textbook of Psychopharmacology, 2nd Edition. Edited by Schatzberg AF, Nemeroff CB. Washington, DC, American Psychiatric Press, 1995, pp 35–36

Chong SA, Tan CH, Lee HS: Atrial ectopics with clozapine-risperidone combination. J Clin Psychopharmacol 17:130–131, 1997

Ciraulo DA, Shader RI, Greenblatt DJ, et al (eds): Drug Interactions in Psychiatry. Baltimore, MD, Williams & Wilkins, 1989, pp 88–126

Ciraulo DA, Shader RI, Greenblatt DJ: Drug interactions in psychopharmacology, in Manual of Psychiatric Therapeutics, 2nd Edition. Edited by Shader RI. Boston, MA, Little, Brown, 1994, pp 143–158

Cole JO, Goldberg SC, Klerman GL: Phenothiazine treatment in acute schizophrenia. Arch Gen Psychiatry 10:246–261, 1964

Cornelius JR, Soloff PH, Perel JM, et al: A preliminary trial of fluoxetine in refractory borderline patients. J Clin Psychopharmacol 11:116–120, 1991

Cornelius JR, Soloff PH, Perel JM, et al: Continuation pharmacotherapy of borderline personality disorder with haloperidol and phenelzine. Am J Psychiatry 150:1843–1848, 1993

Cowdry RW: Psychopharmacology of borderline personality disorder: a review. J Clin Psychiatry 48 (8, suppl):15–22, 1987

Cozza KL, Armstrong SC, Oesterheld JR: Drug Interaction Principles for Medical Practice: Cytochrome P450, UGTs, P-Glycoproteins, 2nd Edition. Washington, DC, American Psychiatric Publishing, 2003, pp 360–367

Csernansky JG, Newcomer JG: Maintenance drug treatment for schizophrenia, in Psychopharmacology: The Fourth Generation of Progress. Edited by Bloom FE, Kupfer DJ. New York, Raven, 1995, pp 1267–1275

Cummings JL, Street J, Masterman D, et al: Efficacy of olanzapine in the treatment of psychosis in dementia with Lewy bodies. Dement Geriatr Cogn Disord 13:67–73, 2002

Daniel DG, Copeland LF, Tamminga C: Ziprasidone, in The American Psychiatric Publishing Textbook of Psychopharmacology, 3rd Edition. Edited by Schatzberg AF, Nemeroff CB. Washington, DC, American Psychiatric Publishing, 2004, pp 507–518

Davis JM, Chen N, Glick ID: A meta-analysis of the efficacy of second-generation antipsychotics. Arch Gen Psychiatry 60:553–564, 2003

DeQuardo JR: Worsened agitation with aripiprazole: adverse effect of dopamine partial agonism? J Clin Psychiatry 65:132–133, 2004

DeVane CL: Pharmacogenetics and drug metabolism of newer antidepressant agents. J Clin Psychiatry 55 (12, suppl):38–45, 1994

Drug Facts and Comparisons. St Louis, MO, Facts and Comparisons, 1995, p 1438

Dubovsky SL, Buzan R: Psychopharmacology, in The American Psychiatric Press Textbook of Geriatric Neuropsychiatry, 2nd Edition. Edited by Coffey EC, Cummings JL. Washington, DC, American Psychiatric Press, 2000, pp 779–827

Dulcan MK, Bregman JD, Weller EB: Treatment of childhood and adolescent disorders, in The American Psychiatric Press Textbook of Psychopharmacology, 2nd Edition. Edited by Schatzberg AF, Nemeroff CB. Washington, DC, American Psychiatric Press, 1995, pp 669–706

Dursun SM, Deakin JFW: Augmenting antipsychotic treatment with lamotrigine or topiramate in patients with treatment-resistant schizophrenia: a naturalistic case-series outcome study. J Psychopharmacol 15:297–301, 2001

Ebenbichler CF, Laimer M, Eder U, et al: Olanzapine induces insulin resistance: results from a prospective study. J Clin Psychiatry 64:1436–1439, 2003

Ellison JM, Adler D: A strategy for the pharmacotherapy of personality disorders. New Dir Ment Health Serv Fall(47):43–63, 1990

Emes C, Millson R: Risperidone-induced priapism (letter). Can J Psychiatry 39:315–316, 1994

Erickson B, Morris D: Clozapine-associated postoperative ileus: case report and review of the literature (letter). Arch Gen Psychiatry 52:508–509, 1995

Falloon IRH, Boyd JL, McGill CW, et al: Family management in the prevention of morbidity of schizophrenia. Arch Gen Psychiatry 42:887–896, 1985

Farde L, Wiesel F-A, Halldin C, et al: Central D_2 dopamine receptor occupancy in schizophrenic patients treated with antipsychotic drugs. Arch Gen Psychiatry 45:71–76, 1988

Fernandez HH, Trieschmann ME, Burke MA, et al: Quetiapine for psychosis in Parkinson's disease versus dementia with Lewy bodies. J Clin Psychiatry 63:513–515, 2002

Fink M: Response to "Neuroleptic malignant-like syndrome due to cyclobenzaprine?" J Clin Psychopharmacol 16:97–98, 1996

Fink M, Bush G, Francis A: Catatonia: a treatable disorder, occasionally recognized. Directions in Psychiatry 13:1–7, 1993

Fontaine CS, Hynan LS, Koch K, et al: A double-blind comparison of olanzapine versus risperidone in the acute treatment of dementia-related behavioral disturbances in extended care facilities. J Clin Psychiatry 64:726–730, 2003

Foster DW: Diabetes mellitus, in Harrison's Principles of Internal Medicine, 14th Edition. Edited by Fauci AS, Braunwald E, Isselbacher KJ. New York, McGraw-Hill, 1998, pp 2060–2081

Frankenburg F, Zanarini MC: Clozapine treatment of borderline patients: a preliminary study. Compr Psychiatry 34:402–405, 1993

Frazier JA, Gordon CT, McKenna K, et al: An open trial of clozapine in 11 adolescents with childhood-onset schizophrenia. J Am Acad Child Adolesc Psychiatry 33:658–663, 1994

Freedman JE, Wirshung WC, Russel AT, et al: Absence status seizures during successful long-term clozapine treatment of an adolescent with schizophrenia. J Child Adolesc Psychopharmacol 4:53–62, 1994

Freudenreich O, McEvoy JP: How much Haldol D does Larry really need? (letter) J Clin Psychiatry 56:331–332, 1995

Freudenreich O, Beebe M, Goff DC: Clozapine-induced sialorrhea treated with sublingual ipratropium spray: a case series. J Clin Psychopharmacol 24:98–100, 2004

Frick A, Kopitz J, Bergemann N: Omeprazole reduces clozapine plasma concentrations: a case report. Pharmacopsychiatry 36:121–123, 2003

Friedman H, Greenblatt DJ: Rational therapeutic drug monitoring. JAMA 256:2227–2233, 1986

Gelenberg A: Clozapine for adolescents? Biological Therapies in Psychiatry Newsletter 17:37–38, 1994

Gelenberg AJ: Bipolar patients. J Clin Psychiatry (Monograph Series) 13 (October):28–29, 1995a

Gelenberg AJ: Risperidone for psychosis of Parkinson's syndrome and Lewy body dementia. Biological Therapies in Psychiatry Newsletter 18:43–44, 1995b

Gelenberg AJ: Fatal risperidone overdose. Biological Therapies in Psychiatry Newsletter 19:34–35, 1996

Gelenberg AJ: IM antipsychotics. Biological Therapies in Psychiatry Newsletter 26:37, 2003a

Gelenberg AJ: Modafinil for sedation. Biological Therapies in Psychiatry Newsletter 26:8, 2003b

Gex-Fabry M, Balant-Gorgia AE, Balant LP: Therapeutic drug monitoring of olanzapine: the combined effects of age gender, smoking, and comedication. Ther Drug Monit 25:46–53, 2003

Ghaemi SN, Hsu DJ: Novel maintenance treatments for bipolar disorder: recent olanzapine and lamotrigine studies. Int Drug Ther Newsl 39:1–8, 2004

Godleski LS, Sernyak MJ: Agranulocytosis after addition of risperidone to clozapine treatment. Am J Psychiatry 153:735–736, 1996

Goff DC: Risperidone, in The American Psychiatric Publishing Textbook of Psychopharmacology, 3rd Edition. Edited by Schatzberg AF, Nemeroff CB. Washington, DC, American Psychiatric Publishing, 2004, pp 495–505

Goff DC, Baldessarini RJ: Antipsychotics, in Drug Interactions in Psychiatry, 2nd Edition. Edited by Ciraulo DA, Shader RI, Greenblatt DJ, et al. Baltimore, MD, Williams & Wilkins, 1995, pp 129–174

Goff DC, Arana GW, Greenblatt DJ, et al: The effect of benztropine on haloperidol-induced dystonia, clinical efficacy, and pharmacokinetics: a prospective, double-blind trial. J Clin Psychopharmacol 11:106–108, 1991

Goff DC, Hennen J, Lyoo IK, et al: Modulation of brain and serum glutamatergic concentrations following a switch from conventional neuroleptics to olanzapine. Biol Psychiatry 51:493–497, 2002

Goldberg SC, Schulz SC, Schulz PM, et al: Borderline and schizotypal personality disorders treated with low-dose thiothixene vs placebo. Arch Gen Psychiatry 43:680–690, 1986

Goldberger AL: Electrocardiography, in Harrison's Principles of Internal Medicine, 14th Edition. Edited by Fauci AS, Braunwald E, Isselbacher KJ. New York, McGraw-Hill, 1998, pp 1237–1247

Goldmann MB, Janecek HM: Adjunctive fluoxetine improves global function in chronic schizophrenia. J Neuropsychiatry Clin Neurosci 2:429–431, 1990

Goodman WK, McDougle CJ, Price LH: Pharmacotherapy of obsessive compulsive disorder. J Clin Psychiatry 53 (4, suppl):29–37, 1992

Grcevich SJ, Findling RL, Schulz SC, et al: Risperidone in the treatment of children and adolescents with psychotic illness: a retrospective review. Poster presented at the 148th annual meeting of the American Psychiatric Association, Miami, FL, May 20–25, 1995

Greenspan A, Eerdekens M, Mahmoud R: Is there an increased rate of cerebrovascular adverse events, including mortality, with risperidone in dementia patients? Poster presented at the annual meeting of the American College of Neuropsychopharmacology, San Francisco, CA, December 7–11, 2003

Gupta S, Sonnenberg SJ, Frak B: Olanzapine augmentation of clozapine. Ann Clin Psychiatry 10:113–115, 1998

Hallward A, Ellison JM: Antidepressants and Sexual Function. London, Harcourt Health Communications/Mosby International, 2001

Harnett DS: Psychotherapy and psychopharmacology, in Handbook of Clinical Psychopharmacology, 2nd Edition. Edited by Tupin JP, Shader RI, Harnett DS. Northvale, NJ, Jason Aronson, 1988, pp 401–424

Harrigan EP, Miceli JJ, Anziano R, et al: A randomized evaluation of the effects of six antipsychotic agents on QTc, in the absence and presence of metabolic inhibition. J Clin Psychopharmacol 24:62–69, 2004

Hayes SG: Long-term use of valproate in primary psychiatric disorders. J Clin Psychiatry 50 (3, suppl):35–39, 1989

Hegarty JD: Antipsychotic drug withdrawal (interview). Current Approaches to Psychoses 5 (July):1–4, 1996

Henderson DC, Goff DC: Risperidone as an adjunct to clozapine therapy in chronic schizophrenics. J Clin Psychiatry 57:395–397, 1996

Heresco-Levy U, Ermilov M, Lichtenberg P, et al: High-dose glycine added to olanzapine and risperidone for the treatment of schizophrenia. Biol Psychiatry 55:165–171, 2004

Hiemke C, Weigmann H, Harter S, et al: Elevated levels of clozapine in serum after addition of fluvoxamine. J Clin Psychopharmacol 14:279–281, 1994

Ho BC, Miller D, Nopoulos P, et al: A comparative effectiveness study of risperidone and olanzapine. J Clin Psychiatry 60:658–663, 1999

Hogarty GE, McEvoy JP, Ulrich RF, et al: Pharmacotherapy of impaired affect in recovering schizophrenic patients. Arch Gen Psychiatry 52:29–41, 1995

Jacobson SA, Pies RW, Greenblatt DJ: Handbook of Geriatric Psychopharmacology. Washington, DC, American Psychiatric Publishing, 2002

Janicak PG, Davis JM, Preskorn SH, et al: Principles and Practice of Psychopharmacotherapy. Baltimore, MD, Williams & Wilkins, 1993, pp 96–115, 164–167, 352–353

Janicak PG, Keck PE, Davis JM, et al: A double-blind, randomized, prospective evaluation of the efficacy and safety of risperidone versus haloperidol in the treatment of schizoaffective disorder. J Clin Psychopharmacol 21:360–368, 2001

Jeanblanc W, Davis YB: Risperidone for treating dementia-associated aggression (letter). Am J Psychiatry 152:1239, 1995

Jenkins SC, Tinsley JA, Van Loon JA: A Pocket Reference for Psychiatrists, 3rd Edition. Washington, DC, American Psychiatric Press, 2001

Jeste DV, Barak Y, Mahusoodanan S, et al: International multisite double-blind trial of the atypical antipsychotics risperidone and olanzapine in 175 elderly patients with chronic schizophrenia. Am J Geriatr Psychiatry 11:638–647, 2003

Jibson MD, Tandon R: A summary of research findings on the new antipsychotic drugs. Directions in Psychiatry 16:1–7, 1996

Kane JM, Marder SR, Schooler NR, et al: Clozapine and haloperidol in moderately refractory schizophrenia. Arch Gen Psychiatry 58:965–972, 2001

Kane J, Eerdekens M, Lindenmayer JP: Long-acting injectable risperidone: efficacy and safety of the first long-acting atypical antipsychotic. Am J Psychiatry 160:1125–1132, 2003a

Kane JM, Leucht S, Carpenter D, et al (eds): Optimizing pharmacologic treatment of psychotic disorders (Expert Consensus Guideline Series). J Clin Psychiatry 64 (suppl 12):1–99, 2003b

Kaplan HI, Sadock BJ, Grebb JA (eds): Synopsis of Psychiatry, 7th Edition. Baltimore, MD, Williams & Wilkins, 1994, pp 933–959

Kapur S, Mamo D: Half a century of antipsychotics and still a central role for dopamine D_2 receptors. Prog Neuropsychopharmacol Biol Psychiatry 27:1081–1090, 2003

Kapur S, Zipursky R, Jones C, et al: A positron emission tomography study of quetiapine in schizophrenia: a preliminary finding of an antipsychotic effect with only transiently high dopamine D_2 receptor occupancy. Arch Gen Psychiatry 57:553–559, 2000

Katz IR, Jeste DV, Mintzer JE, et al: Comparison of risperidone and placebo for psychosis and behavioral disturbances associated with dementia: a randomized, double-blind trial. Risperidone Study Group. J Clin Psychiatry 60:107–115, 1999

Keck PE, Wilson DR, Strakowski SM, et al: Clinical predictors of acute risperidone response in schizophrenia, schizoaffective disorder, and psychotic mood disorders. J Clin Psychiatry 56:466–470, 1995

Keck PE, Buse JB, Dagogo-Jack S, et al: Managing metabolic concerns in patients with severe mental illness. Postgrad Med, December 2003a, pp 7–89

Keck PE Jr, Marcus R, Tourkodimitris S, et al: A placebo-controlled, double-blind study of the efficacy and safety of aripiprazole in patients with acute bipolar mania. Am J Psychiatry 160:1651–1658, 2003b

Keck PE Jr, Versiani M, Potkin S, et al: Ziprasidone in the treatment of acute bipolar mania: a 3-week, placebo-controlled, double-blind, randomized trial. Am J Psychiatry 160:741–748, 2003c

Keith SJ, Schooler NR: Treatment of schizophreniform disorder, in Treatments of Psychiatric Disorders. Edited by Karasu TB. Washington, DC, American Psychiatric Association, 1989, pp 1656–1665

Kelly JF, Berardki A, Raffaele K, et al: Intravenous haloperidol causes greater memory impairment in old compared to young healthy subjects. Presentation at the annual meeting of the American Geriatrics Society, New Orleans, LA, November 1993

Knegtering R, Castelein S, Bous H, et al: A randomized open-label study of the impact of quetiapine versus risperidone on sexual functioning. J Clin Psychopharmacol 24:56–61, 2004

Koran LM: Obsessive-Compulsive and Related Disorders in Adults. Cambridge, UK, Cambridge University Press, 1999, pp 117–118

Koran LM, Ringold AL, Elliott MA: Olanzapine augmentation for treatment-resistant obsessive-compulsive disorder. J Clin Psychiatry 61:514–517, 2000

Kossen M, Selten JP, Kahn RS: Elevated clozapine plasma level with lamotrigine (letter). Am J Psychiatry 158:1930, 2001

Kujawa M, Saha AR, Ingenito CG, et al: Aripiprazole for long-term maintenance treatment of schizophrenia (abstract). Int J Neuropsychopharmacol 5 (suppl 1):S186, 2002

Kukopulos A, Reginaldi D, Laddomada P, et al: Course of the manic-depressive cycle and changes caused by treatments. Pharmakopsychiatr Neuropsychopharmakol 13:156–167, 1980

Lacro JP, Kuczenski R, Roznoski M, et al: Serum haloperidol levels in older psychotic patients. Am J Geriatr Psychiatry 4:229–236, 1996

Lee HS, Kwon KY, Alphs LD, et al. Effect of clozapine on psychogenic polydipsia in chronic schizophrenia. J Clin Psychopharmacol 11:222–223, 1991

Leipzig RM, Mendelowitz A: Adverse psychotropic drug-drug interactions, in Adverse Effects of Psychotropic Drugs. Edited by Kane JM, Lieberman JA. New York, Guilford, 1992, pp 13–76

Leo RJ: Movement disorders associated with the serotonin selective reuptake inhibitors. J Clin Psychiatry 57:449–454, 1996

Leucht S, Wahlbeck K, Hamann J, et al: New generation antipsychotics versus low-potency conventional antipsychotics: a systematic review and meta-analysis. Lancet 361:1581–1589, 2003

Levinson DF, Simpson GM, Singh H, et al: Fluphenazine dose, clinical response, and extrapyramidal symptoms during acute treatment. Arch Gen Psychiatry 47:761–768, 1990

Levinson DF, Umapathy C, Musthaq M: Treatment of schizoaffective disorder and schizophrenia with mood symptoms. Am J Psychiatry 156:1138–1148, 1999

Liberman RP, Mueser RP, Mueser KT, et al: Social skills training for schizophrenic individuals at risk for relapse. Am J Psychiatry 143:523–526, 1986

Lieberman DZ (chairperson), Casey DE, Crismon ML, et al: Special Report: Medication Management Considerations in Schizophrenia. Washington, DC, George Washington University Medical Center/American Pharmaceutical Association, 2002, pp 1–17

Lieberman JA: Aripiprazole, in The American Psychiatric Publishing Textbook of Psychopharmacology, 3rd Edition. Edited by Schatzberg AF, Nemeroff CB. Washington, DC, American Psychiatric Publishing, 2004, pp 487–494

Lindenmayer J-P, Apergi F-S: The relationship between clozapine plasma levels and clinical response. Psychiatr Ann 26:406–412, 1996

Madhusoodanan S, Brenner R, Araujo L, et al: Efficacy of risperidone treatment for psychoses associated with schizophrenia, schizoaffective disorder, bipolar disorder, or senile dementia in 11 geriatric patients: a case series. J Clin Psychiatry 56:514–518, 1995

Manschreck TC: Delusional disorder (interview). Current Approaches to Psychoses 5(April):7–9, 1996

Marder SR, Wirshing DA: Clozapine, in The American Psychiatric Publishing Textbook of Psychopharmacology, 3rd Edition. Edited by Schatzberg AF, Nemeroff CB. Washington, DC, American Psychiatric Publishing, 2004, pp 443–456

Marsden CD, Jenner P: The pathophysiology of extrapyramidal side-effects of neuroleptic drugs. Psychol Med 10:55–72, 1980

Martenyi F, Harangozo J, Mod L: Clonazepam for the treatment of stupor in catatonic schizophrenia (letter). Am J Psychiatry 146:1230, 1989

Martin H, Slyk MP, Deymann S, et al: Safety profile assessment of risperidone and olanzapine in long-term care patients with dementia. J Am Med Dir Assoc 4:183–188, 2003

Mathews M, Mathews M, Mathews J: How to remedy excessive salivation in patients taking clozapine. Current Psychiatry 2:80, 2003

McCarthy RH, Terkelsen KG: Esophageal dysfunction in two patients after clozapine treatment (letter). J Clin Psychopharmacol 14:281–283, 1994

McDougle CJ, Goodman WK, Price LH, et al: Neuroleptic addition in fluvoxamine-refractory obsessive-compulsive disorder. Am J Psychiatry 147:652–654, 1990

McDougle CJ, Fleischmann RL, Epperson CN, et al: Risperidone addition in fluvoxamine-refractory obsessive-compulsive disorder: three cases. J Clin Psychiatry 56:526–528, 1995

McElhatton PR: The use of phenothiazines during pregnancy and lactation. Reprod Toxicol 6:475–490, 1992

McGlashan TH: Schizophrenia: psychosocial treatments and the role of psychosocial factors in its etiology and pathogenesis, in Psychiatry Update: American Psychiatric Association Annual Review, Vol 5. Edited by Frances AJ, Hales RE. Washington, DC, American Psychiatric Press, 1986, pp 96–111

McIntyre R, Traskas K, Lin D, et al: Risk of weight gain associated with antipsychotic treatment: results from the Canadian National Outcomes Measurement Study in Schizophrenia. Can J Psychiatry 48:689–694, 2003

Meehan K, Zhang F, David S, et al: A double-blind, randomized comparison of the efficacy and safety of intramuscular injections of olanzapine, lorazepam, or placebo in treating acutely agitated patients diagnosed with bipolar mania. J Clin Psychopharmacol 21:389–397, 2001

Meltzer HY: Atypical antipsychotic drugs, in Psychopharmacology: The Fourth Generation of Progress. Edited by Bloom FE, Kupfer DJ. New York, Raven, 1995, pp 1277–1286

Meltzer HY: Suicidality in schizophrenia: a review of the evidence for risk factors and treatment options. Curr Psychiatry Rep 4:279–283, 2002

Meltzer HY, Matsubara S, Lee JC: Classification of typical and atypical drugs on the basis of dopamine D_1, D_2 and serotonin$_2$ pK_i values. J Pharmacol Exp Ther 251:238–246, 1989

Millan MJ: Improving the treatment of schizophrenia: focus on serotonin (5HT-1A) receptors. J Pharmacol Exp Ther 295:853–861, 2000

Miyamoto S, Duncan GE, Goff DC, et al: Therapeutics of schizophrenia, in Neuropsychopharmacology: The Fifth Generation of Progress. Edited by Davis KL, Charney DS, Coyle JT, et al. Philadelphia, PA, Lippincott Williams & Wilkins, 2002, pp 775–807

Moller HJ: New (i.e., atypical) neuroleptic agents for negative symptoms of schizophrenia: results and methodological problems of evaluation. Nervenarzt 71:345–353, 2000

Mouly S, Lown KS, Kornhauser D: Hepatic but not intestinal CYP3A4 displays dose-dependent induction by efavirenz in humans. Clin Pharmacol Ther 72:1–9, 2002

Naimark D, Harris J, Jeste DV: Use of atypical neuroleptics in the elderly. Geriatric Psychiatry News 1(September/October):12–13, 1995

Nakane Y, Rapoport J: Childhood-onset schizophrenia (interview). Current Approaches to Psychoses 4(October):1–4, 1995

Navarro V, Pons A, Romero A, et al: Topiramate for clozapine-induced seizures. Am J Psychiatry 158:968–969, 2001

Nemeroff CB, Devane CL, Pollack BG: Summary and review of antidepressants and the cytochrome P450 system. ASCP Progress Notes 6(Fall–Winter):38–40, 1995–1996

Newport DJ, Fisher A, Graybeal S, et al: Psychopharmacology during pregnancy and lactation, in The American Psychiatric Publishing Textbook of Psychopharmacology, 3rd Edition. Edited by Schatzberg AF, Nemeroff CB. Washington, DC, American Psychiatric Publishing, 2004, pp 1109–1146

Nguyen HN, Lalonde P: Clozapine and pregnancy. Encephale 29:119–124, 2003

Oepen G: Polypharmacy in schizophrenia, in Polypharmacy in Psychiatry. Edited by Ghaemi SN. New York, Marcel Dekker, 2002, pp 101–132

Okuma T, Yamashita I, Takahashi R, et al: A double-blind study of adjunctive carbamazepine versus placebo on excited states of schizophrenic and schizoaffective disorders. Acta Psychiatr Scand 80:250–259, 1989

Osser DN: A systematic approach to pharmacotherapy in patients with neuroleptic-resistant psychosis. Hosp Community Psychiatry 40:921–926, 1989

Osser DN, Patterson RD: Pharmacotherapy of schizophrenia, I: acute treatment, in Handbook for the Treatment of the Seriously Mentally Ill. Edited by Soreff SM. Seattle, WA, Hogrefe & Huber, 1996, pp 91–119

Osser DN, Sigadel R: Short-term inpatient pharmacotherapy of schizophrenia. Harv Rev Psychiatry 9:89–104, 2001

Osser DN, Najarian DM, Dufresne RL: Olanzapine increases weight and serum triglyceride levels. J Clin Psychiatry 60:767–770, 1999

Ovsiew F: Bedside neuropsychiatry: eliciting the clinical phenomena of neuropsychiatric illness, in The American Psychiatric Press Textbook of Neuropsychiatry, 2nd Edition. Edited by Yudofsky SC, Hales RE. Washington, DC, American Psychiatric Press, 1992, pp 99–101

Patton SW, Misri S, Corral MR, et al: Antipsychotic medication during pregnancy and lactation in women with schizophrenia: evaluating the risk. Can J Psychiatry 47:959–965, 2002

Pearlman CA: Neuroleptic malignant syndrome: a review of the literature. J Clin Psychopharmacol 6:257–273, 1986

Pearlman C: Clozapine, nocturnal sialorrhea, and choking (letter). J Clin Psychopharmacol 14:283, 1994

Perry PJ, Alexander B, Liskow BI: Psychotropic Drug Handbook. Washington, DC, American Psychiatric Press, 1997

Petersdorf RG: Hypothermia and hyperthermia, in Harrison's Principles of Internal Medicine, 12th Edition. Edited by Wilson JD, Braunwald E, Isselbacher KJ, et al. New York, McGraw-Hill, 1991, pp 2194–2200

Peterson BS: Natural history, pathophysiology, and treatment of Tourette's syndrome. J Clin Psychiatry (Monograph Series) 13(1):17–19, 1995

Phillips KA: Body dysmorphic disorder: the distress of imagined ugliness. Am J Psychiatry 148:1138–1149, 1991

Physicians' Desk Reference, 49th Edition. Montvale, NJ, Medical Economics, 1995, p 2150

Physicians' Desk Reference, 50th edition. Montvale, NJ, Medical Economics, 1996

Physicians' Desk Reference, 58th Edition. Montvale, NJ, Thompson Healthcare, 2004

Pies R: Distinguishing obsessional from psychotic phenomena. J Clin Psychopharmacol 6:345–347, 1984

Pies RW: Clinical Manual of Psychiatric Diagnosis and Treatment. Washington, DC, American Psychiatric Press, 1994, pp 466–469

Pies RW: Combining antipsychotics: risks and benefits. Int Drug Ther Newsl 36:9–13, 2001

Pies RW, Dewan MJ: The difficult-to-treat patient with schizophrenia, in The Difficult-to-Treat Psychiatric Patient. Edited by Dewan MJ, Pies RW. Washington, DC, American Psychiatric Publishing, 2001, pp 41–80

Pies R, Popli AP: Self-injurious behavior: pathophysiology and implications for treatment. J Clin Psychiatry 56:580–588, 1995

Pool D, Bloom W, Mielke DH, et al: A controlled evaluation of Loxitane in seventy-five adolescent schizophrenia patients. Curr Ther Res 19:99–104, 1976

Potkin SG, Saha AR, Kujawa MJ, et al: Aripiprazole, an antipsychotic with a novel mechanism of action, and risperidone vs placebo in patients with schizophrenia and schizoaffective disorder. Arch Gen Psychiatry 60:681–690, 2003

Rapoport JL: Clozapine and child psychiatry. J Child Adolesc Psychopharmacol 4:1–3, 1994

Raskin S, Katz G, Zislin Z, et al: Clozapine and risperidone: combination/augmentation treatment of refractory schizophrenia: a preliminary observation. Acta Psychiatr Scand 101:334–336, 2000

Raskind MA: Treatment of Alzheimer's disease and other dementias, in The American Psychiatric Press Textbook of Psychopharmacology, 2nd Edition, Edited by Schatzberg AF, Nemeroff CB. Washington, DC, American Psychiatric Press, 1995, pp 657–667

Ratey JJ, MacNaughton KL: Beta-blockers, in Drug Interactions in Psychiatry, 2nd Edition. Edited by Ciraulo DA, Shader RI, Greenblatt DJ, et al. Baltimore, MD, Williams & Wilkins, 1995, pp 311–355

Remschmidt H, Schulz E, Martin M: An open trial of clozapine in thirty-six adolescents with schizophrenia. J Child Adolesc Psychopharmacol 4:31–41, 1994

Rhoads E: Polypharmacy of two atypical antipsychotics. J Clin Psychiatry 61:678–679, 2000

Rogers D: The metabolic syndrome (Bipolar Disorder and Impulsive Spectrum letter). Psychiatric Times 20 (suppl):1–4, 2003

Roose SP, Pollock BG, Devanand DP: Treatment during late life, in The American Psychiatric Publishing Textbook of Psychopharmacology, 3rd Edition. Edited by Schatzberg AF, Nemeroff CB. Washington, DC, American Psychiatric Publishing, 2004, pp 1083–1108

Rosebush P, Stuart T: A prospective analysis of 24 episodes of neuroleptic malignant syndrome. Am J Psychiatry 146:717–725, 1989

Rosenblatt JE, Rosenblatt NC: Clinical psychopharmacology online. Currents in Affective Illness 22(October):4, 2003

Rosenheck R, Perlick D, Bingham S, et al: Effectiveness and cost of olanzapine and haloperidol in the treatment of schizophrenia: a randomized controlled trial. JAMA 290:2693–2702, 2003

Roth M: Delusional (paranoid) disorders, in Treatments of Psychiatric Disorders. Edited by Karasu TB. Washington, DC, American Psychiatric Association, 1989, pp 1609–1648

Sachdev P, Loneragan C: Intravenous benztropine and propranolol challenges in acute neuroleptic-induced akathisia. Clin Neuropharmacol 16:324–331, 1993

Sachdev P, Kruk J, Kneebone M, et al: Clozapine-induced neuroleptic malignant syndrome: review and report of new cases. J Clin Psychopharmacol 15:365–370, 1995

Salzman C, Satlin A, Burrows AB: Geriatric psychopharmacology, in The American Psychiatric Press Textbook of Psychopharmacology, 2nd Edition. Edited by Schatzberg AF, Nemeroff CB. Washington, DC, American Psychiatric Press, 1995, pp 803–821

Schexnayder LW, Hirschowitz J, Sautter FJ, et al: Predictors of response to lithium in patients with psychoses. Am J Psychiatry 152:1511–1513, 1995

Schulz SC, Olson S, Kotlyar M: Olanzapine, in The American Psychiatric Publishing Textbook of Psychopharmacology, 3rd Edition. Edited by Schatzberg AF, Nemeroff CB. Washington, DC, American Psychiatric Publishing, 2004, pp 457–472

Seeman P: Dopamine receptors: clinical correlates, in Psychopharmacology: The Fourth Generation of Progress. Edited by Bloom FE, Kupfer DJ. New York, Raven, 1995, pp 295–302

Seeman P: Atypical antipsychotics: mechanism of action. Can J Psychiatry 47:27–38, 2002

Segraves RT: Sexual dysfunction complicating the treatment of depression. J Clin Psychiatry (Monograph Series) 10(1):75–79, 1992

Sensky T, Turkington D, Kingdon D, et al: A randomized controlled trial of cognitive behavioral therapy for persistent symptoms in schizophrenia resistant to medication. Arch Gen Psychiatry 57:165–172, 2000

Shader RI: Dissociative, somatoform, and paranoid disorders, in Manual of Psychiatric Therapeutics, 2nd Edition. Boston, MA, Little, Brown, 1994, pp 15–23

Shader RI: Approaches to the treatment of schizophrenia, in Manual of Psychiatric Therapeutics, 3rd Edition. Philadelphia, PA, Lippincott Williams & Wilkins, 2003a, pp 285–314

Shader RI: Medical evaluation of psychiatric patients and the acute treatment of psychotropic drug overdose, in Manual of Psychiatric Therapeutics, 3rd Edition. Philadelphia, PA, Lippincott Williams & Wilkins, 2003b, pp 17–51

Shelton RC, Tollefson GD, Tohen M, et al: A novel augmentation strategy for treating resistant major depression. Am J Psychiatry 158:131–134, 2001

Sherman C: Adherence problems persist in schizophrenia. Clinical Psychiatry News, June 2004, p 12

Shiloh R, Zemishlany D, Aizenberg D, et al: Sulpiride augmentation in people with schizophrenia partially responsive to clozapine. Br J Psychiatry 171:569–573, 1997

Simpson GM: Postmarketing evaluation of haloperidol decanoate injection: efficacy, safety, and dosing considerations. J Clin Psychiatry 1:1–8, 1988

Skogh E, Reis M, Dahl ML, et al: Therapeutic drug monitoring data on olanzapine and its N-demethyl metabolite in the naturalistic clinical setting. Ther Drug Monit 24:518–526, 2002

Soloff RH, George A, Nathan R, et al: Progress in pharmacotherapy of borderline disorders: a double-blind study of amitriptyline, haloperidol, and placebo. Arch Gen Psychiatry 43:691–697, 1986

Spears NM, Leadbetter RA, Shutty MS: Clozapine treatment in polydipsia and intermittent hyponatremia. J Clin Psychiatry 57:123–128, 1996

Stahl SM: Antipsychotic polypharmacy, Part 1: therapeutic option or dirty little secret? J Clin Psychiatry 60:425–426, 1999

Stanilla JK, Simpson GM: Drugs to treat extrapyramidal side effects, in The American Psychiatric Publishing Textbook of Psychopharmacology, 3rd Edition. Edited by Schatzberg AF, Nemeroff CB. Washington, DC, American Psychiatric Publishing, 2004, pp 519–544

Sternbach H: The serotonin syndrome. Am J Psychiatry 148:705–713, 1991

Stowe ZN, Nemeroff CB: Psychopharmacology during pregnancy and lactation, in The American Psychiatric Press Textbook of Psychopharmacology, 2nd Edition. Edited by Schatzberg AF, Nemeroff CB. Washington, DC, American Psychiatric Press, 1995, pp 823–837

Suppes T, McElroy SL, Gilbert J, et al: Clozapine in the treatment of dysphoric mania. Biol Psychiatry 32:270–280, 1992

Suppes T, Swann AC, Dennehy EB, et al: Texas Medication Algorithm Project: development and feasibility testing of a treatment algorithm for patients with bipolar disorder. J Clin Psychiatry 62:439–447, 2001

Sussman N: Augmentation of antipsychotic drugs with selective serotonin reuptake inhibitors. Primary Psychiatry 4:24–31, 1997

Sylvester B: Olanzapine helps compliance in schizophrenia. Clinical Psychiatry News, January 2004, p 29

Tariot PN, Salzman C, Yeung PP, et al: Long-term use of quetiapine in elderly patients with psychotic disorders. Clin Ther 22:1068–1084, 2000

Theoharides TC, Harris RS, Weckstein D: Neuroleptic malignant-like syndrome due to cyclobenzaprine? J Clin Psychopharmacol 15:79–81, 1995

Thompson JW, Ware MR, Blashfield RK: Psychotropic medication and priapism: a comprehensive review. J Clin Psychiatry 51:430–433, 1990

Tohen M, Sanger TM, McElroy SL, et al: Olanzapine versus placebo in the treatment of acute mania. Olanzapine HGEH Study Group. Am J Psychiatry 156:702–709, 1999

Tohen M, Jacobs TG, Grundy SL, et al: Efficacy of olanzapine in acute bipolar mania: a double-blind, placebo-controlled study. The Olanzapine HGGW Study Group. Arch Gen Psychiatry 57:841–849, 2000

Troster AI, Fields JA, Koller WC: in The American Psychiatric Press Textbook of Geriatric Neuropsychiatry. Edited by Coffey CE, Cummings JL. Washington, DC, American Psychiatric Press, 2000, pp 559–600

Tsang MW, Shader RI, Greenblatt DJ: Metabolism of haloperidol: clinical implications and unanswered questions (editorial). J Clin Psychopharmacol 14:159–161, 1994

Tueth MJ, DeVane CL, Evans DL: Treatment of psychiatric emergencies, in The American Psychiatric Press Textbook of Psychopharmacology, 2nd Edition. Edited by Schatzberg AF, Nemeroff CB. Washington, DC, American Psychiatric Press, 1995, pp 769–781

Tyson SC, DeVane CL, Risch SC: Pharmacokinetic interaction between risperidone and clozapine (letter). Am J Psychiatry 152:1401–1402, 1995

VanderZwaag C, McGee M, McEvoy JP, et al: Response of patients with treatment-refractory schizophrenia to clozapine within three serum level ranges. Am J Psychiatry 153:1579–1584, 1996

Van Putten T, Marder SR, Mintz J: A controlled dose comparison of haloperidol in newly admitted schizophrenic patients. Arch Gen Psychiatry 47:754–758, 1990a

Van Putten T, Marder SR, Wirshing W, et al: Neuroleptic plasma levels in treatment-resistant schizophrenic patients, in The Neuroleptic-Nonresponsive Patient: Characterization and Treatment. Edited by Angrist B, Schulz SC. Washington, DC, American Psychiatric Press, 1990b, pp 69–85

Vazquez E: Sustiva flashbacks. Posit Aware 10:17, 1999

Velamoor VR, Swamy GN, Parmar RS, et al: Management of suspected neuroleptic syndrome. Can J Psychiatry 40:545–550, 1995

Venkatakrishnan K, Shader RI, von Moltke LL, et al: Drug interactions in psychopharmacology, in Manual of Psychiatric Therapeutics, 3rd Edition. Edited by Shader RI. Philadelphia, PA, Lippincott Williams & Wilkins, 2003, pp 441–470

Vieta E, Goikolea JM, Corbella B, et al: Risperidone safety and efficacy in the treatment of bipolar and schizoaffective disorders: results from a 6-month, multicenter, open study. J Clin Psychiatry 62:818–825, 2001

Viguera AC, Baldessarini RJ, Hegarty JM, et al: Clinical risk following abrupt and gradual withdrawal of maintenance neuroleptic treatment. Arch Gen Psychiatry 54:49–55, 1997

Wagner KD: Treatment of childhood and adolescent disorders, in The American Psychiatric Publishing Textbook of Psychopharmacology, 3rd Edition. Edited by Schatzberg AF, Nemeroff CB. Washington, DC, American Psychiatric Publishing, 2004, pp 949–1007

Waldman MD, Safferman AZ: Pregnancy and clozapine (letter). Am J Psychiatry 150:168–169, 1993

Warner JP, Barnes TRE, Henry JA: Electrocardiographic changes in patients receiving neuroleptic medication. Acta Psychiatr Scand 93:311–313, 1996

Webster P, Wijeratne C: Risperidone-induced neuroleptic malignant syndrome (letter). Lancet 344:1228–1229, 1994

Weiden PJ: Establishing therapeutic goals in schizophrenia, in Modern Approach to the Pharmacologic and Psychosocial Treatment of Schizophrenia and Psychosis (Advanced Studies in Medicine, Johns Hopkins University School of Medicine). Somerville, NJ, Galen Publishing, 2003, pp 782–787

Wirshing WC, Marder SR, Van Putten T, et al: Acute treatment of schizophrenia, in Progress in Psychopharmacology: The Fourth Generation of Progress. Edited by Bloom FE, Kupfer DJ. New York, Raven, 1995, pp 1259–1266

Young CR, Bostic JQ, McDanald CL: Clozapine and refractory obsessive-compulsive disorder: a case report. J Clin Psychopharmacol 14:209–210, 1994

Yudofsky SC, Silver JM, Schneider SE: Pharmacologic treatment of aggression. Psychiatr Ann 17:397–406, 1987

Zalsman G, Carmon E, Martin A, et al: Effectiveness, safety, and tolerability of risperidone in adolescents with schizophrenia: an open-label study. J Child Adolesc Psychopharmacol 13:319–327, 2003

Zanarini MC, Frankenburg FR: Olanzapine treatment of female borderline personality disorder patients: a double-blind, placebo-controlled pilot study. J Clin Psychiatry 62:849–854, 2001

Zanarini MC, Silk KN: The difficult-to-treat patient with borderline personality disorder, in The Difficult-to-Treat Psychiatric Patient. Edited by Dewan MJ, Pies RW. Washington, DC, American Psychiatric Publishing, 2001, pp 179–208

Zarate CA, Tohen M, Baldessarini RJ: Clozapine in severe mood disorders. J Clin Psychiatry 56:411–417, 1995

CHAPTER 4

ANXIOLYTICS AND SEDATIVE-HYPNOTICS

Overview

Drug Class

Anxiolytics and hypnotics comprise a wide variety of pharmacological agents, including many "antidepressants" now approved for use in anxiety disorders. Indeed, selective serotonin reuptake inhibitors (SSRIs) and related agents are gradually becoming the drugs of first choice for several anxiety disorders. Nevertheless, in many clinical settings, benzodiazepines (BZDs) are by far the most frequently prescribed anxiolytics and still make up a large percentage of prescribed hypnotic agents. In recent years, however, zolpidem—a non-BZD—has become the most widely prescribed hypnotic in the United States. Other non-BZD hypnotics (e.g., zaleplon, zopiclone) are finding increasing use in the United States and abroad; indeed, *eszopiclone* has received an "approvable letter" from the U.S. Food and Drug Administration (FDA) and is expected to be available shortly.

Although the BZDs are sometimes classified by chemical structure, their clinical use is more directly influenced by pharmacokinetic factors, such as metabolic pathway and $t_{1/2}\beta$. The *azapirone* anxiolytic buspirone has been found effective for use in treating patients with generalized anxiety; at higher doses, this class of agents may have antidepressant properties. Other drugs sometimes used as anxiolytics or hypnotics include some antihistamines, several non-SSRI antidepressants, and the "first generation" agents with high abuse potential, such as chloral hydrate, barbiturates, and meprobamate, which are virtually never used in modern psychiatric practice. *Anti-noradrenergic agents,* including clonidine and guanfacine, are occasionally used to treat various forms of anxiety or agitation, as are beta-blockers. There is growing interest in the *anticonvulsants* as anxiolytic agents (e.g., valproate, lamotrigine, gabapentin, and tiagabine). Although none of these anticonvulsants has FDA-approved labeling for use in anxiety disorders, both clinical and theoretical considerations suggest they may be useful. In selected cases, atypical antipsychotics are also used—usually adjunctively—in treating anxiety disorders.

Given the plethora of potential "anti-anxiety" agents, in this chapter I focus primarily on BZDs; newer antidepressants used as anxiolytics; and several non-BZD hypnotic agents. Details regarding the pharmacokinetics, side effects, drug interactions, and other aspects of antidepressants are discussed in Chapter 2 ("Antidepressants").

Indications

The BZD anxiolytic-hypnotics are used primarily in the treatment of generalized anxiety disorder (GAD) and panic disorder and in the short-term treatment of stress-related insomnia. There is still controversy as to the efficacy and safety of long-term BZD use for chronic insomnia, stemming mainly from a paucity of long-term studies. The BZDs are also the agents of choice in the treatment of alcohol withdrawal, and they may be useful for various kinds of extrapyramidal symptoms, nocturnal myoclonus, and night terrors. In addition, the BZDs have found use as adjunctive agents in the treatment of mania and acute psychosis, usually combined with mood stabilizers and antipsychotics, respectively. There is less convincing evidence for the role of BZDs in the adjunctive treatment of obsessive-compulsive disorder (OCD), social phobia disorder, avoidant personality disorder, posttraumatic stress disorder (PTSD), and depression. The non-BZD anxiolytic buspirone is useful in the treatment of GAD, but not panic disorder.

Recently, a number of newer antidepressants have received FDA-approved labeling for use in various anxiety disorders (see Table 4–6). As of this writing, four SSRIs are now labeled for use in OCD; three for panic disorder; two for PTSD; two for social phobia; and two for GAD. Venlafaxine—often referred to as a *serotonin-norepinephrine reuptake inhibitor,* or SNRI, though it is primarily a serotonergic agent—also has FDA-approved labeling in GAD. We may assume confidently that this list of FDA-approved "anxiolytic antidepressants" will grow in the near future.

Mechanisms of Action

$GABA_A$, a receptor of γ-aminobutyric acid (GABA), is the binding site for BZDs, barbiturates, neurosteroids, and several non-BZD hypnotics, including zolpidem, zaleplon, zopiclone, and eszopiclone. All these agents are GABA agonists, though they may also have other mechanisms of action. They cause an influx of negatively charged chloride ions, leading to hyperpolarization of the neuron and decreased firing rate. The $GABA_A$ receptor consists of five subunits in a rosette—usually two α subunits, two β subunits, and one γ unit. These subunits have variant forms, such as α_1, α_2, β_2, and so forth. GABA itself binds to the β subunit of the $GABA_A$ receptor. BZDs bind to the major binding cleft defined by the *interface* of the α and γ subunits. All standard BZDs bind to receptors containing α_1, α_2, or α_3 subunits. The non-BZD hypnotics zolpidem (Ambien) and zaleplon (Sonata) also bind to the BZD site on the $GABA_A$ receptor; however, they bind with high affinity only to receptors containing the α_1 subunit (termed ω_1 receptors in the older literature). Eszopiclone (Lunesta, formerly Estorra), which was recently approved for the treatment of insomnia, also interacts with the BZD site on the $GABA_A$ receptor but probably binds to different "microdomains" within the γ subunit than do BZDs, zolpidem, and zaleplon (Davies et al. 2000). Since different α receptor subunits are expressed to different degrees in certain brain regions (e.g., cortex, brain stem), these binding properties may have clinical implications for the various BZD and non-BZD hypnotics, for example, with respect to amnestic, sedative, and true hypnotic effects. In contrast to the BZDs, the drug tiagabine (Gabitril) *inhibits reuptake* of GABA, leading to more of it in the synaptic cleft. The mechanism of the azapirone anxiolytic buspirone is completely different from that of BZDs, involving variable effects at serotonin receptors; for example, buspirone is a partial agonist at the postsynaptic serotonin$_{1A}$ (5-HT$_{1A}$) receptor. Buspirone may have antidepressant effects when given in high doses.

The mechanism of action of the SSRIs and other antidepressants has already been described in Chapter 2 ("Antidepressants"). Interestingly, however, some recent research suggests that at least one SSRI, fluoxetine, may actually have GABAergic effects, perhaps by acting through a modulatory site on the GABA$_A$ receptor (Robinson et al. 2003).

Pharmacokinetics

The BZDs may be divided into three main groups—long-, intermediate-, and short-acting—based on their elimination half-lives (McGee and Pies 2002). Most of the *longer-acting* agents share a common active intermediate, *desmethyldiazepam,* which has a $t_{1/2}\beta$ exceeding 60 hours (and generally longer in the elderly). Long-acting BZDs undergo oxidative metabolism, which is sensitive to alterations in hepatic function. Three of the *intermediate-acting* BZDs—*lorazepam, oxazepam,* and *temazepam*—require only *glucuronidation* and are relatively unaffected by alterations in hepatic function. Their use in hepatically impaired patients, or in those receiving various enzyme inhibitors, may be preferable. *Estazolam* (used as a hypnotic agent) and *alprazolam* are intermediate-duration BZDs; both undergo oxidative metabolism but have no active metabolites of significant duration. Another intermediate-acting agent, *clonazepam,* undergoes *nitroreduction* as its primary metabolic step. *Triazolam,* which has a $t_{1/2}$ of only about 3 hours, is the only *short-acting* BZD in general clinical use. (*Midazolam,* which has a $t_{1/2}$ of about 2 hours, is used primarily as a presurgical sedative.) Those BZDs that undergo oxidative metabolism are usually substrates of the cytochrome P450 (CYP) 3A3 (3A3/4) and 2C19 systems.

The non-BZD hypnotics *zolpidem* and *zaleplon* are metabolized in part via CYP 3A4, although zaleplon is metabolized mainly by aldehyde oxidase. *Buspirone* is also metabolized via CYP 3A4. Zopiclone and its *S*-isomer, *eszopiclone,* undergo complex metabolism involving CYP 3A4 (Cozza et al. 2003). The pharmacokinetics of SSRIs and related antidepressants are discussed in Chapter 2 ("Antidepressants").

Main Side Effects

The side effects of BZDs are primarily extensions of their sedative properties. Though generally well tolerated, BZDs can produce drowsiness, fatigue, weakness, lightheadedness, ataxia, respiratory suppression, and falls. Confusion, psychomotor impairment, amnesia, depression, and paradoxical excitation are also seen. Some predisposed individuals can become psychologically and/or physically dependent on BZDs (McGee and Pies 2002). Significant withdrawal effects (e.g., seizures) may be seen if BZDs are suddenly discontinued. *Rebound insomnia* may be seen with sudden discontinuation of short-acting (and to some degree, intermediate-acting) BZDs. Buspirone is generally well tolerated, although it can occasionally produce dizziness, gastrointestinal disturbance, and headache.

Some evidence indicates that non-BZD hypnotics, if taken in recommended doses, are less likely to provoke cognitive and amnestic side effects than are BZDs. However, this may be more the case with zaleplon than with zolpidem (Jacobson et al. 2002). Withdrawal syndromes may be less common following sudden discontinuation of zolpidem, zaleplon, and eszopiclone than following sudden discontinuation of BZD hypnotics.

The antihistamines—often purchased "over-the-counter" as sleep aids—are not true hypnotic agents and rapidly produce tolerance (Richardson et al. 2002). First-generation antihistamines, such as diphenhydramine, may also produce impaired attention and confusion in susceptible individuals (Witek et al. 1995), as well as constipation and urinary retention.

Drug–Drug Interactions

BZDs are generally safe in combination with most other medications. However, a variety of drugs may increase the plasma levels and/or toxicity of oxidatively metabolized BZDs (e.g., cimetidine, ketoconazole, fluvoxamine, nefazodone, fluoxetine, erythromycin, and various protease inhibitors used to treat HIV infection). In contrast, rifampin, phenobarbital, carbamazepine, oxcarbazepine, and phenytoin may decrease the clinical effects of some BZDs, probably via induction of hepatic metabolism. The coadministration of BZDs and anticholinergic agents may lead to greater cognitive impairment than administration of either drug class alone. The combination of BZDs with clozapine has led to severe sedation and/or cardiorespiratory suppression in some individuals. BZDs may increase the neurotoxicity of alcohol, narcotics, and other central nervous system (CNS) depressants. Although the BZDs by themselves have little toxicity in overdose, they may be lethal when combined with alcohol or other CNS depressants.

Buspirone is generally well tolerated in combination with most other drugs, though pharmacodynamic interactions may occur in combination with monoamine oxidase inhibitors (MAOIs) or other agents with serotonergic properties. Drugs that inhibit metabolism of the CYP 3A4 system are likely to elevate blood levels of the non-BZDs buspirone, zolpidem, and zopiclone (Cozza et al. 2003).

Potentiating Maneuvers

Some reports suggest that BZDs may be potentiated by the addition of buspirone, for example, in the treatment of GAD. Beta-blockers may also be used in combination with BZDs, though hypotension may result. BZDs are often used in combination with antidepressants, but the effect of BZDs on depression per se is equivocal. For example, BZDs may sometimes worsen preexisting depression. BZDs are useful in potentiating the effects of antimanic and antipsychotic agents, and may reduce the dosage of antipsychotic medication needed for management of acute mania or psychosis. Recently, a small, open study found benefits from adjunctive use of the GABA reuptake inhibitor tiagabine in PTSD patients (F. B. Taylor 2003).

Use in Special Populations

The use of BZDs during the first trimester of pregnancy is associated with cleft lip or palate and possibly with impaired intrauterine growth. However, the absolute risk of such problems appears small. Infants exposed to BZDs either in the last trimester or at the time of parturition may show a “floppy baby syndrome,” characterized by muscular hypotonicity, lethargy, failure to feed, impaired temperature regulation (hypothermia), poor respiratory effort, and low Apgar scores (Newport et al. 2004). There are insufficient data in humans to determine the risks of using buspirone, zolpidem, and zaleplon during pregnancy.

In elderly and medically ill populations, the use of BZDs is generally best undertaken on a short-term basis. In these populations, BZDs may be associated with cognitive impairment; falls and hip fractures; behavioral disinhibition: confusion (particularly in dementia patients); reduced hepatic metabolism; drug–drug interactions; and “hangover” effects from long-acting hypnotic agents (Jacobson et al. 2002; McGee and Pies 2002). BZDs metabolized via conjugation—lorazepam, oxazepam, and temazepam—are generally preferred in elderly patients (Jacobson et al. 2002). Buspirone is relatively well tolerated in the elderly and medically ill but may cause dizziness and headache. Less sedation and psychomotor impairment is seen with buspirone than with BZDs in older patients (Jacobson et al. 2002).

Wagner (2004) has noted that the pharmacotherapy of most childhood anxiety disorders, with the exception of OCD, is based on open studies, chart reviews, and case reports. There are only a few studies of BZDs for the treatment of GAD and panic disorder in children and adolescents. Most recent research has focused on the use of serotonergic agents (including venlafaxine) in treating childhood anxiety, and BZDs are now recommended only for short-term use in younger populations (Wagner 2004).

Tables

Drug Class

TABLE 4–1. Commonly used benzodiazepine anxiolytics

Agent (brand)	Tablet/capsule strengths (mg)	Usual adult total daily dose (mg)
alprazolam (Xanax)	0.25, 0.5, 1, 2	0.75–4.0[a]
chlordiazepoxide (Librium)	5, 10, 25	15–100
clonazepam (Klonopin)	0.5, 1, 2	0.5–4.0
clorazepate (Tranxene)	3.75, 7.5, 15 (11.25, 22.5 single-dose tabs)	15–60
diazepam (Valium)	2, 5, 10 (15 sustained release)	4–40
halazepam (Paxipam)	20, 40	60–160
lorazepam (Ativan)	0.5, 1, 2	2–6
oxazepam (Serax)	10, 15, 30	30–120
prazepam (Centrax)	5, 10, 20	20–60

[a]Up to 10 mg for panic disorder.

Source. Drug Facts and Comparisons 1995; Shader and Greenblatt 1994b.

TABLE 4–2. Commonly prescribed benzodiazepine and nonbenzodiazepine hypnotics

Agent	Tablet/capsule strengths (mg)	Usual adult total daily dose (mg)
Benzodiazepines		
estazolam (ProSom)	1, 2	1–2
flurazepam (Dalmane)	15, 30	15–30
quazepam (Doral)	7.5, 15	7.5–15
temazepam (Restoril)	7.5, 15, 30	15–30
triazolam (Halcion)	0.125, 0.25	0.125–0.5[a]
Nonbenzodiazepines		
zolpidem (Ambien)	5, 10	5–10[b]
zaleplon (Sonata)	5, 10	5–20
eszopiclone (Lunesta)	1, 2, 3	3[c]

[a]Do not exceed 0.25 mg in elderly patients; see discussion in subsection "Use in Special Populations" in the "Overview" section of this chapter.
[b]5 mg at bedtime recommended in elderly patients.
[c]1 mg at bedtime recommended for initial treatment in elderly patients.

TABLE 4–3. Nonbenzodiazepine anxiolytics and hypnotics

Agent	Comments
Antihistamines (e.g., diphenhydramine, hydroxyzine)	Not as well studied as anxiolytics or hypnotics; anticholinergic effects can be sedating and may cause cognitive impairment in elderly or dementia patients. Diphenhydramine loses its effectiveness after a few days' use. Hydroxyzine occasionally useful as a short-term anxiolytic in agitated psychotic patients and may ameliorate extrapyramidal symptoms. Caution should be used with these drugs in patients with concomitant medical conditions (i.e., glaucoma, constipation, benign prostatic hypertrophy); avoid in dementia patients.
Barbiturates	Effective anxiolytics, but too prone to abuse and lethality (in overdose) to be useful in most cases. Generally no longer appropriate in psychiatric practice.
Buspirone	Azapirone that acts as a serotonin (5-HT) agonist at the presynaptic 5-HT_{1A} receptor, but as a *partial* agonist at postsynaptic 5-HT_{1A} receptors. Causes down-regulation of 5-HT_2 receptors (much as do antidepressants). Has anxiolytic and (in high doses) antidepressant properties. Useful in GAD; possibly useful in social phobia and PTSD; useful for agitated dementia patients and aggressive/self-injurious mentally retarded patients. Does not impair psychomotor performance; has little if any abuse potential and is relatively safe in overdose. Not useful for panic disorder, BZD withdrawal, or OCD. Takes several weeks to become fully effective, so not useful for acute anxiety.
Meprobamate	Structurally, does not resemble BZDs or other psychoactive drugs. Has muscle relaxant and anxiolytic properties. May bind to BZD receptor and competitively inhibit BZD binding; may also potentiate adenosine. Has significant abuse liability, and withdrawal from high doses resembles barbiturate withdrawal. Generally no longer appropriate in psychiatric practice.

TABLE 4–3. Nonbenzodiazepine anxiolytics and hypnotics *(continued)*

Agent	Comments
Zaleplon	Marketed as a hypnotic agent (5–20 mg at bedtime). Non-BZD (pyrazolopyrimidine), but binds with high affinity to BZD receptors containing an α_1 subunit. $t_{1/2}$ of about 1.5 hours; may be taken in middle of night, with little residual effect 4 hours later. Appears to have reduced cognitive and psychomotor impairment, compared with BZDs, but may cause cognitive impairment in some elderly patients. No tolerance to zaleplon over course of 4-week study, and no indications of rebound insomnia or withdrawal symptoms after discontinuation.
Zolpidem	Marketed as hypnotic agent (5–10 mg at bedtime). Non-BZD (imidazopyridine), but binds to BZD type-1 receptors (those with α_1 subunit) with very low affinity for other receptor subtypes. Short $t_{1/2}$ (approximately 3 hours). May be useful for short-term treatment of insomnia; little effect on sleep architecture. Has no muscle relaxant, anxiolytic, or anticonvulsant properties (unlike BZDs). Generally well tolerated and effective in inducing and maintaining sleep in healthy adults, with minimal residual cognitive effects in morning. May have less potential for "rebound" insomnia than BZDs; however, there are reports of rebound insomnia and withdrawal symptoms compared with zaleplon. Less commonly, reports of amnestic and psychotic reactions, hallucinatory phenomena (the last occurring at therapeutic doses). May cause confusion, falls in elderly and dementia patients (generally do not exceed 5 mg at bedtime). Probably carries the same abuse potential as that of BZDs.

TABLE 4–3. Nonbenzodiazepine anxiolytics and hypnotics *(continued)*

Agent	Comments
Zopiclone/eszopiclone	Eszopiclone received FDA approvable letter for treatment of insomnia (approximately 3 mg at bedtime). Zopiclone and eszopiclone (cyclopyrrolones) believed to bind to the BZD receptor at the α–γ subunit interface. Binding is nonspecific (subunit may be α_1, α_2, or α_3). Appears to have relatively "balanced" effects on α_1, α_2, and α_3 subunit receptors vs. zolpidem and zaleplon (both of which have more α_1 affinity). Clinical implications of this not clear, but may influence site of action in brain (e.g., α_3 subunits expressed in brain stem, near reticular formation) and perhaps lead to reduced cognitive side effects with eszopiclone compared with BZDs. $t_{1/2}$ of eszopiclone approximately 6 hours. Preliminary data suggest eszopiclone is safe and effective in chronic nightly use over a 6-month period, but further controlled study is needed.

Note. BZD=benzodiazepine; FDA=U.S. Food and Drug Administration; GAD=generalized anxiety disorder; OCD=obsessive-compulsive disorder; PTSD=posttraumatic stress disorder.
Source. Ayd 1995; Cole and Yonkers 1995; Davies et al. 2000; Fry et al. 2000; Jacobson et al. 2002; Krystal et al. 2003; Ninan and Muntasser 2004; Pies 1995a; Reite 2004.

TABLE 4–4. Dosage and cost of selected benzodiazepines

Agent	Equivalent dose (mg[a])	Cost ($) per equivalent dose (AWP)
alprazolam (Xanax)	0.5[b]	0.95
alprazolam XR	0.5[b]	2.15
chlordiazepoxide (Librium)	10	0.30
clonazepam (Klonopin)	0.25[b]	0.70
clorazepate (Tranxene)	7.5	1.60
diazepam (Valium)	5	0.22
estazolam (ProSom)	2	1.00
flurazepam (Dalmane)	15	0.30
lorazepam (Ativan)	1	0.90
oxazepam (Serax)	15	1.00
temazepam (Restoril)	15	0.73
triazolam (Halcion)	0.25	0.70

Note. AWP = average wholesale price.
[a]Roughly equivalent (anxiolytic/hypnotic effect) to 5 mg of diazepam.
[b]Other sources rate clonazepam and alprazolam as equivalent in potency.
Source. Jenkins et al. 2001; prices obtained from local pharmacy database using AWP cost (December 2004).

Indications

TABLE 4–5. Indications for benzodiazepines (BZDs)

Indication	Database/Comments
Generalized anxiety disorder (GAD)	BZDs are primary pharmacological treatment for GAD. Virtually all BZDs are more effective than placebo during short-term, outpatient treatment. Controlled studies fail to demonstrate superiority of one BZD over another; thus, choice of agent depends heavily on side-effect profile, patient-specific factors, and medical issues. Paroxetine, escitalopram, or venlafaxine may be a preferred agent in many patients (and have FDA-approved labeling for GAD).
Panic disorder	Most data on efficacy of BZDs in panic disorder are derived from studies of alprazolam, showing efficacy significantly greater than placebo in reducing frequency and severity of panic attacks. Alprazolam is FDA-approved for the treatment of panic disorder; however, it is probable that other BZDs, including clonazepam, diazepam, and lorazepam, have comparable efficacy. Clonazepam may provide better "coverage" of panic disorder, with less "breakthrough" of symptoms and perhaps fewer dependency and withdrawal problems than with alprazolam. In general, BZDs are now used as second-line treatments for panic disorder, with SSRIs used as first-line agents (as well as cognitive-behavioral therapy).
Obsessive-compulsive disorder (OCD)	Clonazepam may be modestly effective in treating OCD, based on a few case reports.
Social phobia	In small, uncontrolled studies, alprazolam and clonazepam have been effective in treating social phobia. SSRIs are now considered treatments of choice for social phobia. One controlled study supports use of gabapentin.
Avoidant personality disorder (APD)	Very little systematic investigation of medication for "pure" APD (comorbidity and overlap with social phobia are very high). One study found alprazolam helpful in reducing many symptoms of AVP in a small sample (N=14) of social phobia patients.

TABLE 4–5. Indications for benzodiazepines (BZDs) *(continued)*

Indication	Database/Comments
Posttraumatic stress disorder (PTSD)	Few systematic trials of BZDs in treating PTSD. A small retrospective study (*N*=20) showed that alprazolam (0.5–6 mg/day) reduced many PTSD symptoms in 16 cases; however, disinhibited behavior was seen in 4 patients. A placebo-controlled study of alprazolam showed modest improvement in anxiety and in subjective sense of well-being, but no significant improvement in core PTSD areas of "intrusion" and "avoidance." Because substance abuse is common in PTSD, use of BZDs should be very conservative in this population. SSRIs now regarded as medications of first choice for PTSD.
Insomnia	Nearly all BZDs are effective as short-term (1–4 weeks) hypnotics; use in the long term is still controversial, and problems with dependency and withdrawal must be considered. Use of long-acting BZDs, such as flurazepam, is usually not optimal for most patients with insomnia, owing to "hangover" effects (especially in elderly patients). Very-short-acting agents (such as triazolam) may lead to "breakthrough" insomnia/ early awakening. Triazolam is also associated with higher-than-average cognitive impairment. Some clinicians recommend use of BZDs every second or third night in cases of chronic insomnia in order to reduce tolerance; however, there has been little controlled study of this practice. More recent opinion favors long-term, intermittent use of newer, non-BZD hypnotics for chronic insomnia.
Mania	Lorazepam and clonazepam have both been found useful as antimanic agents and may reduce need for adjunctive neuroleptics during initiation of mood stabilizers. There is some evidence that lorazepam may work more rapidly than clonazepam during the first 2 weeks of an acute manic episode.

TABLE 4–5. Indications for benzodiazepines (BZDs) *(continued)*

Indication	Database/Comments
Depression	With the exception of alprazolam (and possibly clonazepam) there is little evidence that BZDs have antidepressant properties. Some data indicate that BZDs (including clonazepam) can worsen depression. However, during initiation of treatment with "stimulating" antidepressants (e.g., fluoxetine, desipramine, bupropion), a brief period of adjunctive BZD use may be warranted, particularly as a bedtime dose.
Acute psychosis	Short-term use of BZDs, either orally or intramuscularly, can reduce the need for neuroleptics in the management of acute psychosis, particularly when accompanied by agitated or catatonic features. BZDs may be useful for agitated PCP-induced psychosis. Haloperidol and lorazepam may be combined in the same syringe for intramuscular treatment of severe/psychotic agitation.
Akathisia/Dyskinesia	Clonazepam, diazepam, and lorazepam have been reported useful in small, open, short-term studies of neuroleptic-induced akathisia, parkinsonism, and tardive dyskinesia. Very few controlled data in large populations are available. In open studies of tardive dyskinesia, approximately 58% of patients improved with BZDs; in double-blind studies, the rate was 43%.
Nocturnal myoclonus	BZDs reduce periodic leg movements of sleep. Preliminary data suggest BZDs (clonazepam) may also be helpful in REM sleep behavioral disorder.
Night terrors/ Other sleep disorders	Because they suppress delta (stages 3 and 4) sleep, BZDs are useful for night terrors. There is risk of worsening sleep apnea, so this condition should be ruled out prior to BZD use.

TABLE 4–5. Indications for benzodiazepines (BZDs) *(continued)*

Indication	Database/Comments
Substance withdrawal	BZDs are the treatment of choice for alcohol withdrawal. Duration of clinical action of a BZD after a single oral dose is related not to its $t_{1/2}\beta$ but to its distribution in lipid compartments (CNS and extra-CNS). Thus, repeated doses of, say, diazepam may be necessary in initial treatment of delirium tremens. Note the poor intramuscular absorption of all commonly prescribed BZDs except lorazepam.

Note. CNS=central nervous system; FDA=U.S. Food and Drug Administration; PCP=phencyclidine; REM=rapid eye movement; SSRI=selective serotonin reuptake inhibitor; $t_{1/2}\beta$=elimination half-life.

Source. Ballenger 1995; Braun et al. 1990; Cornish et al. 1995; Davidson and Connor 2004; Davidson et al. 1991; Feldmann 1987; Gardos and Cole 1995; Hajak et al. 2003; Hewlett et al. 1990; Janicak et al. 1993; Pagel 1996; Pande et al. 1999; Reich et al. 1989; Shader and Greenblatt 1994a, 1994b; Stanilla and Simpson 1995; Taylor 1995; Walsh et al. 2000.

TABLE 4–6. Selective serotonin reuptake inhibitors (SSRIs) or related antidepressants with FDA-approved labeling for use in treating DSM-IV-TR anxiety disorders

Anxiety disorder	Antidepressants with FDA-approved labeling[a]
Obsessive-compulsive disorder	Fluoxetine, fluvoxamine, paroxetine, sertraline Fluoxetine, fluvoxamine, sertraline (in children)
Panic disorder	Fluoxetine, paroxetine, sertraline
Posttraumatic stress disorder	Paroxetine, sertraline
Generalized anxiety disorder	Paroxetine, escitalopram, venlafaxine
Social phobia (social anxiety disorder)	Paroxetine, sertraline, venlafaxine

Note. FDA=U.S. Food and Drug Administration.
[a]All lists of drugs are for adults unless otherwise noted.
Source. Physicians' Desk Reference 2004.

TABLE 4–7. Off-label uses for beta-blockers and clonidine for anxiety/agitation in selected disorders

Agent	Off-label uses
Beta-blockers	Akathisia
	Aggressive/impulsive behaviors following brain damage
	Performance anxiety
	Tremor (essential, drug-related)
	Alcohol withdrawal (adjunct to BZDs)
	? GAD
	? Panic disorder, agoraphobia
	? Narcotic/BZD withdrawal (adjunctive agent)
	? Management of cocaine intoxication
	? Schizophrenia (adjunctive agent)
	? Mania (adjunctive agent)
Clonidine	ADHD
	Opioid detoxification
	Nicotine dependence
	? PTSD (augmenting agent)
	Tourette's syndrome
	? Panic disorder
	? OCD (augmenting agent)
	? GAD
	? Refractory mania
	? Tricyclic-induced sweating

Note. ? = database is quite limited or contradictory. ADHD = attention-deficit/hyperactivity disorder; BZD = benzodiazepine; GAD = generalized anxiety disorder; OCD = obsessive-compulsive disorder; PTSD = posttraumatic stress disorder.
Source. Ayd 1995; Cornish et al. 1995; Dulcan et al. 1995; Pies and Parks 1996; Yudofsky et al. 1995.

Mechanisms of Action

TABLE 4–8. Effect of various agents on $GABA_A$ receptors

Agent	Effect on receptor
Alcohol	Weakly augments GABA-activated chloride ion conductance, but also inhibits NMDA receptor–mediated depolarization.
Barbiturates	Augment receptor affinity for GABA (as do BZDs), but also directly increase ion channel opening, even in the absence of GABA. Dual mechanism may account for greater toxicity of barbiturates vs. BZDs.
BZDs	Bind to α–γ subunit interface of $GABA_A$ receptor and increase the affinity of the receptor for GABA, an inhibitory neurotransmitter that leads to increased chloride ion conductance. This hyperpolarizes the neuron and leads to decreased excitability. BZDs have no direct effect on chloride channel opening. Most standard BZDs bind to receptors containing α_1, α_2, or α_3 subunits.
Buspirone	$5\text{-}HT_{1A}$ agonist. No effect on GABA–BZD complex.
Zolpidem	Appears to interact with BZD binding site, since effects of zolpidem can be prevented by flumazenil (a BZD-receptor antagonist). Binds with high affinity only to receptors containing the α_1 subunit.
Zaleplon	Binds to the BZD site on the $GABA_A$ receptor; binds with high affinity only to receptors containing the α_1 subunit.
Zopiclone/ Eszopiclone	Interact with the BZD site on the $GABA_A$ receptor, but probably bind to different "microdomains" within the γ subunit than do BZDs, zolpidem, and zaleplon. Act on receptors with α_1, α_2, or α_3 subunits.

Note. BZD=benzodiazepine; $5\text{-}HT_{1A}$=serotonin$_{1A}$ receptor; GABA=γ-aminobutyric acid; NMDA=*N*-methyl-D-aspartate.

Source. Davies et al. 2000; Kaplan et al. 1995; Paul 1995.

TABLE 4–9. Pharmacodynamic aspects of hypnotic agents

Agent	Active at $GABA_A$ receptor	Binds to α_1 subunit receptors[a]	Binds to α_2, α_3, or α_5 subunit receptors[b]	Atypical binding[c]
BZD hypnotics				
temazepam	Yes	++	++	
triazolam	Yes	++	++	
estazolam	Yes	++	++	
flurazepam	Yes	++	++	
quazepam	Yes	+++	+	
Non-BZD hypnotics				
zolpidem	Yes	++	+/–	
zaleplon	Yes	++	+/–	
zopiclone/eszopiclone	Yes	+/–	+/–	+

Note. +/–=none to minimal affinity; +=slight affinity; ++=moderate affinity; +++=high affinity.
BZD=benzodiazepine; GABA=γ-aminobutyric acid.
[a]Old terminology: BZ-1, ω_1.
[b]Old terminology: BZ-2, ω_2.
[c]The only agent with putative atypical binding is zopiclone/eszopiclone.
Source. Davies et al. 2000.

Pharmacokinetics

TABLE 4–10. Pharmacokinetics of orally administered benzodiazepine anxiolytics

Agent	Onset of peak action,[a] hours	Effective $t_{1/2}\beta$,[b] hours	Active metabolites
alprazolam	1.5	12–15	No
chlordiazepoxide	2.0	>50	Yes
clonazepam	1.5	18–50	No
clorazepate	1.5	>50	Yes
diazepam	1.3	>50	Yes
halazepam	2.5	>50	Yes
lorazepam	1.3	12–15	No
oxazepam	3.0	12–15	No
prazepam	5.0	> 50	Yes

$t_{1/2}\beta$ = elimination half-life.

[a]Onset of peak action after oral dosing varies from patient to patient, and the above data reflect the author's experience as well as published data pertaining to peak blood levels.

[b]Includes effect of any long-acting metabolite(s), usually desmethyldiazepam. $t_{1/2}\beta$ may vary with age and hepatic function, with longer half-lives usually found in elderly patients.

Source. Ballenger 1995; Drug Facts and Comparisons 1995; Physicians' Desk Reference 1996; Shader and Greenblatt 1994b.

TABLE 4–11. Pharmacokinetics of benzodiazepine hypnotics

Agent	Onset of peak action,[a] hours	Effective $t_{1/2}\beta$,[b] hours	Active metabolites
estazolam (ProSom)	2.0	10–24	No
flurazepam (Dalmane)	0.5–2.0	>50	Yes
temazepam (Restoril)	1.0–2.0	7–12	No
triazolam (Halcion)	0.5–2.0	2–5	No

$t_{1/2}\beta$ = elimination half-life.
[a]Onset of peak action after oral dosing varies from patient to patient, and the above data reflect the author's experience as well as published data pertaining to peak blood levels.
[b]Includes effects of long-acting active metabolites (e.g., desalkylflurazepam and desalkyl-2-oxoquazepam).
Source. Ballenger 1995; Drug Facts and Comparisons 1995; Physicians' Desk Reference 1996; Shader and Greenblatt 1994a.

TABLE 4–12. Pharmacokinetics of nonbenzodiazepine hypnotics

Agent	Time to peak plasma level, hours	Effective $t_{1/2}\beta$, hours	Active metabolites
zolpidem	0.8–2.0	1.5–3.5	No
zaleplon	1.0	1.0–2.0	No
eszopiclone[a]	1.5	5.0–7.0	No

$t_{1/2}\beta$ = elimination half-life.

[a]Based on values for racemic zopiclone.

Source. Nishino et al. 2004; Physicians' Desk Reference 2004.

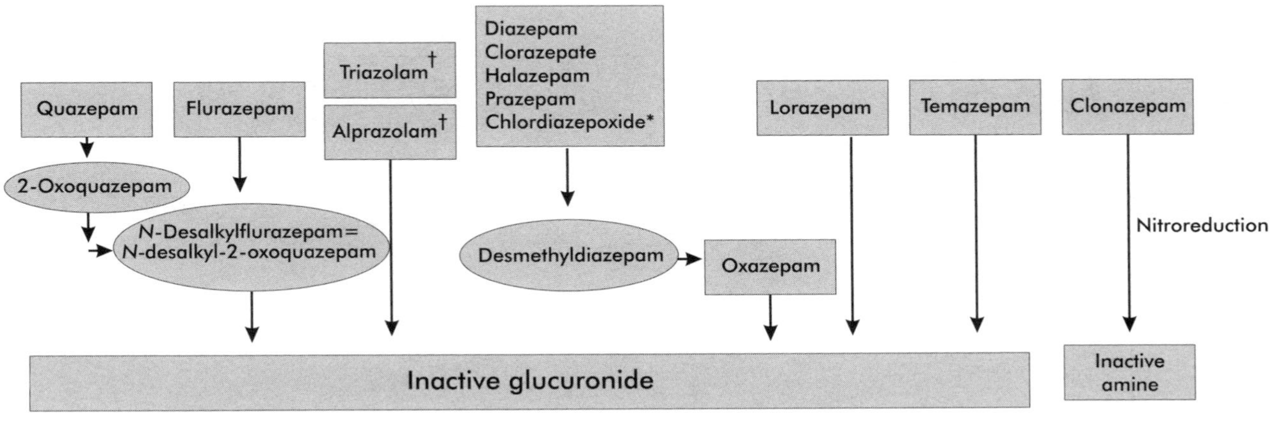

FIGURE 4–1. Simplified metabolic pathways of benzodiazepines.

Note. *Intermediates include desmethylchlordiazepoxide and demoxepam.
†Very transient active metabolites (of little clinical importance).

Main Side Effects

TABLE 4–13. Frequency (%) of benzodiazepine (BZD) and buspirone side effects (average for various BZDs)

Side effect(s)	BZDs	Buspirone
Hypotension	4.7	<1.0
Hypertension	0	<1.0
Dizziness	13.4	13.6
Fainting	3.1	<1.0
Tachycardia	7.7	1.3
Palpitations	7.7	1.0
Bradycardia	<1.0	<1.0
Dyspnea	<1.0	<1.0
Chest pain	—[a]	1.5
Dry mouth/throat	12.6	5.3
Salivation	4.2	<1.0
Nausea, vomiting	7.4	10.8
Diarrhea	7.0	2.5
Constipation	7.1	1.3
Weight gain	2.7	—[a]
Sexual dysfunction	11.0	1.0
Blurry vision	10.6	2.0
Weakness, fatigue	17.7	7.6
Clumsiness	20.0	—[a]
Headache	9.1	10.6
Ataxia, incoordination	17.6	2.5
Confusion, disorientation	6.9	1.4
Insomnia	6.4	6.7
Unusual dreams	—[a]	5.5
Hallucinations	5.5	<1
Paradoxical anxiety, nervousness	4.1	5.0
Irritability, hostility	5.5	2.0
Depression	8.3	1.4

[a]No data available.

Source. Maxmen 1991.

TABLE 4–14. Side effects and management of benzodiazepines (BZDs)

Side effect(s)	Management/Comments
Drowsiness, fatigue, weakness	At fixed dose of BZD, sedation usually subsides after about a week, as anxiolytic action emerges. Dosage reduction and administration mostly at bedtime may reduce the problem.
Lightheadedness, ataxia, falls	Some, but not all, studies show BZDs linked with risk of falls and hip fracture in elderly patients. Whereas some studies suggest less risk of falls with short-acting BZDs, other data suggest that risk of falls and hip fracture is related to rate of dosage increase and total dose. Dosage reduction; patient education about rising slowly from bed.
Slurred speech, double vision	Dosage reduction.
Confusion, psychomotor impairment	Visual-spatial ability (e.g., perception of objects in one's visual field), coordination, and sustained attention may be impaired and may affect driving skills (although there is no conclusive evidence linking BZDs with automobile accidents). Patient not often aware of decreased ability until stopping the BZD. Dysfunction is synergistic with use of alcohol. Elderly patients may be especially susceptible to cognitive decrements. Some cognitive dysfunction may diminish with time and chronic dosing. Use minimal effective dose; avoid sudden dosage increases. Some patients may benefit from a small amount of caffeine.
Memory impairment, anterograde amnesia	All BZDs can cause memory impairment to some degree. Triazolam probably has somewhat greater risk of causing, in a dose-related fashion, amnestic and cognitive symptoms than do other BZD hypnotics. BZD-related confusion and amnesia may be misdiagnosed as dementia in elderly patients. Triazolam may be especially likely to cause memory impairment in the elderly. Avoid triazolam dose >0.125 mg in the elderly.

TABLE 4–14. Side effects and management of benzodiazepines (BZDs) *(continued)*

Side effect(s)	Management/Comments
Depression	When depression occurs after onset of panic disorder, a BZD may be useful for both anxiety and depression. However, with the exception of alprazolam, BZDs generally lack antidepressant properties and may cause or exacerbate depression in some patients.
Paradoxical stimulation/ disinhibition	Can manifest as irritability, increased anxiety, aggression, euphoria, and psychosis. Tends to occur in patients with underlying brain damage or dementia and in some BPD patients. May be more likely with alprazolam on the basis of anecdotal reports, but not all data support this association.
Respiratory suppression	Flurazepam and probably all BZDs may exacerbate sleep apnea. Chlordiazepoxide and probably all BZDs can exacerbate breathing difficulties in patients with chronic lung disease. There are reports of respiratory suppression/arrest when BZDs are combined with clozapine (see subsection "Drug–Drug Interactions" in the "Overview" section of this chapter). Avoid BZDs if possible in patients with sleep-related breathing problems. Avoid high doses of BZDs in other patients at risk; increase dose slowly. SSRIs or buspirone may be a good alternative in anxious patients at risk for respiratory suppression.
Miscellaneous (e.g., GI complaints, dry mouth, urinary hesitancy)	Dosage reduction. Administration with food may reduce GI complaints (may also slow rate of absorption). Urinary hesitancy may respond to bethanechol.

TABLE 4–14. Side effects and management of benzodiazepines (BZDs) *(continued)*

Side effect(s)	Management/Comments
Discontinuation/withdrawal syndromes	Withdrawal of BZDs may lead to continuum of symptoms, ranging from restlessness, headaches, insomnia, and hyperacusis to (rarely) severe depression, myoclonus, involuntary movements, delirium, and seizures. Likelihood of withdrawal reaction is probably related to duration of BZD use and daily dosage, possibly related to use of short-acting BZDs. Alprazolam, and perhaps other triazolo-BZDs, may be especially hard to discontinue. Key management strategy is very slow taper of BZDs over weeks to months. "Coverage" of triazolo-BZD with non-triazolo-BZD (e.g., "covering" a patient withdrawing from alprazolam by using clonazepam) may not be complete.

Note. BPD=borderline personality disorder; GI=gastrointestinal; SSRI=selective serotonin reuptake inhibitor.

Source. Ballenger 1995; Creelman et al. 1989; Herings et al. 1995; Janicak et al. 1993; Jenkins et al. 2001; McGee and Pies 2002; Pies 1992; Smoller 1996; Woods et al. 1995.

Drug–Drug Interactions

TABLE 4–15. Benzodiazepine (BZD) drug interactions

Index drug (added to BZD)	Clinical effect/Other interactions
Cimetidine, isoniazid Disulfiram Oral contraceptives Ketoconazole Metoprolol Propranolol Valproate Propoxyphene Erythromycin Omeprazole	Potential for increased toxicity of diazepam, chlordiazepoxide, other BZDs that undergo *oxidative* hepatic metabolism, due to inhibition of BZD metabolism. Dosage adjustment of BZD may be necessary. Ketoconazole-type agents affect mainly triazolo-BZD metabolism (alprazolam, triazolam, midazolam). Metoprolol and propranolol may inhibit metabolism of demethylated BZDs (e.g., diazepam), but they do not interfere with metabolism of alprazolam, lorazepam, oxazepam, and (probably) temazepam.
Oral contraceptives	Some (but not all) data suggest that oral contraceptives can increase clearance rate and reduce levels of BZDs that undergo *glucuronidation* (lorazepam, oxazepam). In contrast, oral contraceptives *decrease* clearance of diazepam and other BZDs that undergo *oxidative* metabolism. Inhibition of *both* cytochrome P450 (CYP) 3A4 and 2C19 by oral contraceptives is more likely to increase diazepam levels than is inhibition of only one CYP pathway. Diazepam plus oral contraceptive may increase psychomotor/cognitive impairment. Thus, lorazepam dose might need upward adjustment with oral contraceptives, while diazepam dose might need downward adjustment. Alprazolam clearance is probably not affected by oral contraceptives.
Rifampin Phenytoin Carbamazepine	Decreased clinical effect of BZDs due to induction of hepatic metabolism (e.g., phenytoin may increase oxazepam clearance and decrease levels).
Ranitidine	May reduce GI absorption of diazepam; however, does not impair oxidative or conjugative metabolism of diazepam or lorazepam (as may cimetidine).

TABLE 4–15. Benzodiazepine (BZD) drug interactions *(continued)*

Index drug (added to BZD)	Clinical effect/Other interactions
Antacids Anticholinergics	Suspension-type antacids (e.g., magnesium/aluminum hydroxide) may alter the *rate* but usually not the *extent* of GI absorption. Delay in oral absorption and/or onset of effect of BZDs is possible but is probably most relevant after single-dose (rather than chronic) treatment. Biodegradation of clorazepate (pro-drug) to active desmethyldiazepam may be delayed with antacids. The proton-pump inhibitor omeprazole may raise diazepam blood levels modestly (via inhibition of CYP 2C19).
Anticholinergics	Coadministration may produce more cognitive impairment than with either drug alone, particularly in the elderly.
Digoxin	Alprazolam, and perhaps diazepam, may lead to increased digoxin levels (which could lead to toxicity).
Alcohol, narcotics, and other CNS depressants	Increased CNS sedation and toxicity.
TCAs	Increased imipramine and desipramine (but not nortriptyline) levels with concomitant alprazolam administration. Amitriptyline may increase the psychomotor effects of BZDs.
SSRIs	Fluoxetine and fluvoxamine may reduce clearance of some oxidatively metabolized BZDs, including diazepam and alprazolam, leading to increased BZD levels/effects. Fluoxetine does not appear to affect metabolism of glucuronidated BZDs (lorazepam, oxazepam) or clonazepam, but it may raise blood levels of all triazolo-BZDs via inhibition of CYP 3A4 by the fluoxetine metabolite norfluoxetine. Sertraline may slightly increase levels of diazepam; metabolite of sertraline would be expected to affect CYP 3A4 (which metabolizes triazolo-BZDs). Paroxetine is a mild inhibitor of CYP 2C19 and CYP 3A4, so it should not greatly affect diazepam levels. Citalopram should have minimal effect on BZD levels.
Nefazodone	Increased levels of triazolo-BZDs (e.g., alprazolam's $t_{1/2}\beta$ may double).

TABLE 4–15. Benzodiazepine (BZD) drug interactions *(continued)*

Index drug (added to BZD)	Clinical effect/Other interactions
Antipsychotics/Clozapine	BZDs may act synergistically with clozapine to cause severe sedation, hypotension, and respiratory depression (may be related to dose of BZD).
L-Dopa	Possibly decreased effect of L-dopa when BZDs are coadministered.

Note. CNS=central nervous system; CYP=cytochrome P450; GI=gastrointestinal; SSRI=selective serotonin reuptake inhibitor; TCA=tricyclic antidepressant; $t_{1/2}\beta$=elimination half-life.

Source. Abernethy et al. 1982, 1984; Ayd 1995; Cobb et al. 1991; Cozza et al. 2003; Drug Facts and Comparisons 1995; Ellinwood et al. 1984; Pies and Weinberg 1990; Preskorn 1996; Salzman et al. 1986; Sands et al. 1995; Venkatakrishnan et al. 2003.

TABLE 4–16. Nonbenzodiazepine (non-BZD) hypnotic drug interactions

Agent	Drug added	Effect on non-BZD hypnotic blood level
zaleplon	Inhibitors of aldehyde oxidase (e.g., cimetidine, hydralzine, methadone) or of CYP 3A4	Increased
	Rifampin and other CYP 3A4 inducers	Decreased
zolpidem	Ritonavir, ketoconazole, sertraline, nefazodone, and other CYP 3A4 inhibitors	Increased
	Rifampin and other CYP 3A4 inducers	Decreased
zopiclone eszopiclone[a]	Ritonavir, ketoconazole, sertraline, nefazodone, and other CYP 3A4 inhibitors	Increased
	Rifampin and other CYP 3A4 inducers	Decreased

Note. CYP = cytochrome P450.

[a]Data are preliminary and extrapolated from experience with racemic zopiclone.

Source. Cozza et al. 2003.

Potentiating Maneuvers

TABLE 4–17. Agents used in combination with benzodiazepines (BZDs) for augmentation of effect

Agent combined with BZD	Rationale/Comment
Anticholinergic/ antiparkinsonian agents	BZDs may augment antiparkinsonian effect of benztropine and similar agents in treatment of neuroleptic-induced tremor, muscle rigidity, and akathisia. **Note:** anticholinergics may slow BZD absorption.
Antidepressants	BZDs may provide early relief of agitation and insomnia in patients with depression or panic disorder, before primary (coadministered antidepressant) treatment has become effective. Some clinicians use BZD during first days of SSRI treatment in panic disorder patients, then gradually taper off the BZD as SSRI becomes effective. Some patients with primary depression may become more depressed with continued use of BZDs.
Antipsychotics	Antipsychotics and BZDs (e.g., lorazepam) may work synergistically in acute psychosis. BZDs may also be of help for catatonic features.
Buspirone	Buspirone may augment the anxiolytic effect of BZDs in panic disorder and may facilitate discontinuation of BZDs.
Mood stabilizers	Clonazepam and lorazepam potentiate the antimanic effect of valproate, lithium, and perhaps other mood stabilizers.

Note. SSRI = selective serotonin reuptake inhibitor.

Source. Cole and Yonkers 1995; Coplan and Gorman 1990; Fawcett 1990; Gastfriend and Rosenbaum 1989; Lenox and Manji 1995; Tueth et al. 1995.

Use in Special Populations

TABLE 4–18. Potential concerns of benzodiazepine (BZD) use during pregnancy

Cleft lip and palate	Recent evidence suggests small absolute risk from BZD exposure during first trimester (<1%) but higher risk than in the general population (0.06%). Thus, informed consent and discussion with mother and obstetrician are indicated. If possible, minimize or avoid BZD use during first trimester.
"Floppy baby syndrome"	Infants exposed to BZDs either in the last trimester or at the time of parturition may show muscular hypotonicity, lethargy, failure to feed, impaired temperature regulation (hypothermia), poor respiratory effort, and low Apgar scores.
Impaired intrauterine growth and various dysmorphic birth defects	Data mostly derived from one group (Laegreid et al. 1992); informed consent and discussion with mother and obstetrician are indicated; if possible, minimize or avoid use during first trimester.
Increased duration of labor	Consult with obstetrician in advance of expected delivery date.
Withdrawal symptoms in neonate	May be manifest as tremulousness, hypertonicity, irritability, hyperactivity, disturbed sleep, and tremors. Avoid high doses of short-acting BZDs. Do not discontinue BZDs suddenly during pregnancy, but, rather, taper slowly as delivery approaches.
Appearance of BZDs in breast milk	Use lowest effective BZD dose during lactation; however, amount of BZD in breast milk appears to be very small percentage of maternal dose and is unlikely to pose a threat to the nursing infant. Discontinue breastfeeding if infant experiences sedation or other signs of BZD toxicity, regardless of maternal dose.

Source. Altshuler et al. 1996; Ayd 1995; Laegreid et al. 1992; Newport et al. 2004; Pies 1995b; Stowe and Nemeroff 1995.

TABLE 4–19. Risks of benzodiazepine (BZD) use in elderly and/or dementia patients

Risk/Problem	Management
Cognitive dysfunction/ amnesia	Use lowest effective dose; intermediate-duration agents with no active metabolites may be preferable. If triazolam is used, avoid dose >0.125 mg (triazolam generally not recommended in the elderly). Reassess rationale for long-term BZD use periodically. If BZD is used as a hypnotic, consider use of a non-BZD, such as zaleplon or eszopiclone.
Falls and hip fractures	Use lowest effective dose; avoid sudden increases in dose; instruct patient to rise slowly; check blood pressure supine and standing after dose increases. Reassess rationale for long-term BZD use periodically. ? Avoid long-acting BZDs (conflicting data).
Behavioral disinhibition	Avoid BZDs for most agitated dementia patients (most likely to become disinhibited or confused); if a BZD must be used, prescribe the lowest effective dose for limited duration. ? Avoid alprazolam (data are weak, but clinical experience suggests caution).
Reduced hepatic metabolism	Use intermediate-duration agents that do not undergo oxidative metabolism (e.g., oxazepam, lorazepam, temazepam); agents metabolized by cytochrome P450 (CYP) 3A4 may be prone to drug interactions.
Drug–drug interactions	Be aware of metabolic route of coprescribed agents, and avoid those that specifically inhibit CYP 2C19 and/or CYP 3A4 (see Table 4–15 and subsection "Drug–Drug Interactions" in the "Overview" section of this chapter).
"Hangover effect" from hypnotic	Avoid long-acting agents (e.g., flurazepam, any BZD with desmethyldiazepam metabolite) when treating simple insomnia (without daytime anxiety). Reassess rationale for long-term BZD use periodically, and consider use of non-BZD, such as zaleplon or eszopiclone.

Source. Dubovsky 1994; Jacobson et al. 2002; McGee and Pies 2002.

Questions and Answers

Drug Class

Q. What are the main factors determining the choice of one benzodiazepine (BZD) versus another for any given indication?

A. Since all the BZDs are probably equal in efficacy for their principal indications, the choice of agent is dictated mainly by pharmacokinetic considerations (Arana and Hyman 1991; McGee and Pies 2002). The onset of action, distribution in body compartments, metabolic pathway, potential drug interactions, and $t_{1/2}\beta$ are more important factors than the specific chemical structure of the BZD (see Tables 4–10 and 4–11). For example, in patients with cirrhosis, lorazepam or oxazepam may be an agent of choice, owing to their elimination route (glucuronidation). In some cases, pharmacodynamic factors may be relevant. Thus, the chemical structure of triazolo-BZDs may confer somewhat atypical properties—for example, high potency and antidepressant effects (the latter having been demonstrated in some studies of alprazolam). This qualitative difference between triazolo- and nontriazolo-BZDs may also make it difficult to "cover" a patient withdrawing from alprazolam with another (nontriazolo) BZD such as clonazepam. Some patients will continue to complain of withdrawal symptoms as the alprazolam is tapered, despite equipotent doses of clonazepam or other long-acting BZDs.

Another factor in choosing a BZD is the potential for interaction with other medications (see subsection "Drug–Drug Interactions" in the "Overview" section of this chapter). Triazolo-BZDs are metabolized mainly by the cytochrome P450 (CYP) 3A4 system. For example, nefazodone, fluvoxamine, and sertraline/desmethylsertraline all have inhibitory effects on CYP 3A4 and might elevate blood levels of triazolo-BZDs. Sertraline is also known to inhibit glucuronidation and thus might elevate blood levels of BZDs undergoing only phase II metabolism (e.g., lorazepam, oxazepam, and temazepam) (Cozza et al. 2003; Kaufman and Gerner 1998). In practice, FDA-approved labeling may also influence BZD prescribing decisions, but the decision to use a certain medication based on such labeling is rarely a consequence of well-founded clinical differences among agents.

Q. Can BZDs be administered sublingually?

A. Lorazepam, alprazolam, and triazolam are well absorbed sublingually. Although the time to peak plasma levels is only modestly reduced for sublingual versus oral alprazolam (roughly 1.2 vs. 1.7 hours; Scavone et al. 1987), the sublingual route may be preferable in acutely anxious patients who cannot swallow pills or who have a full stomach, which would slow absorption (Arana and Hyman 1991). Dry mouth may interfere with the sublingual route.

Q. Are BZDs ever used intravenously in psychiatry?

A. The intravenous route is rarely used, except as preoperative sedation and in treating seizures; however, intravenous diazepam, lorazepam, or midazolam may be used to treat neuroleptic-induced laryngeal dystonia if anticholinergics are not effective (Arana and Hyman 1991). Occasionally, intravenous midazolam or lorazepam may be used in the treatment of severe alcohol withdrawal (Ciraulo et al. 1994; Saitz et al. 2003). The intravenous route carries a substantial risk of respiratory suppression or arrest and should not be attempted without adequate medical support.

Indications

Q. How effective are BZDs in the psychic versus the somatic aspects of generalized anxiety disorder (GAD), and how long do beneficial effects last?

A. Most studies of two commonly used BZDs—chlordiazepoxide and diazepam—have found evidence of global effectiveness in treating GAD or similar conditions when compared with placebo; however, few such studies have distinguished psychic from somatic aspects of relief (Hollister et al. 1993). In a study of diazepam, Pourmotabbed et al. (1996) found that somatic symptoms of GAD are more responsive to diazepam than are psychic symptoms. But superiority of diazepam over placebo was seen only for the first 3 weeks, after which time the placebo group continued to improve. Pourmotabbed et al. suggested that diazepam be used to treat symptoms of GAD for only a few weeks; however, their results do not indicate that diazepam is *ineffective* for GAD after the first 3 weeks, and the author has seen some patients with GAD who appear to benefit from—and, indeed, require—longer use of BZDs. One study of diazepam noted that the improvement obtained by the sixth week was sustained when medication was continued for 22 weeks (Rickels et al. 1983).

Q. How do the indications for BZDs differ from those of buspirone?

A. Buspirone, an azapirone anxiolytic that does not interact with brain BZD receptors, differs from BZDs in its pharmacodynamic profile (Janicak et al. 1993). First, buspirone's clinical effect takes several weeks to accrue, so it is not useful in treating an acute episode of anxiety. Second, buspirone is not useful when taken on an as-needed ("prn") basis, in contrast to BZDs (for some patients). Third, buspirone has not been shown effective in treating panic attacks or panic disorder; nor is buspirone capable of "covering" BZD withdrawal symptoms. Finally, buspirone—in doses greater than 60 mg/day—has demonstrated antidepressant properties in double-blind studies (Rickels et al. 1990). In contrast, with the exception of alprazolam and possibly clonazepam, BZDs have minimal antidepressant activity and may sometimes be associated with treatment-emergent depression (Janicak et al. 1993; Tesar 1990). Buspirone may be useful for patients with generalized anxiety who cannot tolerate respiratory suppression or sedation. However, it is the clinical impression of some psychiatrists that buspirone is not perceived as very helpful among patients who have been exposed to long-term BZD use.

Q. Are serotonergic antidepressants now the drugs of first choice for most types of anxiety—in preference to BZDs? What about long-term treatment of anxiety?

A. Current practice guidelines tend to support this position. For obsessive-compulsive disorder (OCD), BZDs are not particularly useful, whereas selective serotonin reuptake inhibitors (SSRIs) are considered agents of first choice for both acute and long-term treatment (Greist et al. 2003). Similarly, the World Council of Anxiety (WCA) recommendations now identify SSRIs as first-choice agents in the treatment of panic disorder, with or without agoraphobia (Pollack et al. 2003). For posttraumatic stress disorder (PTSD), WCA guidelines note that "while the selective serotonin inhibitors sertraline, paroxetine, and fluoxetine have shown efficacy in acute treatment trials, sertraline is the only one for which long-term efficacy has been demonstrated" (Stein et al. 2003, p. 31). This, of course, does not prove that other SSRIs are *ineffective* as maintenance agents. SSRIs are also considered drugs of first choice for the treatment of social phobia (Van Ameringen et al. 2003). Although three SSRI/serotonin-norepinephrine reuptake inhibitors (SNRIs)—paroxetine, sertraline, and venlafaxine—have FDA-approved labeling for social phobia, one placebo-controlled study (Davidson et al. 2004) found that controlled-release fluvoxamine (at dosages of up to 300 mg/day) was also effective.

The situation is more complex with respect to the treatment of GAD. WCA guidelines observe that "benzodiazepines have been commonly used as the first-line acute treatment for GAD…[but] their use is limited by several factors related to long-term use…" (Allgulander et al. 2003, p. 56), such as the risk of physical dependence and tolerance. On the other hand, these same authors cite a prospective, double-blind study of clorazepate versus buspirone in the long-term treatment of patients with GAD (N= 134) (Rickels et al. 1988). Both treatments demonstrated efficacy during the trial, and there was no evidence of tolerance development with either drug. Indeed, in the author's experience, some patients seem able to continue taking their dose of BZD for several years without evidence of substantial tolerance developing. Allgulander et al. (2003) concluded that "more research is needed to determine the usefulness of the selective serotonin reuptake inhibitors in the treatment of GAD, and the best approach for the long-term treatment of the disorder" (p. 53). Thus, in theory, antidepressants with FDA-approved labeling for GAD (i.e., paroxetine, escitalopram, venlafaxine) may be the agents of first choice in treating patients with GAD. In clinical practice, however, some patients may not be able to tolerate the gastrointestinal (GI), sexual, and other side effects of these agents; nor will all severely anxious patients be willing to wait 2–3 weeks for these agents to "kick in." Thus, some clinicians may opt for combined BZD/SSRI treatment for the first few weeks, with gradual taper and discontinuation of the BZD after a month or so. Patients must be carefully prepared for this strategy, however, since some will find BZD discontinuation either physiologically or psychologically difficult. In short, a careful risk–benefit assessment is required in determining the agent of first choice for any given patient with GAD, including, of course, ruling out any history of alcohol or substance abuse. (Local Boards of Registration in Medicine have taken a rather hard line on physicians who prescribe BZDs to known alcohol or substance abusers.) Finally, the clinician should bear in mind that cognitive-behavioral therapy (CBT) has a prominent role in the treatment of nearly all the anxiety disorders (Pollack et al. 2003; Van Ameringen et al. 2003). Since concurrent BZD treatment may interfere with the acquisition of CBT principles, at least in phobic individuals (Marks 1983), the timing of medication with respect to psychotherapy should be considered carefully (see Ellison 1996 for general principles of integrated treatment).

Q. Should BZDs be considered useless in the treatment of OCD?

A. There are few controlled studies bearing on this question, but clinical and research experience has generally not supported use of BZDs for OCD (Greist et al. 2003). However, Hewlett et al. (1990) reported on three patients who met DSM-III-R criteria for OCD (American Psychiatric Association 1987) and who responded well to clonazepam (3–5 mg/day) over a 1-year period. One patient showed reductions in obsessions and compulsions that were equal to or greater than those seen with clomipramine treatment, and also experienced improvement in depressive symptoms. The authors noted that clonazepam does have complex effects on serotonin metabolism. In the present author's experience treating patients with OCD, clonazepam may sometimes be a useful adjunct to an SSRI.

Q. How are BZDs employed in the treatment of acute psychosis or severe agitation in the emergency setting?

A. Most experience has been gained with lorazepam, which is the only conventional BZD (excluding midazolam) that is reliably absorbed via the intramuscular route. For the agitated, psychotic patient, lorazepam 1–2 mg po or im may be given alone, every 0.5–2 hours, up to 6–12 mg over a 24-hour period. Lorazepam is often coprescribed with variable amounts of an antipsychotic. Alternatively, lorazepam (2–4 mg) may be *combined in the same syringe* with haloperidol (2.5–5 mg) and administered every 1–2 hours, up to five times or so in a 24-hour period. The disadvantage of such a "cocktail" is that when adverse reactions (including allergic ones) occur, it is difficult to determine which agent was responsible. On the other hand, some data suggest that this combination may be superior to either agent alone in the acute setting (Garza-Trevino et al. 1989). Keep in mind that elderly patients may experience hypotension from intramuscular lorazepam and that some patients with underlying brain damage may become disinhibited with BZD administration.

Q. Are BZDs useful in the long-term management of schizophrenia?

A. Since BZDs appear to inhibit dopamine neurotransmission and decrease presynaptic dopamine release, there is some theoretical justification for their use in schizophrenia (Pies and Dewan 2001; Wolkowitz and Pickar 1991). Of 16 double-blind studies assessing adjunctive use of BZDs in schizophrenia, 7 reported positive results, while 4 reported mixed or transiently positive results. The overall response rate in such patients is about 40% (Ayd 1995; Wolkowitz and Pickar 1991). Wolkowitz and Pickar (1991) noted "rapid (within 1–2 weeks) and occasionally striking improvements in social relatedness, affability, spontaneity, humor, and interest in family and social life in some benzodiazepine-treated patients" (p. 720). However, some patients appear to lose therapeutic response within a few weeks. BZDs may be useful in ameliorating neuroleptic-induced extrapyramidal effects, and this may secondarily improve psychotic features. Patients with high initial anxiety, psychosis, or motor disturbance (e.g., catatonic features) may be most likely to respond to adjunctive BZDs (Wolkowitz and Pickar 1991). A more recent review (Janicak et al. 2001) noted that BZDs have shown some benefit for both amelioration of anxiety and tension and reduction of auditory hallucinations in patients with chronic schizophrenia. However, these authors rightly concluded that the effects of BZDs in schizophrenia "range from deterioration, to no change in most patients, to striking improvement in a rare patient when using BZDs either as the sole agent or as adjunct to antipsychotics" (Janicak et al. 2001, p. 146).

Q. Are BZDs indicated in the long-term treatment of chronic insomnia?

A. Opinion differs on this controversial issue. Historically, most experts have counseled that BZDs are indicated primarily for the short-term (<1 month) treatment of insomnia (Janicak et al. 1993). This approach seems prudent, in general, because there are few studies showing hypnotic efficacy of BZDs beyond 12 weeks (Janicak et al. 1993) and because these agents carry the risk of cognitive impairment, tolerance, withdrawal, and exacerbation of sleep-related breathing disorders. On the other hand, as Hollister et al. (1993) cogently put it, "the labeling of benzodiazepine hypnotic drugs typically recommends that prescriptions should not exceed 1 month. Such statements have been widely interpreted as reflecting evidence that the drugs lose efficacy after these periods of time. *In fact, they reflect only that there have simply not been enough studies of long-term efficacy from which to draw definitive conclusions*" (p. 138; emphasis added). Moreover, some sleep laboratory data have documented continued benefits for up to 6 months after the start of regular BZD use (Hollister et al. 1993). One study spanning 12 years found that long-term nightly treatment of sleep disorders with BZDs *was* effective and did not lead to dosage escalation or drug abuse in the vast majority of patients (Schenck and Mahowald 1996). In the author's experience, there is a small subgroup of patients with mixed anxiety and depression whose chronic insomnia does respond well to low doses of BZDs, over a period of months to years, with no evidence of tolerance, abuse, or cognitive impairment. (Almost always, the BZD is an adjunct to ongoing antidepressant therapy.) Nevertheless, prudence would dictate use of alternative treatments, including behavioral modification, whenever possible (Lenhart and Buysse 2001). Trazodone or (in selected cases) small amounts of doxepin may be useful for chronic, intractable insomnia that is not amenable to behavioral methods, though controlled evidence supporting use of these agents is quite limited in well-defined insomniac populations. Other clinicians suggest that if BZDs are used chronically for insomnia without complicating anxiety, the patient try to take the hypnotic every second or third night. To the author's knowledge, however, this method has not been compared with every-night dosing in a controlled study. Zammit (1999) has summarized both the controversy and the more recent perspective of some sleep experts. Zammit noted that in some cases, insomnia is undertreated, owing to physicians' concerns that the patient will become "addicted" to the hypnotic medication. Nevertheless, some people with insomnia truly need the chronic use of a hypnotic agent, and most of these individuals do not show signs of "addiction," such as use of escalating or excessive doses of hypnotics (Zammit 1999). In summary, the issue of long-term BZD hypnotic therapy has not been settled by appropriately controlled studies but may be indicated in carefully selected patients (McGee and Pies 2002).

Q. What about the long-term use of non-BZD hypnotics?

A. Here, too, the controlled data are limited. Randomized, controlled, *nightly* dosing trials with zolpidem have not exceeded 4 weeks. However, *intermittent* use of zolpidem has shown longer-term efficacy in several treatment regimens and study designs (Hajak et al. 2003; Walsh et al. 2000). Walsh and colleagues

(2000) carried out a placebo-controlled, 8-week study of intermittent zolpidem use (10 mg at least three, and no more than five, times per week), using subjective measures of efficacy. Zolpidem was more effective than placebo in initiating and maintaining sleep on nights it was taken, with no evidence of rebound insomnia on the "off" nights. Randomized controlled studies with zaleplon have not exceeded 4 weeks. However, a recent, 36-center, open-label, long-term study (6–12 months) found zaleplon useful in the long-term treatment of primary insomnia (Ancoli-Israel et al. 2003). Preliminary data suggest eszopiclone is safe and effective in chronic nightly use over a 6-month period (Krystal et al. 2003).

Q. What BZDs are employed in the treatment of periodic leg movements of sleep (PLMS)?

A. While most BZDs could be used for PLMS, clonazepam (1 mg at bedtime) is probably the most commonly used agent for this purpose, owing to its intermediate $t_{1/2}$. This allows it to provide "coverage" of PLMS for 6–8 hours (Nofzinger and Reynolds 1996). However, as with all BZDs, adaptation or tolerance to the effects of clonazepam may develop, and BZDs must be used cautiously in the presence of obstructive sleep apnea (Nofzinger and Reynolds 1996). Alternative treatments for more severe or persistent PLMS and restless leg syndrome (e.g., dopamine agonists such as pergolide) may also be worth considering (Earley and Allen 1996).

Q. What is the role of BZDs in the management of bipolar disorder?

A. BZDs may be very useful as adjunctive agents in the management of acute mania and mixed bipolar states (American Psychiatric Association 2002; Chouinard 1987; McElroy and Keck 1995). In one controlled study comparing lorazepam with haloperidol as adjuncts to lithium in acute mania, the two treatments were comparable (Lenox et al. 1992). Typically, clonazepam 0.5–2.0 mg q 2–6 hours is used, until the patient is calm or sedated. The maximum daily dose is usually less than 6 mg (Sachs 1996), although higher dosages (>12 mg/day) may be employed. One study (Bradwejn et al. 1990) found lorazepam superior to clonazepam during the first 2 weeks of treatment, but these differences may diminish with time. After 2–3 weeks—and usually after the primary mood-stabilizing agents have achieved control of the mania—

the BZD can often be tapered and discontinued. However, some bipolar patients, particularly those with comorbid anxiety disorders, may benefit from longer-term BZD treatment. Contraindications to BZD maintenance include a history of BZD-induced behavioral dyscontrol/paradoxical response and substance abuse (Sachs 1996). Although one study found neurotoxicity when clonazepam was combined with lithium (Koczerginski et al. 1989), the patients were also taking neuroleptics, which may have contributed to this problem (Sarid-Segal et al. 1995).

Q. What about the use of BZDs in the *depressed* phase of bipolar illness?

A. Anxiety may intensify dysphoria and insomnia during bipolar depression, and loss of sleep is a risk factor for the "switch" into mania. Therefore, brief periods of BZD use may be warranted in depressed bipolar patients with anxiety and/or insomnia (Sachs 1996). Since alprazolam may occasionally induce mania, use of lorazepam or clonazepam is probably preferable. Although one study of clonazepam (1.5–6.0 mg/day) showed that it improved depression in bipolar depressed patients (Kishimoto et al. 1988), the evidence that clonazepam has significant antidepressant properties is weak. BZDs may also be associated with treatment-emergent depression in patients with some anxiety disorders (Janicak et al. 1993; Tesar 1990). The American Psychiatric Association (2002) revised guideline for the treatment of bipolar disorder does not include BZDs among the preferred agents for acute bipolar depression. Thus, the use of BZDs for bipolar depression must be carefully considered.

Q. Are BZDs effective in the treatment of unipolar depression?

A. In a review of 20 controlled studies of the use of BZDs in treating patients with depressive disorders, Schatzberg and Cole (1978) concluded that BZDs may significantly relieve anxiety and insomnia but that they do not have significant impact on core depressive symptoms (e.g., psychomotor retardation, diurnal mood variation). There was little evidence for efficacy in severe depression unless prominent anxiety was also present (Janicak et al. 1993).

Some data suggest that BZDs may aggravate depression and/or suicidality (Klerman 1986). Alprazolam, however, may be an exception, and in one study, alprazolam showed antidepressant properties equal to those of imipramine (Feighner 1982). Another study (Jonas and Hearron 1996) of alprazolam in patients with major depression compared its effects on suicidality with those of both placebo and various "active comparator" medications (including several tricyclics). Alprazolam-treated patients showed greater improvement in suicidality than did placebo-treated patients, though the improvement was somewhat less than patients treated with active comparator drugs. The authors interpreted the results to indicate that "although alprazolam may have efficacy in mild-to-moderate depression, standard antidepressants are more effective in severe depression" (p. 211). In a recent review of suicide in persons with treatment-refractory depression, Fawcett and Harris (2001) concluded that in extremely anxious depressed patients, "the aggressive treatment of this anxiety with potent, short-acting benzodiazepines (except in some borderline patients who may experience disinhibition or dissociation, resulting in an increase of impulsive, self-destructive behaviors) can reduce acute suicide risk so that antidepressant therapy can have the required time to relieve the depressive symptoms" (p. 480). This may be the case, but there are few if any controlled data bearing on this approach.

Q. Are there any appropriate indications for barbiturates in modern clinical psychiatry?

A. In the author's opinion, there are virtually no good reasons to use barbiturates in preference to safer agents, such as BZDs and antidepressants, in the treatment of anxiety. Amobarbital (50–100 mg im) is sometimes used in emergency settings to control agitation; however, laryngospasm and respiratory depression may occur, and intramuscular lorazepam may be just as effective (Kaplan et al. 1995). Amobarbital has been used, historically, for diagnostic purposes (the so-called Amytal interview), but both clinical and medicolegal considerations make this use problematic; for example, the *Ramona v. Ramona* (1991) case, in California, has cast suspicion on the amobarbital interview, owing to fears of "implanted memories."

Q. What about the use of chloral hydrate for insomnia?

A. Chloral hydrate (500–1,000 mg at bedtime) may rarely be indicated in the *short-term* treatment (two or three nights) of insomnia if BZDs are not effective or cannot be tolerated. However, the lethal dose of chloral hydrate is only 5–10 times the "therapeutic" dose, giving this drug a very narrow therapeutic index. Moreover, symptoms of intoxication, dependence, and withdrawal may be associated with chloral hydrate, and tolerance develops after only 2 weeks of treatment (Kaplan et al. 1995). GI side effects (e.g., gastritis and gastric ulceration) are also common. Aside from its use in painful pediatric procedures, the role of chloral hydrate is quite limited in modern medical practice.

Q. What is *guanfacine,* and what are its indications in psychiatry?

A. Guanfacine is an α_2-adrenergic agonist, similar to clonidine in its reduction of autonomic arousal. Guanfacine also suppresses REM sleep. It has been used in lieu of clonidine in the treatment of attention-deficit/hyperactivity disorder, and occasionally in Tourette's syndrome (Wagner 2004). Guanfacine appeared to be of benefit in one case of PTSD-related "nightmares" (Horrigan and Barnhill 1996). Guanfacine is usually given at a dosage of 2–4 mg/day. Because it has a longer $t_{1/2}\beta$ than clonidine, guanfacine may have some advantages in various disorders of autonomic arousal or REM sleep. Controlled studies are needed to establish guanfacine's indications, benefits, and risks.

Q. What is the role of older and newer anticonvulsants in the treatment of anxiety?

A. None of the older or newer anticonvulsants have FDA-approved labeling for use in any of the anxiety disorders. However, there is some evidence—mainly from open studies—that several of these agents have anxiolytic effects (Davidson and Connor 2004; Lydiard 2003). Valproate, for example, showed benefit in a small (N= 12) open, 6-week study of patients with panic disorder, in which an initial valproate dosage of 500 mg/day was used (Woodman and Noyes 1994). Measures of panic attacks and anxiety improved more quickly and robustly than did measures of phobic avoidance. Eleven of the 12 patients showed sustained improvement at 6-month follow-up. A case series of patients with panic disorder and agoraphobia (Zwanzger et al. 2001) found that tiagabine (15 mg/day) improved these symptoms within 2–4 weeks; however, one patient experienced sedation and vertigo, requiring discontinuation. Some psychiatrists have raised questions about tiagabine's safety, given reports of dizziness, tremor, abnormal thinking, nervousness, nonconvulsive status epilepticus (absence stupor), and emotional lability in some epileptic populations

(French et al. 2004). In any case, given better-validated options, it is premature to recommend tiagabine for routine use in psychiatry.

Gabapentin, though not validated for use as monotherapy in bipolar disorder, was shown to be useful in a controlled study of social phobic disorder. Pande et al. (1999) carried out a randomized, double-blind, placebo-controlled, parallel-group study involving 69 patients with social phobia. Patients were randomly assigned to receive either gabapentin (900–3,600 mg/day in three divided doses) or placebo for 14 weeks. There was a significant reduction in symptoms of social phobia among patients taking gabapentin, compared with those receiving placebo, based on several clinician- and patient-rated scales. Curiously, the drug–placebo difference was smaller for women than for men. No serious adverse events were reported in the gabapentin group, though dizziness and dry mouth were significantly more common than in the placebo group. Response rates were somewhat lower than seen in placebo-controlled studies of social phobia utilizing clonazepam or phenelzine.

With respect to PTSD, valproate, topiramate, and lamotrigine have shown some benefit (Davidson and Connor 2004). However, an 8-week, open study of valproate monotherapy in civilian patients ($N=10$) with non-combat-related PTSD did not demonstrate valproate's efficacy (Otte et al. 2004). One placebo-controlled study of 15 outpatients with PTSD (Hertzberg et al. 1999) found that lamotrigine (200–500 mg/day) led to a response rate of 50% (compared with 25% with placebo). Intrusive and avoidance symptoms responded most robustly.

Finally, there is increasing interest in *pregabalin,* a drug that—contrary to its name—does not appear to have direct effects on γ-aminobutyric acid (GABA) or GABA receptors, but that may *reduce calcium influx* in nerve terminals (Pande et al. 2004). Some controlled evidence suggests that pregabalin is rapidly effective in treating the psychic and somatic symptoms of GAD (Lydiard et al. 2003) and may also be effective in treating social phobia at a dosage of 600 mg/day (Pande et al. 2004). Somnolence and dizziness may be side effects of pregabalin, and further research is needed before this agent may be recommended for routine psychiatric use.

Taken in total, these data suggest that anticonvulsants may play a useful role in several anxiety disorders but that more controlled studies are needed.

Q. Is there a role for atypical antipsychotics (APs) in treating anxiety disorders?

A. In general, atypical APs would be considered second- or third-line agents, or, in some cases, adjunctive treatments for very refractory cases of anxiety. The long-term risks of AP medication—including neuroleptic malignant syndrome, tardive dyskinesia, and metabolic syndromes—generally argue against use of these agents in most cases of nonpsychotic anxiety. However, there are case reports and open data favoring the use of atypical APs for PTSD and for refractory OCD. For example, Petty et al. (2001) found that olanzapine was useful for ameliorating PTSD symptoms in an open-label study. However, in a 10-week, double-blind, placebo-controlled evaluation of 15 patients randomized to either olanzapine or placebo, olanzapine was no more effective than placebo (Butterfield et al. 2001). In a placebo-controlled study of PTSD-related symptoms in combat veterans, Monnelly et al. (2003) found that adjunctive risperidone (0.5–2.0 mg/day) was superior to placebo for reduction of irritability and intrusive thoughts. Adjunctive quetiapine (average dosage = 100 mg/day) also reduced PTSD symptoms in a 6-week, open study of combat veterans with PTSD and was generally well tolerated (Hamner et al. 2003). Finally, a small (*N* = 6) retrospective case study of clozapine treatment of chronic PTSD in adolescents found the drug useful at dosages up to 800 mg/day; however, these subjects had psychotic symptoms (Wheatley et al. 2004).

As discussed in Chapter 3 ("Antipsychotics"), there are open studies finding that adjunctive atypical APs may be useful in OCD (Bourgeois and Klein 1996; Koran et al. 2000; McDougle et al. 1995). In addition, Hollander et al. (2003) performed an 8-week, double-blind, placebo-controlled study of risperidone augmentation of SSRI treatment in adult subjects with treatment-resistant OCD. Four patients taking risperidone (40%) and none (0%) receiving placebo were responders, and risperidone was generally well tolerated. (Note, however, possible drug–drug interactions between some SSRIs and atypical agents.) The effects of olanzapine in OCD have been equivocal.

In summary, there may be a limited role for atypical APs in anxiety disorders, but more controlled studies are needed before these agents can be recommended for routine use.

Q. Is there a role for tricyclic antidepressants (TCAs) and/or trazodone in the treatment of anxiety disorders? What about monoamine oxidase inhibitors (MAOIs)?

A. There are certainly controlled data supporting the use of the TCAs (mainly imipramine and clomipramine) for treatment of OCD, panic disorder, and GAD (Allgulander et al. 2003; Greist et al. 2003; Pollack et al. 2003). Both TCAs and MAOIs have also shown efficacy in PTSD (Stein et al. 2003). However, given the numerous side effects and risks associated with TCAs and MAOIs, these agents are usually reserved for refractory cases or as adjunctive treatment. Trazodone does have antianxiety properties and has been used successfully for generalized anxiety and OCD; however, controlled data have been negative for trazodone's anti-obsessional effects (Golden et al. 2004; Pigott et al. 1992).

Mechanisms of Action

Q. *Baclofen,* like BZDs, is also active at GABA receptors. Does baclofen have anxiolytic properties?

A. Baclofen is active at $GABA_B$ receptors, whose activation results in an increase in potassium channel conductance and hyperpolarization of the neuron. Baclofen is not active at $GABA_A$ receptors (the site of action of BZDs) and seems to have primarily antispasmodic properties (Paul 1995). However, baclofen does have sedative properties and can lead to somnolence, tolerance, and respiratory depression (Drug Facts and Comparisons 1995). One recent, open study found baclofen (at a dosage up to 80 mg/day in divided doses) helpful in a small group ($N=14$) of male veterans with PTSD (Drake et al. 2003). Both anxious and depressive symptoms appeared responsive. Larger, controlled studies are needed to validate this interesting finding.

Q. Do BZDs have effects on other neurotransmitters besides GABA?

A. In animal studies, BZDs have been shown to decrease nigrostriatal dopamine release and turnover; block stress-induced activation in cortical dopamine turnover; and augment the chronic decreases in dopamine turnover seen with neuroleptics (Wolkowitz and Pickar 1991). It has also been hypothesized that the antipanic properties of BZDs relate to their inhibitory effects on noradrenergic function in the locus coeruleus (Charney and Heninger 1985). Clonazepam, perhaps more so than other BZDs, may have significant effects on serotonin (Kishimoto et al. 1988).

Q. What is buspirone's mechanism of action, and how does this relate to its clinical use?

A. Buspirone has no effect on the GABA–BZD receptor complex; rather, it is an agonist or partial agonist at the serotonin$_{1A}$ (5-HT$_{1A}$) receptor. Buspirone may also have activity at serotonin$_2$ (5-HT$_2$) and dopamine$_2$ (D$_2$) receptors, but the clinical significance of these effects is not clear (Kaplan et al. 1995). Buspirone's action at the 5-HT$_{1A}$ receptor is complex, depending on whether the receptor is pre- or postsynaptic. It appears that buspirone acts as an agonist at presynaptic 5-HT$_{1A}$ receptors but as a *partial* agonist at postsynaptic 5-HT$_{1A}$ receptors. This pharmacodynamic "flexibility" may permit buspirone to act as either an anxiolytic or an antidepressant, depending on the concentration of "ambient" serotonin (Eison 1990; Pies 1993). In anxiety states, buspirone's net effect may be to reduce serotonergic function in some brain regions, via effects on the (presynaptic) 5-HT$_{1A}$ autoreceptor; however, in depressive conditions characterized by *low ambient 5-HT levels,* buspirone (at a dosage of 50 mg/day or more) may enhance serotonergic function by acting as a "stand-in" for endogenous 5-HT (Eison 1990; Pies 1993; Rickels et al. 1990).

Q. How do zolpidem, zaleplon, and zopiclone/eszopiclone work?

A. All three of these non-BZDs are, nevertheless, active at the BZD receptor (α–γ subunit interface) of the GABA$_A$ receptor. Zolpidem (Ambien) and zaleplon (Sonata) bind with high affinity only to receptors containing the α_1 subunit (termed "ω_1" receptors in the older literature). Eszopiclone (Lunesta)—recently approved for the treatment of insomnia—also interacts with the BZD site on the GABA$_A$ receptor but probably binds to different "microdomains" within the γ subunit than do BZDs, zolpidem, and zaleplon (Davies et al. 2000). Moreover, eszopiclone is active at BZD receptors containing α_1, α_2, or α_3 subunits. Presumably, allosteric modulation of the BZD receptor by all three drugs leads to influx of chloride ions, thus hyperpolarizing the neuron and making it less likely to fire. Differences in receptor subunits, and their variable expression in different brain regions, may confer different clinical properties—and, to some degree, side-effect profiles—on these agents. For example, α_1 subunit receptors may mediate *sedative* and *amnestic* effects of BZD receptor ligands, whereas α_2 subunit receptors may mediate *anxiolysis* and *muscle relaxation.* α_3 subunit receptors are in high concentration in the brain stem/reticular activating system, where they may interact with neurotransmitter pathways for serotonin and norepinephrine—perhaps affecting sleep. The clinical implications of these differences are still not entirely clear, but subunit binding may influence how much a BZD ligand promotes sedation versus true sleep, anxiolysis, and so forth (Low et al. 2000; Mohler et al. 2002).

Pharmacokinetics

Q. What issues arise regarding absorption (GI, intramuscular) of BZDs?

A. With the exception of clorazepate, all BZDs are absorbed unchanged from the GI tract. Clorazepate is converted in the GI tract to desmethyldiazepam, and this requires an acidic medium. Thus, concomitant administration of antacids may impair absorption of clorazepate, at least acutely (see subsection "Drug–Drug Interactions" in the "Overview" section of this chapter). The BZDs differ in their rates of absorption from the GI tract; for example, lorazepam is rapidly absorbed, whereas oxazepam is slowly absorbed. The rate of absorption largely determines onset of clinical action after oral dosing, but other factors are involved (see next question). Oral absorption may be affected by the presence of food; for example, patients who take a BZD with a snack at bedtime may experience a slower onset of hypnotic activity than if the same drug had been taken several hours after a meal (Janicak et al. 1993). Lorazepam is the only commonly used BZD that is well absorbed *intramuscularly;* thus, intramuscular administration of other BZDs (e.g., for the treatment of delirium tremens) is unlikely to be reliable. Midazolam, which is also well absorbed intramuscularly, is a BZD usually used as a preanesthetic agent (e.g., prior to surgical procedures) and in some emergency situations in which rapid sedation is desired.

Q. What is the relationship between how lipophilic a BZD is and its onset of clinical action?

A. All other things being equal, more lipophilic compounds would cross the blood–brain barrier more rapidly than less lipophilic ones and would, in principle, have a more rapid onset of action (Greenblatt 1991). This has been demonstrated with intravenously administered BZDs, such as the highly lipophilic diazepam (which has an almost immediate onset) and the less lipophilic lorazepam (which has a more delayed onset). However, after oral dosage, the rate-limiting step in onset of clinical action is the drug's *rate of absorption from the GI tract* (Greenblatt 1991).

Q. What are the specific metabolic pathways for BZD metabolism?

A. Three BZDs—lorazepam, oxazepam, and temazepam—require only *glucuronidation* and are relatively unaffected by alterations in hepatic function, as in cirrhosis. Most of the other BZDs—including diazepam, chlordiazepoxide, flurazepam, and the triazolo-BZDs—undergo *oxidative metabolism* ("Phase I" reaction). Clonazepam undergoes *nitroreduction* as its primary metabolic step, which is also sensitive to alterations in hepatic function (Sands et al. 1995). Most Phase I oxidative metabolism is mediated by the CYP system; in the case of BZDs, the 3A4 (3A3/4) and 2C19 systems appear to be primarily involved. Thus, the triazolo-BZDs—alprazolam, midazolam, and triazolam—are metabolized via CYP 3A4. Diazepam has a complex route of demethylation, involving both CYP 2C19 and 3A4 (Sands et al. 1995).

Q. What is "single-dose kinetics," and in what clinical situations involving BZDs is this important?

A. *Single-dose kinetics* refers to the distribution and accumulation of a drug after a single oral or parenteral dose. Single-dose kinetics with respect to BZDs is governed mainly by the distribution of the agent in particular body compartments (e.g., blood, central nervous system [CNS] lipids, or lipid stores outside the CNS). The $t_{1/2}\beta$ of a BZD becomes important only after *repeated* dosing. Single-dose kinetics applies in situations such as a single night's treatment of insomnia or "jet lag"; emergency treatment of alcohol withdrawal; status epilepticus; preoperative sedation; and induction of anesthesia (Arana and Hyman 1991; Greenblatt 1991) (see also question on antacid–BZD interaction in subsection "Drug–Drug Interactions" in this "Questions and Answers" section).

Main Side Effects

Q. What are the most common BZD side effects and their frequency?

A. BZD side effects tend to be "extensions" of their sedative properties (e.g., drowsiness or lightheadedness). Using lorazepam as a prototypical agent, one might expect the following common side-effect frequency: sedation (15.9%); dizziness (6.9%); weakness (4.2%); and unsteadiness (3.4%) (Physicians' Desk Reference 1996). For alprazolam, a triazolo-BZD, the *placebo-adjusted* rate of side effects is as follows: drowsiness (19.4%); hypotension (2.5%); increased salivation (1.8%); dry mouth (1.4%); lightheadedness (1.5%); and dizziness (1%). It is important to note that some side effects actually occur more frequently in the placebo group than in the BZD group; thus, side effects reported less frequently in the alprazolam group ($n=565$) than in the placebo group ($n=505$) include depression, headache, confusion, insomnia, nervousness, constipation, diarrhea, tachycardia, rigidity, and tremor (Physicians' Desk Reference 1996). With the hypnotic agent quazepam, placebo-adjusted side effects were as follows: daytime drowsiness (8.7%); headache (2.3%); and fatigue (1.9%) (Physicians' Desk Reference 1996) (see also Table 4–13).

Q. What effects do BZDs have on memory, and do these effects differ among agents?

A. All BZDs may cause varying degrees of memory impairment. If we divide memory into several components—*acquisition, retention, consolidation,* and *retrieval*—it is clear that BZDs impair memory at the level of consolidation; that is, when data are transferred from short- to long-term memory (American Psychiatric Association 1990). Thus, a person who has taken a BZD will recall something told to him or her after 1–2 minutes but will be unable to recall this information after 15–20 minutes. Anterograde amnesia associated with BZDs—difficulty in learning material presented after drug administration—may be seen even after a single oral dose of a BZD and is not correlated with degree of psychomotor impairment and sedation (Roache and Griffiths 1985).

Some data suggest that high-potency, short-$t_{1/2}$ BZDs (e.g., triazolam) impair memory more than low-potency, short-$t_{1/2}$ agents (e.g., oxazepam) at comparable therapeutic doses (American Psychiatric Association 1990; Scharf et al. 1987). It should be borne in mind, however, that even over-the-counter sedative-hypnotics (mainly antihistamines) can also impair memory, probably via their anticholinergic effects (Pies 1992). In the author's experience, elderly or dementia patients may show persistent cognitive deficits in some cases.

Q. What is the abuse liability of BZDs?

A. The question of abuse liability of BZDs is almost always a source of controversy among mental health professionals, depending on their philosophy and background (Pies 1991). Clinicians with a "12-step" orientation sometimes take the view that BZDs are widely abused, and discourage their long-term use. Unfortunately, the literature on "substance abuse" often uses terms that are either poorly defined, overlapping in meaning, or misunderstood, such as "addiction," "physical dependency," "psychological dependency," "tolerance," and "withdrawal" (McGee and Pies 2002; Raj and Sheehan 2004). Such confusion may lead some clinicians to conclude, for example, that any agent associated with a withdrawal syndrome must also be highly "addicting" (Raj and Sheehan 2004), which is not necessarily the case. (Even beta-blockers may produce withdrawal phenomena if abruptly discontinued.) Raj and Sheehan (2004) argue that true "abuse" is present if the drug is taken 1) in order to get "high"; 2) to further psychological regression; 3) in doses higher than those prescribed; and 4) after the medical indication has passed. Using one or more of these criteria, *actual BZD abuse seems to occur primarily in persons who abuse other drugs* (Schweizer et al. 1995). The reinforcing properties of BZDs, compared with those of other drugs of abuse, appear to be fairly low in nonaddict populations. There is some evidence suggesting that diazepam (and perhaps alprazolam and lorazepam) is more likely to be abused than other BZDs in "at-risk" populations (Griffiths and Wolf 1990; Schweizer et al. 1995). In contrast, oxazepam, halazepam, and possibly chlordiazepoxide have a relatively low abuse potential (Griffiths and Wolf 1990). Keep in mind that "abuse liability" as determined by clinical studies of euphoria, interviews with addicted individuals, and so forth is not necessarily related to *actual rates of abuse.* The latter has to do with factors such as overall availability of a drug and its cost "on the street." Thus, while lorazepam and alprazolam constitute a small percentage of illicit "drug traffic," they may still have a high abuse potential for a given individual (Griffiths and Wolf 1990). The bottom line is that BZDs should be used very conservatively, if at all, in patients with known histories of substance abuse and/or dependence; and only when other alternatives (such as a sedating antidepressant or an SSRI) have been exhausted. *Nevertheless, appropriately diagnosed individuals who are not at high risk should not be denied BZDs for short- or long-term use if these agents provide demonstrable and enduring therapeutic benefits.* In all such cases, of course, periodic monitoring and documentation of efficacy, pattern of use, and justification for continued BZD treatment are essential (McGee and Pies 2002).

Q. What is the abuse liability of BZDs in relatives of substance/alcohol abusers?

A. Several studies now indicate that subjective response to alprazolam and diazepam differs in subjects who have first-degree relatives with alcoholism compared with subjects who do not. Thus, Ciraulo et al. (1996) found that both the sons and daughters of alcoholic patients had "positive mood responses" to alprazolam more often than control subjects, despite similar alprazolam plasma levels. These authors concluded that their data are consistent with greater risk of alprazolam (and possibly ethanol) abuse in the siblings of alcoholic individuals, though these subjects themselves did not suffer from alcohol abuse or dependence.

Q. Do the BZDs differ in their tendency to produce discontinuation/withdrawal syndromes?

A. While controlled research studies are lacking, the American Psychiatric Association (1990) Task Force on Benzodiazepine Dependency noted that "anecdotal reports and clinical experience…have increasingly noted severe discontinuance with the high-potency, short $t_{1/2}$ benzodiazepines alprazolam, lorazepam, and triazolam.…there have also been suggestions that high-potency, short $t_{1/2}$ benzodiazepines have been associated with a higher incidence of seizures following abrupt withdrawal" (p. 30). Thus, discontinuation should be very gradual with these agents.

Q. What are the main symptoms of BZD withdrawal, and how are they managed?

A. Discontinuation of BZDs may result in *recurrence* or *relapse* symptoms (return of the original symptoms for which BZDs were prescribed); *rebound* symptoms (symptoms such as anxiety or insomnia that are more intense than at baseline); and true *withdrawal* symptoms (probably representing the reaction of the CNS to loss of GABA) (Jenkins et al. 2001; Shader and Greenblatt 1994a). These three types of symptoms can often be difficult to distinguish in a given patient. However, a study of diazepam discontinuation (Pourmotabbed et al. 1996) found that discontinuation of clinical doses produced *rebound anxiety* rather than physical withdrawal symptoms in women with GAD. Most of these rebound symptoms (anxiety, insomnia, GI symptoms) were mild and transient. Withdrawal symptoms can include anxiety, agitation, tachycardia, palpitations, anorexia, blurred vision, muscle cramps, insomnia, nightmares, hyperacusis (increased sensitivity to noise), and seizures (Ayd 1995; Jenkins et al. 2001). Various non-BZD agents have been used to manage BZD withdrawal (e.g., phenobarbital, carbamazepine), but the best approach is to avoid the syndrome in the first place by very slow tapering of BZDs—particularly short-acting agents (Shader and Greenblatt 1994a). One approach is the "quarter per week" method, in which the daily dose of, say, alprazolam is reduced by 25% once per week. Thus, a patient taking 4 mg/day of alprazolam would reduce the daily dose to 3 mg in week one, 2 mg in week two, 1 mg in week three, then discontinue it completely (Shader and Greenblatt 1994a). However, this may be too abrupt for many patients, and the last 0.5–1.0 mg of alprazolam may be particularly difficult to discontinue. Thus, extending the tapering schedule to 6–8 weeks, with very small decrements, may be necessary (Shader and Greenblatt 1994a).

Q. How do the non-BZD hypnotic agents compare in terms of rebound insomnia and withdrawal?

A. Zaleplon has been compared with zolpidem in outpatients with primary insomnia (Fry et al. 2000). No tolerance to zaleplon developed over the course of the 4-week study, and there were no indications of rebound insomnia or withdrawal symptoms after discontinuation. In contrast, zolpidem (10 mg) had significantly greater incidence of withdrawal symptoms and a "suggestion" of sleep difficulty after treatment discontinuation (rebound insomnia). The 6-month study of eszopiclone (Krystal et al. 2003) found no evidence of tolerance over the entire study period.

Q. What is the abuse liability of the non-BZD hypnotics zolpidem and zopiclone?

A. Using worldwide prescription data and case reports in the literature (1966–2002), Hajak et al. (2003) examined the abuse and dependence potential for zolpidem and zopiclone. A total of 36 cases of zolpidem dependence and 22 cases of zopiclone dependence were uncovered. Considering the number of prescriptions written worldwide for these agents, the authors concluded that "the relative incidence of dependence and abuse appears extremely low." However, individuals with a history of substance abuse may be at higher risk for abuse of these agents. Furthermore, individual reports of zolpidem abuse, tolerance, and withdrawal are occasionally seen (Aragona 2000).

Drug–Drug Interactions

Q. What are the most common and serious drug–drug interactions involving BZDs?

A. The most common and serious drug–drug interactions occur with alcohol and other sedative-hypnotics (American Psychiatric Association 1990), often producing severe CNS toxicity and/or respiratory suppression. BZDs also augment the euphoric effects of opiates. There have also been reports of cardiovascular symptoms, respiratory distress, or delirium when BZDs are used concomitantly with clozapine; however, similar symptoms have been reported with clozapine monotherapy (Cobb et al. 1991; Cozza et al. 2003). Adverse reactions seem to occur within 1–2 days of starting high doses of clozapine in patients taking long-acting BZDs (Ayd 1995; Grohmann et al. 1989). In the author's experience, initiation of low-dose BZD treatment (e.g., 0.25–0.5 mg of clonazepam or the equivalent) is usually tolerated in otherwise healthy patients taking moderate doses of clozapine (250–400 mg/day). However, vital signs should be monitored for the first few weeks of treatment, and the rationale for use of BZDs (as well as known risks) should be clearly documented in the medical record.

Q. Is there a clinically significant decrement in the effectiveness of BZDs when antacids are taken simultaneously?

A. With the exception of single-dose treatment, the basic answer is no. While antacids may slow the *rate* of BZD absorption, the *completeness* of absorption and resultant steady-state concentration are not affected. Since slowed absorption may affect subjective antianxiety effects, however, use of a BZD with an antacid may be undesirable if the patient requires rapid onset of anxiolytic action. It is also possible that somewhat lower plasma levels (due to slowed absorption) may decrease efficacy in some patients (Creelman et al. 1989).

Q. What is the effect of taking BZDs with food?

A. As with the use of antacids, food *delays* absorption of BZDs without diminishing the *completeness* of absorption ("area under the curve," or AUC, when one plots plasma level of the drug vs. time); thus, overall bioavailability is not reduced. When rapid anxiolysis is necessary, BZDs should be administered on an empty stomach (Creelman et al. 1989).

Q. How important is protein binding displacement (e.g., by warfarin-type anticoagulants) in treating a patient with a BZD?

A. Although heparin can cause a rapid rise in the free concentration of diazepam, this increase is probably transient and rapidly compensated for by increased exposure of the free BZD to hepatic metabolism. Thus, such interactions are unlikely to be of enduring clinical significance (Ayd 1995; Sands et al. 1995).

Q. Which antidepressants are best to avoid when prescribing concomitant BZDs?

A. As noted earlier (see subsection "Pharmacokinetics" in the "Overview" section of this chapter), the CYP 3A4 and CYP 2C19 systems appear to be primarily involved in BZD metabolism. The triazolo-BZDs—alprazolam, midazolam, and triazolam—as well as clonazepam, are metabolized via CYP 3A4. Diazepam has a complex route of demethylation, involving both CYP 2C19 and CYP 3A4 (Sands et al. 1995). Thus, antidepressants that are *strong* inhibitors of CYP 3A4 (e.g., nefazodone) or CYP 2C19 (e.g., fluvoxamine) should be used with caution when coadministering BZDs (Preskorn 1996; Shader et al. 1996). Norfluoxetine (the active metabolite of fluoxetine), sertraline and its metabolite desmethylsertraline, and fluvoxamine can all have *moderate* degrees of inhibition on CYP 3A4 (Shader et al. 1996). It appears from in vivo studies that fluoxetine and fluvoxamine are likely to increase diazepam and alprazolam levels. Fluoxetine can elevate levels of both these BZDs 25%–50%, and fluvoxamine can lead to increases in levels of these BZDs of 100%–300% (Preskorn 1996). Sertraline may slightly increase diazepam levels, whereas paroxetine appears unlikely to have major effects on BZD metabolism. Venlafaxine appears to have little effect on CYP 3A4, 2C9, or 2C19 and thus should have little effect on BZD metabolism (Cozza et al. 2003; Shader et al. 1996). Citalopram and escitalopram—both mild inhibitors of CYP 2D6—should have little effect on BZD metabolism (Cozza et al. 2003). With respect to TCAs, increased imipramine and desipramine (but not nortriptyline) levels may be seen with concomitant alprazolam administration. Moreover, amitriptyline may increase the psychomotor effects of BZDs (Sands et al. 1995).

Q. What drug–drug interactions can occur with buspirone?

A. Buspirone is metabolized chiefly by CYP 3A4; hence, any strong inhibitor of this enzyme (e.g., ketoconazole, nefazodone, and even grapefruit juice) may lead to elevated levels of buspirone (Cozza et al. 2003). Buspirone and MAOI combinations (according to the manufacturer of buspirone) may lead to hypertension, though not all patients will experience this effect; still, a 2-week washout should follow discontinuation of an MAOI prior to initiation of buspirone. Buspirone has been implicated in cases of the "serotonin syndrome" (see Chapter 2, "Antidepressants") and thus may have pharmacodynamic interactions with other serotonergic agents.

Q. What is the preferred method of switching someone from a BZD to buspirone?

A. Because buspirone is not cross-reactive with BZDs, BZD withdrawal symptoms may occur during the "switch," unless the BZD is slowly tapered. Most clinicians would add buspirone to the BZD regimen, stabilize the dose of buspirone, then very gradually taper the BZD (Arana and Hyman 1991;

Ninan and Muntasser 2004; Schatzberg and Cole 1991). Remember that some patients who have taken BZDs for many years may not experience much subjective relief from buspirone and will require several months to be "weaned" from the BZD. A subgroup of chronically anxious patients who cannot tolerate serotonergic agents may need to be maintained indefinitely on a small BZD dose, sometimes in combination with buspirone.

Potentiating Maneuvers

Q. Is it useful to combine buspirone with a BZD in cases of GAD or panic disorder?

A. Some small-sample reports suggest improvement when buspirone is added to a BZD (Cole and Yonkers 1995; Udelman and Udelman 1990). Thus, while buspirone dose *not* block BZD withdrawal symptoms, it may reduce anxiety in patients undergoing withdrawal from alprazolam (Udelman and Udelman 1990). Gastfriend and Rosenbaum (1989) also described four patients with panic disorder, incompletely controlled with BZDs, who had reduced generalized and anticipatory anxiety after the addition of buspirone.

Q. Can BZDs be used to potentiate the primary effects of mood stabilizers and antidepressants?

A. BZDs are routinely used in combination with mood stabilizers in the treatment of manic patients, and BZD hypnotic agents are often recommended for insomniac bipolar patients who are taking lithium (Lenox and Manji 1995). As indicated in Chapter 5 ("Mood Stabilizers"), BZDs are useful adjunctive agents in the management of acute mania (American Psychiatric Association 2002). The issue of BZDs in depression is less clear. Fawcett (1990) found that in patients with major depression and severe anxiety, "aggressive treatment with a benzodiazepine anxiolytic is indicated for immediate relief of anxiety" (p. 42), since antidepressants may take 3–6 weeks to reach peak effectiveness. Fawcett further stated that "the rapid action of benzodiazepines in relieving symptoms of anxiety increases the likelihood that the patient will continue therapy long enough to feel the effects of the antidepressant. As the antidepressant becomes fully effective, benzodiazepine therapy may be discontinued in slowly tapered doses…" (p. 42). Similarly, in patients with comorbid panic disorder and depressive symptoms, Coplan and Gorman (1990) noted that relief of panic is usually more rapid (1–2 weeks) with the concomitant use of a high-potency BZD and an antidepressant, as compared with an antidepressant alone (4–6 weeks). On the other hand, several BZDs may have pharmacokinetic interactions with antidepressants such as fluoxetine and nefazodone (see "Drug–Drug Interactions" subsection above; see also Table 4–15). Moreover, in some susceptible patients, BZDs may worsen depression or increase antidepressant side effects. Thus, it is the author's preference to begin treatment of an anxious depressed patient with a *single agent* possessing both anxiolytic/hypnotic and antidepressant properties, if possible. Nefazodone appears to be a good candidate in this respect (Zajecka 1995), but with its "black box warning" regarding hepatic dysfunction, nefazodone is no longer considered a first-line agent. (The brand Serzone is no longer produced or marketed in the United States, though generic versions may still be available.) Mirtazapine may be an alternative in anxious depressed patients, particularly those with insomnia, but controlled data are lacking (Davidson and Connor 2004). Some extremely anxious patients may require coprescription of an SSRI and—for the first 2 weeks or so—a BZD. The patient should understand at the outset that the BZD is a temporary measure. In the author's experience, patients who are not good candidates for adjunctive BZDs may benefit from a low dose of gabapentin (100–300 mg), especially at bedtime.

Q. Do BZDs potentiate the effects of antipsychotic agents?

A. BZDs either as sole or as adjunctive agents in psychotic patients may ameliorate superimposed anxiety, auditory hallucinations, and perhaps negative symptoms in a few schizophrenic patients; however, sedation, ataxia, and cognitive impairment may occur (Janicak et al. 1993). A number of BZDs (lorazepam, clonazepam, diazepam) have proved useful in catatonic patients, including some with catatonic schizophrenia (Martenyi et al. 1989) (see Chapter 3, "Antipsychotics"). BZD augmentation of neuroleptics may help control agitation during exacerbations of schizophrenia (Tueth et al. 1995); however, a small subset of psychotic patients may experience increased arousal or aggression when treated with BZDs (Arana et al. 1986; Janicak et al. 1993).

Q. What adjunctive role does tiagabine play in the treatment of anxiety disorders?

A. Tiagabine, a selective GABA reuptake inhibitor, appears to have antianxiety properties and has shown benefit in some preliminary reports of patients with PTSD, panic disorder, and generalized anxiety (Lydiard 2003; F.B. Taylor 2003). One recent open study (*N*=7) used tiagabine (4–12 mg/day) as an "add-on" agent in patients with PTSD (F.B. Taylor 2003). Patients were taking a variety of agents prior to addition of tiagabine, including SSRIs, buspirone, BZDs, and valproic acid. PTSD symptoms (including intrusive recollections, avoidance, and arousal) improved in six of the seven patients over the course of just 2 weeks, and tiagabine appeared to be well tolerated. Sleep quality also improved. Nevertheless, the small number of patients, the open design, and the use of multiple agents all mean that these findings are preliminary at best.

Use in Special Populations

Q. What are the teratogenic and behavioral risks to the fetus during exposure to BZDs in utero? What about buspirone?

A. In the 1970s and 1980s, diazepam (Valium) was found to be associated with cleft lip and palate in the fetus, and other BZDs were suspected of this association. In addition, one Swedish group (Laegreid et al. 1992) found a link between maternal use of BZDs during pregnancy and both impaired intrauterine growth and various dysmorphic birth defects. In a more recent review, Altshuler et al. (1996) concluded that the available data "indicate a positive association between first-trimester in utero exposure to BZDs and a specific anomaly, oral cleft" (p. 598). Diazepam may double the risk of oral cleft, while alprazolam may increase the risk by more than 11-fold. However, most available data suggest that BZDs do not markedly increase the *absolute risk* of cleft palate or other congenital abnormalities in exposed fetuses. Thus, the baseline risk of cleft palate is about 6 in 10,000. With alprazolam exposure during the first trimester, the risk may rise to 7 in 1,000—still less than 1 in 100 (Altshuler et al. 1996). The teratogenicity of lorazepam (Ativan) is less clear. Clonazepam (Klonopin) has not been evaluated for teratogenesis in controlled studies of human subjects; however, on the basis of animal data, clonazepam seems to have low teratogenic potential (Altshuler et al. 1996). The presence of alcohol and other substance abuse in pregnant women using BZDs complicates interpretation of the data. However, a matched case–control study of more than 60,000 women (Eros et al. 2002) found that treatment with five different BZDs studied during early pregnancy did not present detectable teratogenic risk to the fetus in humans. Nevertheless, infants exposed to BZDs either in the last trimester or at the time of parturition may show muscular hypotonicity, failure to feed, impaired temperature regulation, apnea, and low Apgar scores. There is also some evidence that BZDs may increase duration of labor and lead to prolonged withdrawal symptoms in the neonate, when mothers have been maintained on these agents throughout pregnancy. Withdrawal effects may be more likely when high doses of short-acting BZDs have been used. BZDs should not be stopped suddenly during pregnancy, but rather tapered slowly as delivery approaches (Stowe and Nemeroff 1995). The data on BZD-related "behavioral teratogenicity" and developmental delay are inconclusive (Altshuler et al. 1996; Newport et al. 2004). Finally, the non-BZD anxiolytic buspirone (BuSpar) has been shown to increase the number of stillbirths in rats, when given in high doses; however, there are insufficient data in humans to determine the risks of buspirone during pregnancy. The same may be said of the non-BZD hypnotics zolpidem and zaleplon (Newport et al. 2004).

Q. Given the risks described in the answer to the previous question, are BZDs contraindicated during pregnancy?

A. There is no absolute contraindication; rather, the modest risks of BZD exposure must be weighed against the severity of the patient's condition, the risks of no medication, and the risks of alternative medications. For example, inadequately treated panic attacks may themselves pose a risk to the fetus (Cohen et al. 1989). TCAs or fluoxetine (and perhaps other SSRIs) may be reasonable alternatives to BZDs for the treatment of panic disorder during pregnancy (see Chapter 2, "Antidepressants"). CBT may also be helpful in a variety of anxiety disorders and may reduce the need for psychotropic drugs during pregnancy (Altshuler et al. 1996).

Q. What are the risks of breastfeeding when the nursing mother is taking a BZD?

A. While there is evidence that several BZDs (e.g., diazepam, lorazepam, oxazepam) are excreted into breast milk, the actual levels of BZDs detected in breast milk seem to be fairly low, and the consequent risk to the infant quite small (McElhatton 1994; Newport et al. 2004; Pons et al. 1994). Lorazepam seems to have minimal accumulation in the fetus, and the percentage of the maternal dose of lorazepam to which a nursing infant is exposed is roughly 2.2% (Summerfield and Nielsen 1985). Thus, use of low-dose lorazepam in the nursing mother—particularly on a prn or short-term basis—is probably safe for the infant. However, if the infant should show signs of neurobehavioral toxicity, breastfeeding should be discontinued. The excretion of buspirone into human breast milk has not been adequately studied.

Q. What are the risks of falls and fractures in elderly patients treated with BZDs?

A. BZD use seems to increase the risk of falls among elderly patients from 1.5–3 times over baseline, with a 60% increase in risk of femur fracture (Gelenberg 1996; Herings et al. 1995). There is some controversy as to whether these effects are more likely with *long-acting* BZDs. Although such risk was found in some studies (e.g., Ray et al. 1989), Herings et al. (1995) found that *short-half-life* BZDs were actually associated with a slightly greater risk for falls and fractures than long-acting agents. Risk was increased further when short- and long-acting agents were used together. *Sudden increase in BZD dose* and *total dose* were more important in predicting falls than the pharmacokinetics of the agent. A recent review of 11 epidemiological studies (Cumming and Le Couteur 2003) found that the use of BZDs was associated with an increased risk of hip fracture of between 50%–110% in the elderly; however, there was no evidence that risk differed between short- and long-acting agents. There was some preliminary evidence that in "very old" individuals, BZDs that undergo oxidative metabolism may be associated with a higher risk of hip fracture than other BZDs. The authors concluded that BZDs should "rarely be prescribed" in older populations.

Q. What are the risks of respiratory suppression when prescribing BZDs for patients with chronic lung or other respiratory problems? Are other agents preferable for treating anxiety in these populations?

A. Although early reports suggested that BZDs may actually improve dyspnea in patients with chronic obstructive pulmonary disease (COPD), other reports have shown that BZDs may depress respiration and worsen carbon dioxide (CO_2) retention in these populations (Smoller 1996). In general, BZDs should be used very conservatively in patients with COPD, with shorter-acting agents preferable. Nevertheless, when used in low doses, BZDs may be useful in some anxious patients with COPD (Harnett 2001). Preliminary data from Smoller (1996; Smoller et al. 1998) suggest that sertraline has a beneficial effect on dyspnea and overall well-being in COPD patients and is effective for treatment of panic attacks. (There is also some evidence that serotonergic agents may block panic attacks by decreasing CO_2 sensitivity; see Klein 1993.) Although buspirone is not effective for panic attacks, it may be useful in some COPD patients with generalized anxiety and does not reduce ventilatory drive (Garner et al. 1989; Smoller 1996).

Q. What is the role of BZDs versus serotonergic agents in the treatment of childhood and adolescent anxiety disorders? How does dosing differ in these younger populations compared with adults?

A. Comprehensive reviews of this burgeoning topic are provided by Wagner (2004) and Oesterheld and colleagues (2003). In brief, the role of BZDs for childhood and adolescent anxiety disorders appears to be increasingly limited. If BZDs are used, they should be started at low daily doses (e.g., lorazepam 0.25 mg or diazepam 0.5 mg) and generally used for no more than a few weeks (Wagner 2004). The SSRIs (and venlafaxine) are fast becoming the medications of choice for most of the anxiety disorders of childhood and adolescence; however, there are few comparative, controlled studies with respect to specific agents. For citalopram, fluoxetine, and paroxetine, the medication is usually initiated at a dosage of 5–10 mg/day; for sertraline, 25–50 mg/day (Wagner 2004). The dosage range is similar to that in adults. For OCD, SSRIs are now the agents of first choice, as in adults. Fluoxetine, fluvoxamine, and sertraline have FDA-approved labeling for OCD in children. In GAD, venlafaxine and sertraline have the best controlled research support, though buspirone (15–40 mg/day) is supported by some open data. For social phobic anxiety, paroxetine has been shown to have some efficacy in a 16-week, double-blind, placebo-controlled trial (*N*=319) (Wagner et al. 2002). For childhood PTSD, there are few controlled studies; however, open data suggest efficacy for citalopram (20 mg/day), clonidine, and guanfacine. Panic disorder in children and adolescents has been found, on the basis of open studies, to respond to most SSRIs at doses similar to those used in adults (Wagner 2004).

In general, side effects from SSRIs in younger populations are similar to those seen in adults (e.g., nausea, headache, sedation, and insomnia). Increasing concerns about the safety of SSRIs in younger depressed populations (e.g., higher risk of suicidal ideation or behavior) warrant a very careful informed-consent process, or use of alternative agents, even though a causal link with suicide has not been demonstrated in either depressed or anxious child and adolescent populations treated with SSRIs. The need to rule out an *underlying bipolar disorder* in "anxious" children or adolescents treated with antidepressants is critical, in the author's view. Failure to do so may result in antidepressant-related dysphoria, agitation, or behavioral disinhibition, as may be seen in bipolar adults (Ghaemi et al. 2000; Mota-Castillo 2002; Perlis 2003).

Vignettes/Puzzlers

Q. Lorazepam has a $t_{1/2}\beta$ of about 10 hours. Diazepam has a $t_{1/2}\beta$ exceeding 50 hours, if one includes the effects of its metabolite, desmethyldiazepam. An acutely psychotic patient in the emergency room is given 1 mg of lorazepam orally, becomes less agitated, and remains so for about 4 hours. Another acutely psychotic, agitated patient is given an equipotent dose of oral diazepam (5 mg), becomes less agitated, but remains so for only 2 hours. Given the elimination half-lives of these agents, how do you account for these findings?

A. Clinical effects after single doses of BZDs are not related to elimination half-lives, but to the *lipophilicity* and *volume of distribution* of the agent (see subsection "Pharmacokinetics" in the "Questions and Answers" section of this chapter). Diazepam, which is highly lipophilic, rapidly crosses the blood–brain barrier and produces its clinical effect. However, it very rapidly exits the CNS lipids and moves into extra-CNS lipids (e.g., in the thighs)—often a very large volume of distribution. This translocation rapidly terminates diazepam's *single-dose* effect. In contrast, lorazepam is less lipophilic and takes slightly longer to have its clinical effect, but also has a smaller volume of distribution. It is thus longer-acting than diazepam after a *single* oral dose (Arana and Hyman 1991; Greenblatt 1993). These factors become less important after chronic dosing, during which, for example, diazepam generates a long-acting, less-lipophilic metabolite (desmethyldiazepam).

Q. A 73-year-old woman living in a nursing home has been successfully treated for major depression with generic nefazodone at a dosage of 300 mg/day. Her one residual symptom is significant initial insomnia, for which her physician adds triazolam 0.25 mg at bedtime. When, 2 nights after the triazolam is begun, the patient awakens at 3 A.M., the nursing staff reports that she is "totally out of it," disoriented to place and date, as well as ataxic and dysarthric. What is the likely explanation?

A. Nefazodone is an inhibitor of the CYP 3A4 system, which metabolizes the triazolo-BZDs. It is likely that the nefazodone raised plasma levels of the triazolam, which is itself associated with confusional states in older patients.

There may also have been pharmacodynamic synergism between the nefazodone (which can cause dose-related cognitive impairment in some elderly patients) and the triazolam (Gelenberg 1995; van Laar et al. 1995).

Q. A 70-year-old man's parkinsonism has been under good control while taking L-dopa and benztropine. Because he complains of acute situational anxiety, chlordiazepoxide 50 mg/day is prescribed. The patient's parkinsonism worsens significantly 2 days later. What is the likely mechanism?

A. Most likely, the GABA agonist effect of BZDs has reduced dopaminergic "outflow" in the basal ganglia, and this is interfering with the effects of L-dopa (Sands et al. 1995; Yosselson-Superstine and Lipman 1982).

Q. A 35-year-old woman with panic disorder has been maintained for 1 year on alprazolam 1 mg po tid. Over the past 3 weeks, the patient has begun to use more alprazolam, on a more frequent basis, in order to control "breakthrough" panic attacks. Her psychiatrist decides to switch her to the longer-acting agent clonazepam, at an initial dosage of 0.75 mg bid (one-half the total prescribed dose of alprazolam). After 2 weeks, the patient's panic attacks are well controlled on clonazepam alone, but she begins to complain of increasing depression. Why?

A. Most patients appear to tolerate the alprazolam-to-clonazepam switch quite well (Herman et al. 1987); however, there is some evidence that clonazepam may induce depression more often than does alprazolam (Janicak et al. 1993). Cohen and Rosenbaum (1987) reported that 5.5% of clonazepam-treated patients developed depression, versus only 0.7% of patients taking alprazolam. The latter medication may also have intrinsic antidepressant properties, and in the vignette, alprazolam may have been treating an undiagnosed, comorbid depressive disorder.

Q. **A 25-year-old man with panic disorder has been stable while taking clonazepam 1.0 mg bid. He suffers a manic episode and is prescribed carbamazepine 200 mg tid, with resultant plasma levels of 8 μg/mL (therapeutic range = 5–12 μg/mL). The patient's manic symptoms abate after 1 week, but his panic disorder worsens. What mechanism accounts for this change?**

A. Carbamazepine is a powerful inducer of hepatic metabolism and is known to decrease clonazepam levels by as much as 37% (Creelman et al. 1989). When these drugs are coadministered, some patients may need an upward adjustment of their clonazepam dose.

Q. **A patient with chronic alcohol abuse and dependence who has been successfully maintained on disulfiram 250 mg/day complains of "leg muscle spasms" that are interfering with his sleep. A polysomnogram confirms the presence of nocturnal myoclonus (PLMS). A trial of valproate is attempted, but the patient cannot tolerate the GI side effects. Chlordiazepoxide 25 mg hs is prescribed, with good control of the PLMS on the first 2 nights. By the third night, however, the patient complains of feeling "groggy" and "hungover." What is the problem, and is there an alternative treatment?**

A. Disulfiram inhibits metabolism of oxidatively metabolized BZDs (see Table 4–15), leading, in this case, to increased levels of chlordiazepoxide. Use of short-acting BZDs that undergo glucuronidation (e.g., lorazepam, oxazepam) may be a viable option (Creelman et al. 1989; Sands et al. 1995).

Q. **A patient presents with increased complaints of anxiety, despite receiving citalopram 40 mg qd and trazodone 50 mg hs. In an attempt to help alleviate her anxiety, the clinician prescribes buspirone 5 mg bid and increases the dosage to 10 mg bid over the next 3 weeks. At the end of the fourth week, the patient presents to the emergency room with hyperthermia (100.4°F), mild hypomanic symptoms, tremors, shivering, diarrhea, and hyperreflexia. Infectious causes are ruled out. What is the most likely etiology of this presentation?**

A. Theoretically, as a partial agonist at postsynaptic 5-HT$_{1A}$ receptors (Golden et al. 2004), buspirone would be expected to have a "protective" effect against states of excessive 5-HT activity, as might exist in someone taking both an SSRI and trazodone (whose metabolite, *m*-chlorophenylpiperazine, or m-CPP, has strong 5-HT agonist effects). Nevertheless, several case reports describe drug–drug interactions involving buspirone, apparently resulting in a "serotonin syndrome" (Manos 2000; Spigset and Adielsson 1997). This appears to have been the case in the example above. Although buspirone may augment SSRIs and related agents, the possibility of pharmacodynamically based adverse reactions should be kept in mind.

Q. A 34-year-old pregnant woman presents to the emergency room with new-onset visual hallucinations, which started early that morning. Her only medications were a prenatal vitamin, a calcium supplement, and zolpidem 10 mg hs prn. She has used the zolpidem "off and on" for the past week. Physical examination reveals essentially no abnormalities, and the patient denies any illicit drug use. All laboratory studies, including "toxic screen," are within normal limits. What could explain the patient's hallucinations?

A. There have been several reports of delirium, sensory distortions, and visual hallucinations associated with the use of zolpidem (Pies 1995a; Tsai et al. 2003). Most of these reactions have occurred in women and have been associated with "off and on again" zolpidem use. Presumably, the drug is altering BZD receptor function in some unexplained way. Although zolpidem is said to be in a "safer" risk category than are BZDs with respect to pregnancy (Category B vs. D), actual studies of zolpidem in pregnant populations are sorely lacking (Newport et al. 2004).

References

Abernethy DR, Greenblatt DJ, Divoll M, et al: Impairment of diazepam metabolism by low-dose estrogen–containing oral contraceptive steroids. N Engl J Med 306: 791–792, 1982

Abernethy DR, Greenblatt DJ, Eshelman FN, et al: Ranitidine does not impair oxidative or conjugative metabolism: noninteraction with antipyrine, diazepam and lorazepam. Clin Pharmacol Ther 35:188–192, 1984

Allgulander C, Bandelow B, Hollander E, et al: WCA recommendations for the long-term treatment of generalized anxiety disorder. CNS Spectr 8 (suppl 1):53–61, 2003

Altshuler LL, Cohen L, Szuba MP, et al: Pharmacologic management of psychiatric illness during pregnancy: dilemmas and guidelines. Am J Psychiatry 153:592–606, 1996

American Psychiatric Association: Diagnostic and Statistical Manual of Mental Disorders, 3rd Edition, Revised. Washington, DC, American Psychiatric Association, 1987

American Psychiatric Association: Benzodiazepine Dependence, Toxicity, and Abuse: A Task Force Report. Washington, DC, American Psychiatric Association, 1990

American Psychiatric Association: Diagnostic and Statistical Manual of Mental Disorders, 4th Edition, Text Revision. Washington, DC, American Psychiatric Association, 2000

American Psychiatric Association: Practice guideline for the treatment of patients with bipolar disorder (revision). Am J Psychiatry 159 (4, suppl):1–50, 2002

Ancoli-Israel S, Richardson GS, Mangano RM: Long-term exposure to zaleplon is safe and effective in younger-elderly and older-elderly patients with primary insomnia (abstract). Sleep 26:A77, 2003

Aragona M: Abuse, dependence, and epileptic seizures after zolpidem withdrawal: review and case report. Clin Neuropharmacol 23:281–283, 2000

Arana GW, Hyman SE: Handbook of Psychiatric Drug Therapy, 2nd Edition. Boston, MA, Little, Brown, 1991, pp 128–161

Arana GW, Ornsteen ML, Kanter F, et al: The use of benzodiazepines for psychotic disorders: a literature review and preliminary clinical findings. Psychopharmacol Bull 22:77–87, 1986

Ayd FJ Jr: Lexicon of Psychiatry, Neurology, and the Neurosciences. Baltimore, MD, Williams & Wilkins, 1995, pp 68–76, 153

Ballenger JC: Benzodiazepines, in The American Psychiatric Press Textbook of Psychopharmacology. Edited by Schatzberg AF, Nemeroff CB. Washington, DC, American Psychiatric Press, 1995, pp 215–230

Bourgeois JA, Klein M: Risperidone and fluoxetine in the treatment of pedophilia with comorbid dysthymia (letter). J Clin Psychopharmacol 16:257–258, 1996

Bradwejn J, Shriqui C, Koszycki D, et al: Double-blind comparison of the effects of clonazepam and lorazepam in acute mania. J Clin Psychopharmacol 10:403–408, 1990

Braun P, Greenberg D, Dasberg H, et al: Core symptoms of posttraumatic stress disorder unimproved by alprazolam treatment. J Clin Psychiatry 51:236–238, 1990

Butterfield MI, Becker ME, Connor KM, et al: Olanzapine in the treatment of posttraumatic stress disorder: a pilot study. Int Clin Psychopharmacol 16:197–203, 2001

Charney DS, Heninger GR: Noradrenergic function and the mechanism of action of antianxiety treatment, I: the effect of long-term alprazolam treatment. Arch Gen Psychiatry 42:458–467, 1985

Chouinard G: Clonazepam in the acute and maintenance treatment of bipolar affective disorder. J Clin Psychiatry 48 (suppl 10):29–36, 1987

Ciraulo DA, Shader RI, Ciraulo AM, et al: Alcoholism and its treatment, in Manual of Psychiatric Therapeutics, 2nd Edition. Edited by Shader RI. Boston, MA, Little, Brown, 1994, pp 181–210

Ciraulo DA, Sarid-Segal O, Knapp C, et al: Liability to alprazolam abuse in daughters of alcoholics. Am J Psychiatry 153:956–958, 1996

Cobb CD, Anderson CB, Seidel D: Possible interaction between clozapine and lorazepam. Am J Psychiatry 148:1606–1607, 1991

Cohen LS, Rosenbaum JF: Clonazepam: new uses and potential problems. J Clin Psychiatry 48 (10, suppl):50–55, 1987

Cohen LS, Rosenbaum J, Heller VL: Panic attack–associated placental abruption: a case report. J Clin Psychiatry 50:266–267, 1989

Cole JO, Yonkers KA: Nonbenzodiazepine anxiolytics, in The American Psychiatric Press Textbook of Psychopharmacology. Edited by Schatzberg AF, Nemeroff CB. Washington, DC, American Psychiatric Press, 1995, pp 231–244

Coplan JD, Gorman JM: Treatment of anxiety disorder in patients with mood disorders. J Clin Psychiatry 51 (10, suppl):9–13, 1990

Cornish JW, McNicholas LF, O'Brien CP: Treatment of substance-related disorders, in The American Psychiatric Press Textbook of Psychopharmacology. Edited by Schatzberg AF, Nemeroff CB. Washington, DC, American Psychiatric Press, 1995, pp 707–724

Cozza KL, Armstrong SC, Oesterheld JR: Concise Guide to Drug Interaction Principles for Medical Practice: Cytochrome P450s, UGTs, P-Glycoproteins, 2nd Edition. Washington, DC, American Psychiatric Publishing, 2003

Creelman W, Sands BF, Ciraulo DA: Benzodiazepines, in Drug Interactions in Psychiatry. Edited by Ciraulo DA, Shader RI, Greenblatt DJ, et al. Baltimore, MD, Williams & Wilkins, 1989, pp 158–180

Cumming RG, Le Couteur DG: Benzodiazepines and risk of hip fractures in older people: a review of the evidence. CNS Drugs 17:825–837, 2003

Davidson JRT, Connor KM: Treatment of anxiety disorders, in The American Psychiatric Publishing Textbook of Psychopharmacology, 3rd Edition. Edited by Schatzberg AF, Nemeroff CB. Washington, DC, American Psychiatric Publishing, 2004, pp 913–934

Davidson JRT, Ford SM, Smith RD, et al: Long-term treatment of social phobia with clonazepam. J Clin Psychiatry 51:16–20, 1991

Davidson J, Yaryura-Tobias J, DuPont R, et al: Fluvoxamine-controlled release formulation for the treatment of generalized social anxiety disorder. J Clin Psychopharmacol 24:118–125, 2004

Davies M, Newell JG, Derry JM, et al: Characterization of the interaction of zopiclone with gamma-aminobutyric acid type A receptors. Mol Pharmacol 58:756–762, 2000

Drake RG, Davis LL, Cates MR, et al: Baclofen treatment for chronic posttraumatic stress disorder. Ann Pharmacother 37:1177–1181, 2003

Drug Facts and Comparisons. St Louis, MO, Facts and Comparisons, 1995, pp 1356–1383

Dubovsky SL: Geriatric neuropsychopharmacology, in The American Psychiatric Press Textbook of Geriatric Neuropsychiatry. Edited by Coffey CE, Cummings JL. Washington, DC, American Psychiatric Press, 1994, pp 596–631

Dulcan MK, Bregman JD, Weller EB, et al: Treatment of childhood and adolescent disorders, in The American Psychiatric Press Textbook of Psychopharmacology. Edited by Schatzberg AF, Nemeroff CB. Washington, DC, American Psychiatric Press, 1995, pp 669–706

Earley CJ, Allen RP: Pergolide and carbidopa/levodopa treatment of the restless legs syndrome and periodic leg movements in sleep in a consecutive series of patients. Sleep 19:801–810, 1996

Eison MS: Serotonin: a common neurobiologic substrate in anxiety and depression. J Clin Psychopharmacol 10(suppl):26–30, 1990

Ellinwood EH, Easter ME, Linnoila M, et al: Effects of oral contraceptives on diazepam-induced psychomotor impairment. Clin Pharmacol Ther 35:360–366, 1984

Ellison JM (ed): Integrative Treatment of Anxiety Disorders. Washington, DC, American Psychiatric Press, 1996

Eros E, Czeizel AE, Rockenbauer M, et al: A population-based case-control teratologic study of nitrazepam, medazepam, tofisopam, alprazolam and clonazepam treatment during pregnancy. Eur J Obstet Gynaecol Reprod Biol 101:147–154, 2002

Fawcett J: Targeting treatment in patients with mixed symptoms of anxiety and depression. J Clin Psychiatry 51 (11, suppl):40–43, 1990

Fawcett J, Harris SG: Suicide in treatment-refractory depression, in Treatment-Resistant Mood Disorders. Edited by Amsterdam JD, Hornig M, Nierenberg AA. Cambridge, England, Cambridge University Press, 2001, pp 479–488

Feighner JP: Benzodiazepines as antidepressants: a triazolobenzodiazepine used to treat depression, in Modern Problems of Pharmacopsychiatry, Vol 18. Edited by Ban TA, Hollender MH. Basel, Switzerland, S Karger, 1982, pp 196–212

Feldmann TB: Alprazolam in the treatment of posttraumatic stress disorder. J Clin Psychiatry 48:216–217, 1987

French JA, Kanner AM, Bautista J, et al: Efficacy and tolerability of the new antiepileptic drugs, II: treatment of refractory epilepsy. Neurology 62:1261–1273, 2004

Fry J, Scharf M, Mangano R, et al: Zaleplon improves sleep without producing rebound effects in outpatients with insomnia. Int Clin Psychopharmacol 15:141–145, 2000

Gardos G, Cole JO: The treatment of tardive dyskinesia, in Psychopharmacology: The Fourth Generation of Progress. Edited by Bloom FE, Kupfer DJ. New York, Raven, 1995, pp 1503–1511

Garner SJ, Eldridge FL, Wagner PG, et al: Buspirone, an anxiolytic drug that stimulates respiration. Am Rev Respir Dis 139:946–950, 1989

Garza-Trevino ES, Hollister LE, Overall JE, et al: Efficacy of combinations of intramuscular antipsychotics and sedative-hypnotics for control of psychotic agitation. Am J Psychiatry 146:1598–1601, 1989

Gastfriend DR, Rosenbaum JF: Adjunctive buspirone in benzodiazepine treatment of four patients with panic disorder. Am J Psychiatry 146:914–916, 1989

Gelenberg A: The P450 family. Biological Therapies in Psychiatry Newsletter 18:29–31, 1995

Gelenberg A: Benzodiazepine use and hip fractures in the elderly. Biological Therapies in Psychiatry Newsletter 19:3, 1996

Ghaemi SN, Boiman EE, Goodwin FK: Diagnosing bipolar disorder and the effect of antidepressants: a naturalistic study. J Clin Psychiatry 61:804–808, 2000

Golden RN, Dawkins K, Nicholas L: Trazodone and nefazodone, in The American Psychiatric Publishing Textbook of Psychopharmacology, 3rd Edition. Edited by Schatzberg AF, Nemeroff CB. Washington, DC, American Psychiatric Publishing, 2004, pp 315–325

Greenblatt DJ: Benzodiazepine hypnotics: sorting the pharmacokinetic facts. J Clin Psychiatry 52 (9, suppl):4–10, 1991

Greenblatt DJ: Basic pharmacokinetic principles and their application to psychotropic drugs. J Clin Psychiatry 54 (suppl 9):8–13, 1993

Greist JH, Bandelow B, Hollander E, et al: WCA recommendations for the long-term treatment of obsessive-compulsive disorder in adults. CNS Spectr 8 (suppl 1):7–16, 2003

Griffiths RR, Wolf B: Relative abuse liability of different benzodiazepines in drug abusers. J Clin Psychopharmacol 10:237–243, 1990

Grohmann R, Ruther E, Sassim N, et al: Adverse effects of clozapine. Psychopharmacology (Berl) 99(suppl):101–104, 1989

Hajak G, Muller WE, Wittchen H-U, et al: Abuse and dependence potential for the nonbenzodiazepine hypnotics zolpidem and zopiclone: a review of case reports and epidemiological data. Addiction 98:1371–1378, 2003

Hamner MB, Deitsch SE, Brodrick PS, et al: Quetiapine treatment in patients with posttraumatic stress disorder: an open trial of adjunctive therapy. J Clin Psychopharmacol 23:15–20, 2003

Harnett DS: The difficult-to-treat psychiatric patient with comorbid medical illness, in The Difficult-to-Treat Psychiatric Patient. Edited by Dewan NJ, Pies RW. Washington, DC, American Psychiatric Publishing, 2001, pp 325–357

Herings RMC, Stricker BHC, de Boer A, et al: Benzodiazepines and the risk of falling leading to femur fractures: dosage more important than elimination half-life. Arch Intern Med 155:1801–1807, 1995

Herman JB, Rosenbaum JF, Brotman AW: The alprazolam to clonazepam switch for the treatment of panic disorder. J Clin Psychopharmacol 7:175–178, 1987

Hertzberg MA, Butterfield MI, Feldman ME, et al: A preliminary study of lamotrigine for the treatment of posttraumatic stress disorder. Biol Psychiatry 45:1226–1229, 1999

Hewlett WA, Vinogradov S, Agras WS: Clonazepam treatment of obsessions and compulsions. J Clin Psychiatry 51:158–161, 1990

Hollander E, Rossi NB, Sood E, et al: Risperidone augmentation in treatment-resistant obsessive-compulsive disorder: a double-blind, placebo-controlled study. Int J Neuropsychopharmacol 6:397–401, 2003

Hollister LE, Muller-Oerlinghausen, Rickels K, et al: Clinical uses of benzodiazepines. J Clin Psychopharmacol 13 (suppl 1):1–169, 1993

Horrigan JP, Barnhill LJ: The suppression of nightmares with guanfacine (letter). J Clin Psychiatry 57:371, 1996

Jacobson SA, Pies RW, Greenblatt DJ: Handbook of Geriatric Psychopharmacology. Washington, DC, American Psychiatric Publishing, 2002

Janicak PG, Davis JM, Preskorn SH, et al: Principles and Practice of Psychopharmacotherapy. Baltimore, MD, Williams & Wilkins, 1993, pp 405–448, 508–512

Janicak PG, Davis JM, Preskorn SH, et al: Principles and Practice of Psychopharmacotherapy, 3rd Edition. Philadelphia, PA, Lippincott Williams & Wilkins, 2001 p 146

Jenkins SC, Tinsley JA, Van Loon JA: A Pocket Reference for Psychiatrists, 3rd Edition. Washington, DC, American Psychiatric Press, 2001, pp 135–136

Jonas JM, Hearron AE: Alprazolam and suicidal ideation: a meta-analysis of controlled trials in the treatment of depression. J Clin Psychopharmacol 16:208–211, 1996

Kaplan HI, Sadock BJ, Grebb JA (eds): Synopsis of Psychiatry, 7th Edition. Baltimore, MD, Williams & Wilkins, 1995

Kaufman KR, Gerner R: Lamotrigine toxicity secondary to sertraline. Seizure 7:163–165, 1998

Kishimoto A, Kamata K, Sugihara T, et al: Treatment of depression with clonazepam. Acta Psychiatr Scand 77:81–86, 1988

Klein DF: False suffocation alarms, spontaneous panics, and related conditions: an integrative hypothesis. Arch Gen Psychiatry 50:306–317, 1993

Klerman GL: The use of benzodiazepines in the treatment of depression. Int Drug Ther Newsl 21:37–38, 1986

Koczerginski D, Kennedy SH, Swinson RP: Clonzapepam and lithium—a toxic combination in treatment of mania? Int Clin Psychopharmacol 4:195–199, 1989

Koran LM, Ringold AL, Elliott MA: Olanzapine augmentation for treatment-resistant obsessive-compulsive disorder. J Clin Psychiatry 61:514–517, 2000

Krystal A, Walsh J, Roth T, et al: The sustained efficacy and safety of eszopiclone over six months of nightly treatment: a placebo-controlled study in patients with chronic insomnia. Presentation at the annual meeting of the American College of Clinical Pharmacy, Atlanta, GA, November 2–5, 2003

Laegreid L, Hagberg G, Lundberg A: The effect of benzodiazepines on the fetus and the newborn. Neuropediatrics 23:18–23, 1992

Lenhart SE, Buysse DJ: Treatment of insomnia in hospitalized patients. Ann Pharmacother 35:1449–1457, 2001

Lenox RH, Manji HK: Lithium, in The American Psychiatric Press Textbook of Psychopharmacology. Edited by Schatzberg AF, Nemeroff CB. Washington, DC, American Psychiatric Press, 1995, pp 303–349

Lenox RH, Newhouse PA, Creelman WL, et al: Adjunctive treatment of manic agitation with lorazepam vs haloperidol: a double-blind study. J Clin Psychiatry 53:47–52, 1992

Low K, Crestani F, Keist R, et al: Molecular and neuronal substrate for the selective attenuation of anxiety. Science 290:131–134, 2000

Lydiard RB: The role of GABA in anxiety disorders. J Clin Psychiatry 64 (suppl 3):21–27, 2003

Lydiard B, Bielski RJ, Zornberg GL, et al: Efficacy of pregabalin in treating psychic and somatic symptoms in generalized anxiety disorder (GAD) (NR773), in 2003 New Research Program and Abstracts, American Psychiatric Association 156th Annual Meeting, San Francisco, CA, May 17–22, 2003

Manos GF. Possible serotonin syndrome associated with buspirone added to fluoxetine. Ann Pharmacother 34:871–874, 2000

Marks IM: Comparative studies on benzodiazepines and psychotherapies. Encephale 9 (suppl 2):23B–30B, 1983

Martenyi F, Harangozo J, Mod L: Clonazepam for the treatment of stupor in catatonic schizophrenia (letter). Am J Psychiatry 146:1230, 1989

Maxmen JS: Psychotropic Drugs: Fast Facts, New York, WW Norton, 1991, pp 177–215

McDougle CJ, Fleischmann RL, Epperson CN, et al: Risperidone addition in fluvoxamine-refractory obsessive-compulsive disorder: three cases. J Clin Psychiatry 56:526–528, 1995

McElhatton PR: The effects of benzodiazepine use during pregnancy and lactation. Reprod Toxicol 8:461–475, 1994

McElroy SL, Keck PE: Antiepileptic drugs, in The American Psychiatric Press Textbook of Psychopharmacology. Edited by Schatzberg AF, Nemeroff CB. Washington, DC, American Psychiatric Press, 1995, pp 351–375

McGee M, Pies R: Benzodiazepines in primary practice: risks and benefits. Resid Staff Physician 48:42–49, 2002

Mohler H, Fritschy JM, Rudolph U: A new benzodiazepine pharmacology. J Pharmacol Exp Ther 300:2–8, 2002

Monnelly EP, Ciraulo DA, Knapp C. et al: Low-dose risperidone as adjunctive therapy for irritable aggression in posttraumatic stress disorder. J Clin Psychopharmacol 23:193–196, 2003

Mota-Castillo M: Five red flags that rule out ADHD in children. Current Psychiatry 4:56, 2002

Newport DJ, Fisher A, Graybeal S, et al: Psychopharmacology during pregnancy and lactation, in The American Psychiatric Publishing Textbook of Psychopharmacology, 3rd Edition. Edited by Schatzberg AF, Nemeroff CB. Washington, DC, American Psychiatric Publishing, 2004, pp 1109–1146

Ninan PT, Muntasser S: Buspirone and gepirone, in The American Psychiatric Publishing Textbook of Psychopharmacology, 3rd Edition. Edited by Schatzberg AF, Nemeroff CB. Washington, DC, American Psychiatric Publishing, 2004, pp 391–404

Nishino S, Mishima K, Mignot E, et al: Sedative-hypnotics, in The American Psychiatric Publishing Textbook of Psychopharmacology, 3rd Edition. Edited by Schatzberg AF, Nemeroff CB. Washington, DC, American Psychiatric Publishing, 2004, pp 651–670

Nofzinger EA, Reynolds CF: Sleep impairment and daytime drowsiness in later life. Am J Psychiatry 153:941–943, 1996

Oesterheld JR, Shader RI, Parmelee DX, et al: Approaches to the psychopharmacologic treatment of children and youth, in Manual of Psychiatric Therapeutics, 3rd Edition. Edited by Shader RI. Philadelphia, PA, Lippincott Williams & Wilkins, 2003, pp 315–345

Otte C, Wiedemann K, Yassouridis A, et al: Valproate monotherapy in the treatment of civilian patients with non-combat-related posttraumatic stress disorder: an open-label study. J Clin Psychopharmacol 24:106–108, 2004

Pagel JF: Disease, psychoactive medication, and sleep states. Primary Psychiatry 1:47–51, 1996

Pande AC, Davidson JR, Jefferson JW, et al: Treatment of social phobia with gabapentin: a placebo-controlled study. J Clin Psychopharmacol 19:341–348, 1999

Pande AC, Feltner DE, Jefferson JW, et al: Efficacy of the novel anxiolytic pregabalin in social anxiety disorder: a placebo-controlled, multicenter study. J Clin Psychopharmacol 24:141–149, 2004

Paul SM: GABA and glycine, in Psychopharmacology: The Fourth Generation of Progress. Edited by Bloom FE, Kupfer DJ. New York, Raven, 1995, pp 87–94

Perlis RH: Child proof: first, do no harm? Paroxetine and suicide. Curbside Consultant (Massachusetts General Hospital) 2(October/November):1, 2003

Petty F, Brannan S, Casada J, et al: Olanzapine treatment for posttraumatic stress disorder: an open-label study. Int Clin Psychopharmacol 16:331–337, 2001

Physicians' Desk Reference, 50th Edition. Montvale, NJ, Medical Economics, 1996

Physicians' Desk Reference, 58th Edition. Montvale, NJ, Thomson Healthcare, 2004

Pies R: Benzodiazepine abuse: how real, how serious? Psychiatric Times 8:13–14, 1991

Pies R: Halcion: is a balanced view possible? Psychiatric Times 8:28–30, 1992

Pies R: The azapirones: broad-spectrum psychotropics? Psychiatric Times 9:30–31, 1993

Pies R: Dose-related sensory distortions with zolpidem (letter). J Clin Psychiatry 66:35–36, 1995a

Pies R: Psychotropic medication during pregnancy and postpartum. Clinical Advances in the Treatment of Psychiatric Disorders 9:4–7, 1995b

Pies RW, Dewan MJ: The difficult-to-treat patient with schizophrenia, in The Difficult-to-Treat Psychiatric Patient. Edited by Dewan MJ, Pies RW. Washington, DC, American Psychiatric Publishing, 2001, pp 41–80

Pies R, Parks A: Beta-blockers in neuropsychiatry: an update. Horizon Physician Quarterly 2:1–10, 1996

Pies R, Weinberg AD: Quick Reference Guide to Geriatric Psychopharmacology. Branford, CT, American Medical Publishing, 1990

Pigott TA, L'Heureux F, Rubenstein CS, et al: A double-blind, placebo-controlled study of trazodone in patients with obsessive-compulsive disorder. J Clin Psychopharmacol 12:156–62, 1992

Pollack MH, Allgulander C, Bandelow B, et al: WCA recommendations for the long-term treatment of panic disorder. CNS Spectr 8 (suppl 1):17–30, 2003

Pons G, Rey E, Matheson I: Excretion of psychoactive drugs into breast milk: pharmacokinetic principles and recommendations. Clin Pharmacokinet 27:270–289, 1994

Pourmotabbed T, McLeod DR, Hoehn-Saric R, et al: Treatment, discontinuation, and psychomotor effects of diazepam in women with generalized anxiety disorder. J Clin Psychopharmacol 16:202–207, 1996

Preskorn SH: Clinical Pharmacology of Selective Serotonin Reuptake Inhibitors. Caddo, OK, Professional Communications, 1996

Raj A, Sheehan D: Benzodiazepines, in The American Psychiatric Publishing Textbook of Psychopharmacology, 3rd Edition. Edited by Schatzberg AF, Nemeroff CB. Washington, DC, American Psychiatric Publishing, 2004, pp 371–404

Ramona v. Ramona: Superior Court, County of Napa, California, Case No. C61898, September 12, 1991

Ray WA, Griffin MR, Downey M: Benzodiazepines of long and short elimination half-life and the risk of hip fracture. JAMA 262:3303–3307, 1989

Reich J, Noyes R, Yates W: Alprazolam treatment of avoidant personality traits in social phobic patients. J Clin Psychiatry 50:91–95, 1989

Reite M: Treatment of insomnia, in The American Psychiatric Publishing Textbook of Psychopharmacology, 3rd Edition. Edited by Schatzberg AF, Nemeroff CB. Washington, DC, American Psychiatric Publishing, 2004, pp 1147–1166

Richardson GS, Roehrs TA, Rosenthal L, et al: Tolerance to daytime sedative effects of H1 antihistamines. J Clin Psychopharmacol 22:511–515, 2002

Rickels K, Case WG, Downing RW, et al: Long-term diazepam therapy and clinical outcome. JAMA 250:767–771, 1983

Rickels K, Schweizer E, Csanalosi I, et al: Long-term treatment of anxiety and risk of withdrawal: prospective comparison of clorazepate and buspirone. Arch Gen Psychiatry 45:444–450, 1988

Rickels K, Amsterdam J, Clary C, et al: Buspirone in depressed outpatients: a controlled study. Psychopharmacol Bull 26:163–167, 1990

Roache JD, Griffiths RR: Comparison of triazolam and pentobarbital: performance impairment, subjective effects, and abuse liability. J Pharmacol Exp Ther 234: 120–133, 1985

Robinson RT, Drafts BC, Fisher JL: Fluoxetine increases GABA(A) receptor activity through a novel modulatory site. J Pharmacol Exp Ther 304:978–984, 2003

Sachs GS: Bipolar mood disorder: practical strategies for acute and maintenance phase treatment. J Clin Psychopharmacol 16 (suppl 1):32S–47S, 1996

Saitz R, Ciraulo DA, Shader RI. et al: Treatment of alcohol withdrawal, in Manual of Psychiatric Therapeutics, 3rd Edition. Edited by Shader RI. Philadelphia, PA, Lippincott Williams & Wilkins, 2003, pp 143–168

Salzman C, Green AI, Rodriqez-Villa F, et al: Benzodiazepines combined with neuroleptics for management of severe disruptive behavior. Psychosomatics 27:17–21, 1986

Sands, BF, Creelman WL, Ciraulo DA, et al: Benzodiazepines, in Drug Interactions in Psychiatry. Edited by Ciraulo DA, Shader RI, Greenblatt DJ, et al. Baltimore, MD, Williams & Wilkins, 1995, pp 214–248

Sarid-Segal O, Creelman W, Shader RI: Lithium, in Drug Interactions in Psychiatry, 2nd Edition. Edited by Ciraulo DA, Shader RI, Greenblatt DJ, et al. Baltimore, MD, Williams & Wilkins, 1995, pp 175–213

Scavone JM, Greenblatt DJ, Shader RI: Alprazolam kinetics following sublingual and oral administration. J Clin Psychopharmacol 7:332–334, 1987

Scharf MB, Saskin P, Fletcher K: Benzodiazepine-induced amnesia: clinical laboratory findings. J Clin Psychiatry (Monograph Series) 5:14–17, 1987

Schatzberg AF, Cole JO: Benzodiazepines in depressive disorders. Arch Gen Psychiatry 24:509–514, 1978

Schatzberg AF, Cole JO: Manual of Clinical Psychopharmacology, 2nd Edition. Washington, DC, American Psychiatric Press, 1991

Schenck C, Mahowald M: Long-term, nightly benzodiazepine treatment of injurious parasomnias and other disorders of disrupted nocturnal sleep in 170 adults. Am J Med 100:333–337, 1996

Schweizer E, Rickels K, Uhlenhuth EH: Issues in the long-term treatment of anxiety disorders, in Psychopharmacology: The Fourth Generation of Progress. Edited by Bloom FE, Kupfer DJ. New York, Raven, 1995, pp 1349–1359

Shader RI, Greenblatt DJ: Approaches to the treatment of anxiety states, in Manual of Psychiatric Therapeutics, 2nd Edition. Edited by Shader RI. Boston, MA, Little, Brown, 1994a, pp 275–298

Shader RI, Greenblatt DJ: Treatment of transient insomnia, in Manual of Psychiatric Therapeutics, 2nd Edition. Edited by Shader RI. Boston, MA, Little, Brown, 1994b, pp 211–216

Shader RI, von Moltke LL, Schmider J, et al: The clinician and drug interactions—an update. J Clin Psychopharmacol 16:197–201, 1996

Smoller JW: Panic-anxiety in patients with respiratory disease. American Society of Clinical Psychopharmacology Progress Notes 7:4–5, 1996

Smoller JW, Pollack MH, Systrom D, et al: Sertraline effects on dyspnea in patients with obstructive airways disease. Psychosomatics 39:24–29, 1998

Spigset O, Adielsson G: Combined serotonin syndrome and hyponatremia caused by a citalopram-buspirone interaction. Int Clin Psychopharmacol 12:61–63, 1997

Stanilla JK, Simpson GM: Drugs to treat extrapyramidal side effects, in The American Psychiatric Publishing Textbook of Psychopharmacology, 3rd Edition. Edited by Schatzberg AF, Nemeroff CB. Washington, DC, American Psychiatric Publishing, 2004, pp 519–544

Stein DJ, Bandelow B, Hollander E, et al: WCA recommendations for the long-term treatment of posttraumatic stress disorder. CNS Spectr 8 (suppl 1):31–39, 2003

Stowe ZN, Nemeroff CB: Psychopharmacology during pregnancy and lactation, in American Psychiatric Press Textbook of Psychopharmacology. Edited by Schatzberg AF, Nemeroff CB. Washington, DC, American Psychiatric Press, 1995, pp 823–837

Summerfield RJ, Nielsen MS: Excretion of lorazepam into breast milk. Br J Anaesth 57:1042–1043, 1985

Taylor CB: Treatment of anxiety disorders, in The American Psychiatric Press Textbook of Psychopharmacology. Edited by Schatzberg AF, Nemeroff CB. Washington, DC, American Psychiatric Press, 1995, pp 641–655

Taylor FB: Tiagabine for posttraumatic stress disorder: a case series of 7 women. J Clin Psychiatry 64:1421–1425, 2003

Tesar GE: High potency benzodiazepines for short-term management of panic disorder: the U.S. experience. J Clin Psychiatry 51(suppl):4–10, 1990

Tsai MJ, Huang YB, Wu PC: A novel clinical pattern of visual hallucinations after zolpidem use. J Toxicol Clin Toxicol 41:869–872, 2003

Tueth MJ, DeVane CL, Evans DL: Treatment of psychiatric emergencies, in The American Psychiatric Press Textbook of Psychopharmacology. Edited by Schatzberg AF, Nemeroff CB. Washington, DC, American Psychiatric Press, 1995, pp 769–781

Udelman HD, Udelman DL: Concurrent use of buspirone in anxious patients during withdrawal from alprazolam therapy. J Clin Psychiatry 51 (9, suppl):46–50, 1990

Van Ameringen M, Allgulander C, Bandelow B, et al: WCA recommendations for the long-term treatment of social phobia. CNS Spectr 8 (suppl 1):40–52, 2003

van Laar MW, van Willigenburg APP, Volkerts ER: Acute and subchronic effects of nefazodone and imipramine on highway driving, cognitive functions, and daytime sleepiness in healthy adult and elderly subjects. J Clin Psychopharmacol 15:30–40, 1995

Venkatakrishnan K, Shader RI, von Moltke LL, et al: Drug interactions in psychopharmacology, in Manual of Psychiatric Therapeutics, 3rd Edition. Edited by Shader RI. Philadelphia, PA, Lippincott Williams & Wilkins, 2003, pp 441–470

Wagner KD: Treatment of childhood and adolescent disorders, in The American Psychiatric Publishing Textbook of Psychopharmacology, 3rd Edition. Edited by Schatzberg AF, Nemeroff CB. Washington, DC, American Psychiatric Publishing, 2004, pp 949–1007

Wagner KD, Stein M, Berard R, et al: Efficacy of paroxetine in childhood and adolescent social anxiety disorder. Poster presented at the 49th annual meeting of the American Academy of Child and Adolescent Psychiatry, San Francisco, CA, October 2002

Walsh JK, Roth T, Randazzo A, et al: Eight weeks of non-nightly use of zolpidem for primary insomnia. Sleep 23:1087–1096, 2000

Wheatley M, Plant J, Reader H, et al: Clozapine treatment of adolescents with posttraumatic stress disorder and psychotic symptoms. J Clin Psychopharmacol 24:167–173, 2004

Witek TJ Jr, Canestrari DA, Miller RD, et al: Characterization of daytime sleepiness and psychomotor performance following H1 receptor antagonists. Ann Allergy Asthma Immunol 74:419–426, 1995

Wolkowitz OM, Pickar D: Benzodiazepines in the treatment of schizophrenia: a review and reappraisal. Am J Psychiatry 148:714–726, 1991

Woodman CL, Noyes R Jr: Panic disorder: treatment with valproate. J Clin Psychiatry 55:134–136, 1994

Woods JH, Katz JL, Winger G: Abuse and therapeutic use of benzodiazepines and benzodiazepine-like drugs, in Psychopharmacology: The Fourth Generation of Progress. Edited by Bloom FE, Kupfer DJ. New York, Raven, 1995, pp 1777–1791

Yosselson-Superstine S, Lipman AG: Chlordiazepoxide interaction with levodopa. Ann Intern Med 96:259–260, 1982

Yudofsky SC, Silver J, Hales RE: Treatment of aggressive disorders, in The American Psychiatric Press Textbook of Psychopharmacology. Edited by Schatzberg AF, Nemeroff CB. Washington, DC, American Psychiatric Press, 1995, pp 735–752

Zajecka JM: Treatment strategies for depression complicated by anxiety disorders. Presentation at the 8th Annual U.S. Psychiatric and Mental Health Congress, New York, NY, November 16, 1995

Zammit G: Insomnia interventions. Clinical Geriatrics 7 (suppl):11–13, 1999

Zwanzger P, Baghai TC, Schule C, et al: Tiagabine improves panic and agoraphobia in panic disorder patients. J Clin Psychiatry 62:656–657, 2001

CHAPTER 5

MOOD STABILIZERS

Overview

Drug Class

Mood stabilizers remain the mainstay of treatment for bipolar disorder. However, it is not easy to list the members of this class, since the very definition of "mood stabilizer" remains controversial (American Psychiatric Association [APA] 2002; Ketter and Calabrese 2002). One "broad" definition of mood stabilizer is *an agent that is effective for one or the other phase of bipolar disorder (mania or depression) and does not worsen the other phase or the overall course of illness.* This definition is so broad as to encompass many different agents, some of which do not have U.S. Food and Drug Administration (FDA)–approved labeling for use in bipolar disorder. For example, most conventional (typical) antipsychotics (neuroleptics) are useful in treating *mania* and may not worsen depression or the overall course of illness in bipolar disorder patients. (Some studies *do* suggest that classical neuroleptics increase the risk of bipolar depression, however.)

A more "stringent" definition of a mood stabilizer is an agent that is effective, as monotherapy, in treating both manic and depressive episodes in bipolar disorder, as well as for bipolar prophylaxis. This definition is so strict that it eliminates most available agents, with the probable exception of *lith-*

ium (Eskalith), and perhaps *carbamazepine* (CBZ), *valproate,* and *lamotrigine* (Lamictal). Indeed, using the most stringent criteria for mood stabilization, a recent review concluded that lithium remains the first-line treatment for bipolar disorder, despite many alternatives (Bauer and Mitchner 2004). It is somewhat easier to speak of "drugs for the treatment of bipolar disorder," which include, but are not necessarily limited to, lithium; valproate (divalproex); CBZ and its keto-congener, oxcarbazepine; lamotrigine; other anticonvulsants (including *topiramate, levetiracetam,* and *zonisamide*); and several atypical antipsychotics, already discussed in Chapter 3 ("Antipsychotics"). As of this writing, there are 10 agents with FDA-approved labeling for treatment of some phase or type of bipolar disorder: lithium, valproate, lamotrigine, *olanzapine, risperidone, quetiapine, aripiprazole, ziprasidone,* extended-release carbamazepine (ERC [Equetro]), and OFC (olanzapine/fluoxetine combination [Symbyax]). However, this list is soon likely to include other agents. There is active interest, for example, in the metabolite of oxcarbazepine as a mood stabilizer. Although *gabapentin* has been widely used in treating bipolar disorder, the evidence supporting its role as a mood stabilizer is decidedly lacking (Maidment 2001). With respect to maintenance treatment in bipolar disorder, the FDA recently approved lamotrigine for the maintenance of bipolar I disorder "to delay the time to occurrence of mood episodes" in patients treated for acute mood episodes with standard therapy. However, lamotrigine appears to be more useful in bipolar depression than in mania (Bowden et al. 2003).

Other agents sometimes used adjunctively in bipolar disorder include *thyroxine* (T_4); calcium channel blockers, such as *nimodipine*; *bupropion*; various selective serotonin reuptake inhibitors (SSRIs); and, to some degree, benzodiazepines such as *clonazepam* and *lorazepam.* The use of antidepressants in bipolar disorder continues to be a source of confusion and controversy (Altshuler et al. 2003; Amsterdam et al. 1998; Ghaemi et al. 2000).

Indications

The indications for the various agents used in bipolar disorder are summarized in Tables 5–2 through 5–6, based primarily on the revised APA (2002) practice guideline. The APA guideline lists lithium as a first-line agent for essentially every type and phase of bipolar disorder, with perhaps one exception: for "mixed" manic episodes, valproate may be preferred over lithium. Contrary to a widely held view, this preference for valproate is *not* repeated with respect to *rapid cycling,* for which the initial treatment may be either lithium or valproate (American Psychiatric Association 2002; Pies 2002b). For the initial treatment of an acute depressive episode in bipolar disorder, the APA guideline recommends either lithium or lamotrigine. With respect to maintenance (prophylaxis) of bipolar disorder, the APA guideline notes that the medications with the best empirical evidence to support their use in maintenance treatment are lithium and valproate. However, the case for use of valproate as a prophylactic agent is not as well established as the use of lithium.

For the treatment of *euphoric mania/hypomania,* the Texas Medication Algorithm (Suppes et al. 2002) recommends lithium, divalproex, or olanzapine (though reportedly, there was some dissent among panel members regarding olanzapine's role). For *mixed or dysphoric mania/hypomania,* divalproex or olanzapine is the initial drug of choice in the Texas Medication Algorithm. For *psychotic mania,* lithium, divalproex, or olanzapine is the recommended agent. In the initial treatment of *bipolar I depression,* the Texas Medication Algorithm recommends that mood-stabilizing medications (unspecified) should be initiated or optimized prior to use of an antidepressant. In the next stage of treatment of bipolar depression, an antidepressant or lamotrigine should be considered for partial responders or nonresponders. The issue of "matching" a particular bipolar patient to a particular mood stabilizer (Gelenberg and Pies 2003) is discussed later in the "Indications" subsection of the "Questions and Answers" section.

Lithium, valproate, other anticonvulsants, and atypical antipsychotics have found many other uses in psychiatry besides the treatment of bipolar disorder—though not necessarily on the basis of well-designed, controlled studies (Table 5–2). For example, lithium, valproate, olanzapine, and CBZ have been found to have utility in the treatment of various excited psychotic states, schizoaffective disorder, and conditions characterized by impulsive aggression or self-injurious behavior. To a more limited degree, these agents have been useful in some cases of posttraumatic stress disorder (PTSD) and borderline personality disorder (BPD). Outside of their use in bipolar disorder, however, most of the evidence for use of lithium, valproate, and CBZ is anecdotal or uncontrolled.

Mechanisms of Action

The precise mechanisms of action for most putative mood stabilizers remain unknown (Gould et al. 2004; Wang et al. 2003). Lithium has numerous actions on neurotransmitters, secondary messengers, and membrane transport mechanisms (the various ion channels and "pumps" that maintain the resting potential across the cell membrane). Effects on serotonin transmission, dopamine formation, norepinephrine turnover, cholinergic transmission, phosphoinositide turnover, and adenylyl cyclase are but a few of the ways lithium may act on the brain. Recently, lithium's role as an inhibitor of the enzyme glycogen synthase kinase–3 (GSK-3) has been emphasized (Gould et al. 2004).

In general, most anticonvulsant mood stabilizers increase the ratio of γ-aminobutyric acid (GABA) to glutamate to varying degrees and via differing mechanisms (Wang et al. 2003). Valproate, a simple branched-chain carboxylic acid, may produce both antiepileptic and antimanic effects by increasing the concentration of GABA, the main inhibitory neurotransmitter in the mammalian central nervous system (CNS). Valproate also has some antiglutamatergic effects; blocks sodium channels; and may decrease dopamine turnover, possibly accounting for its modest antipsychotic effects. Lamotrigine leads to blockade of voltage-dependent sodium channels, which in turn may prevent excessive release of glutamate and aspartate (excitatory neurotransmitters). Two anticonvulsants, gabapentin and pregabalin (neither of which has clear efficacy in bipolar disorder) apparently act on calcium channels to normalize excessive activation (Stahl 2004). Olanzapine and other atypical antipsychotics act on a multitude of neurotransmitter receptors. The efficacy of atypical antipsychotics in mania—and perhaps in bipolar depression—may be related to their complex pattern of dopamine receptor blockade, their serotonin$_2$ (5-HT$_2$) receptor antagonism, and perhaps their effects on glutamatergic activity.

Pharmacokinetics

Lithium is one of the only psychotropic agents in common use that does not undergo hepatic metabolism; rather, it is eliminated almost entirely via the kidneys. Lithium is not protein-bound, and it has a $t_{1/2}\beta$ of approximately 24 hours, implying that steady-state levels are usually reached after 4–6 days on a fixed dose (Janicak et al. 1993). Exposure time to peak lithium levels may be reduced via once-daily dosing, and this may have beneficial effects on some aspects of treatment (see "Main Side Effects" subsection). Lithium retention and excretion may be affected by sodium (salt) restriction or "loading."

Valproate metabolism is quite complex, mediated via two hepatic pathways (one mitochondrial, one microsomal) and glucuronidation (Cozza et al. 2003). One valproate metabolite appears to be hepatotoxic. Valproate has a $t_{1/2}\beta$ of roughly 12 hours (range: 5–20 hours), which may be altered by drugs that affect mitochondrial and/or microsomal enzymes (McElroy and Keck 1995). Some data indicate a mild "autoinduction" of valproate oxidative metabolism, but not glucuronidation, with chronic use (McLaughlin et al. 2000).

CBZ also undergoes complex metabolism, with production of a 10,11-epoxide being of greatest significance for both pharmacological activity and neurotoxicity. At least one portion of CBZ's metabolism is thought to go through cytochrome P450 (CYP) 3A4 (Cozza et al. 2003; DeVane 1994), a pathway that is inhibited by nefazodone, ketoconazole, and other drugs. CBZ's $t_{1/2}\beta$ ranges from 18 to 55 hours, and autoinduction (i.e., induction of its own metabolism) occurs during the first few months of treatment; this may reduce $t_{1/2}$ to 5–26 hours and may also reduce plasma levels (McElroy and Keck 1995). Autoinduction also occurs after each dose increase. CBZ has been shown to decrease the plasma levels of many medications, including various psychotropics. The keto-congener of CBZ, oxcarbazepine, is also metabolized in part via CYP 3A4. However, its main metabolic pathway is via a non-CYP enzyme that is not inducible; thus, oxcarbazepine does not significantly induce its own metabolism, and it has somewhat more limited effects than CBZ on most CYP enzymes (Hellewell 2002). However, oxcarbazepine may still affect plasma levels of other medications (Cozza et al. 2003).

Lamotrigine is metabolized mainly via glucuronidation and does show some autoinduction. Though lamotrigine does not typically affect plasma levels of other anticonvulsants, valproate may significantly increase lamotrigine levels, thus increasing the risk of serious rash (Cozza et al. 2003; Physicians' Desk Reference 2004).

The pharmacokinetic properties of the atypical antipsychotics were detailed in Chapter 1 ("Introduction to Pharmacodynamics and Pharmacokinetics") and Chapter 3 ("Antipsychotics"). Occasionally, there may be drug–drug interactions between some atypicals and anticonvulsant mood stabilizers.

Main Side Effects

Lithium commonly produces increased urination with associated thirst and increased water intake (polyuria/polydipsia); mild gastrointestinal (GI) problems (e.g., loose stools); and mild tremor. Most of these side effects may be mitigated by reducing the dose and/or peak plasma levels. Hypothyroidism may be found in roughly 5%–10% of patients, particularly in women (who also have a higher intrinsic rate of thyroid disease) (Lenox and Manji 1995; Pies 1995b). Dose-related cognitive dulling or slowed thinking related to lithium may be a source of poor medication compliance. Frank nephrogenic diabetes insipidus is uncommon with lithium, as is significant glomerular dysfunction (Lenox and Manji 1995); however, a small subgroup of lithium-treated patients may experience insidious decrements in glomerular function.

Valproate generally produces fewer side effects than lithium, with the main exception being dose/plasma level–related GI disturbance (McElroy and Keck 1995). Some patients may develop significant weight gain, transient hair loss, or tremor, and thrombocytopenia is not uncommon in elderly patients. There appears to be an association between valproate and both menstrual dysfunction and polycystic ovarian disease, though a causal relationship is hard to confirm. Divalproex has three "black box warnings" that clinicians must consider carefully before they prescribe any form of valproate: *hepatotoxicity, pancreatitis,* and *teratogenicity* (e.g., spina bifida). There have been reports of hyperammonemic encephalopathy associated with valproate (Oechsner et al. 1998).

Lamotrigine is usually well tolerated but may cause transient headache early in treatment; unlike many anticonvulsants, lamotrigine is not associated with weight gain (Wang et al. 2003). Lamotrigine has a black box warning regarding the development of severe rash, including Stevens-Johnson syndrome and toxic epidermal necrolysis. When titrated appropriately, lamotrigine is very rarely associated with severe rash. The incidence is roughly 0.1%–0.3% in adults; however, this may rise to about 1% in pediatric patients (Messenheimer et al. 2000; Wang et al. 2003). Incidence of rash is increased with rapid escalation of dose and with the coadministration of valproic acid derivatives (particularly when valproate is added to lamotrigine).

CBZ may be associated with side effects in roughly 40% of patients, including fatigue, gait instability, headache, lightheadedness, and rash (Shader 1994). However, CBZ may produce less weight gain, hair loss, and tremor than valproate, and less memory impairment than lithium (Andrews et al.

1990; Mattson et al. 1992). Transient leukopenia occurs in about 10% of CBZ-treated patients but is usually benign. The much-feared complication of aplastic anemia is exceedingly rare with CBZ (roughly 1 in 125,000). Hyponatremia (SIADH [syndrome of inappropriate antidiuretic hormone]), altered liver functions, and cardiac conduction abnormalities may sometimes be seen with CBZ. Oxcarbazepine is generally better tolerated than CBZ and is not associated with hematological complications; however, it induces hyponatremia in about 3% of cases.

Drug–Drug Interactions

Clinically significant drug–drug interactions with lithium include those with nonsteroidal anti-inflammatory agents (NSAIDs) such as ibuprofen; thiazide diuretics; indapamide (a nonthiazide diuretic); and tetracyclines. All of these interactions may lead to increased lithium levels and potential toxicity (Janicak et al. 1993). Theophylline, caffeine, verapamil, and carbonic anhydrase inhibitors can all increase lithium excretion, thus reducing lithium levels. Valproate tends to be a mild *inhibitor* of hepatic oxidative metabolism and thus may increase plasma levels of CBZ and its epoxide metabolite; phenobarbital; phenytoin; tricyclic antidepressants (TCAs); and (to a small degree) antipsychotics (McElroy and Keck 1995). Caution should be used when valproate and lamotrigine are administered together. Lamotrigine levels may be increased as a result of valproate's inhibition of glucuronidation (Cozza et al. 2003), thus increasing the risk of rash. Cimetidine, salicylates, and chlorpromazine may decrease valproate clearance, thus raising valproate levels. Fluoxetine (Prozac) may also raise valproate concentrations (Sovner and Davis 1991). As a general rule, CBZ tends to be a strong *inducer* of hepatic metabolism, generally reducing levels of other hepatically metabolized drugs. Thus, CBZ reduces valproate levels but may *raise* levels of valproate's hepatotoxic metabolite. CBZ significantly reduces levels of haloperidol and other antipsychotics, as well as levels of TCAs, benzodiazepines, warfarin, prednisone, theophylline, and oral contraceptives. CBZ metabolism may be reduced (and CBZ increased to potentially toxic levels) by verapamil, diltiazem, erythromycin, valproate, and other agents (McElroy and Keck 1995). Oxcarbazepine—though probably associated with fewer drug interactions than CBZ—may induce CYP 3A4 and inhibit CYP 2C19. This may lead, respectively, to reduced blood levels of oral contraceptives and increased blood levels of CYP

2C19 substrates such as phenytoin (Cozza et al. 2003).

In addition to the pharmacokinetic interactions discussed above, numerous *pharmacodynamic* interactions may occur between the mood stabilizers and other agents acting on the CNS (leading to, e.g., increased sedation, cognitive effects, cerebellar dysfunction, or extrapyramidal effects).

Potentiating Maneuvers

In the treatment of refractory bipolar disorder, mood stabilizers and putative mood stabilizers are often used in various combinations (Pies 2002a). A valproate–lithium combination is often used in patients with mixed or rapid-cycling mania who do not respond to valproate (or lithium) alone. Patients whose symptoms remain refractory may have CBZ added to this regimen, though pharmacokinetic and pharmacodynamic interactions may be problematic. Hence, oxcarbazepine is sometimes used instead (American Psychiatric Association 2002). The addition of lamotrigine to other mood stabilizers has become more common in refractory cases, particularly in bipolar depression. Both classical neuroleptics and atypical antipsychotics may play an important adjunctive role during the first few weeks of severe, acute mania, before the primary mood stabilizer has become fully effective (efficacy may occur more rapidly with valproate than with lithium; McElroy and Keck 1995). Atypical antipsychotics appear to be useful in treating severe mania, even in the absence of psychotic features. In addition, atypical antipsychotics are rapidly becoming first-line or primary agents in the acute and long-term management of bipolar disorder. Lorazepam and clonazepam are often used as adjunctive antimanic agents, with some data suggesting that lorazepam has a more rapid onset (Bradwejn et al. 1990). Thyroid hormones (mainly T_4), calcium channel blockers, beta-blockers, and clonidine have all been used as adjunctive treatments of mania or rapid cycling, with varying degrees of success.

Use in Special Populations

There is good evidence that lithium use during early pregnancy is associated with the development of cardiac abnormalities, especially *Ebstein's anomaly*—a severe, sometimes fatal malformation involving a downward displacement of the tricuspid valve into the right ventricle. However, the actual likelihood of lithium-related cardiac malformations appears to be lower than previously believed. In utero exposure to CBZ is associated with higher-than-expected rates of craniofacial defects, developmental delay, and spina bifida. There is also a 1% rate of spina bifida in infants exposed in utero to valproate (divalproex; Depakote). Some experts now regard lithium as the "safest" of the major mood stabilizers in the treatment of bipolar disorder during the first trimester.

Lithium is the mood stabilizer most commonly used in children and adolescents, though few double-blind, placebo-controlled studies of its efficacy exist for this population. Valproate and valproate–lithium combinations appear to be effective in pediatric bipolar populations, but again, there are few controlled studies to support their use (Wagner 2004). There is limited experience with lamotrigine in pediatric bipolar populations, perhaps reflecting the increased risk of serious rash in this age group. Controlled data on the use of atypical antipsychotics in younger bipolar cohorts are also quite limited, though uncontrolled data suggest that olanzapine is useful as primary or adjunctive treatment (Wagner 2004).

Although all the commonly prescribed mood stabilizers have been used in elderly bipolar patients, there are few well-controlled studies. Lithium may have an increased likelihood of neurotoxicity in elderly and dementia populations and must be used cautiously in patients with reduced renal function (e.g., the elderly and medically ill). Valproate appears to be relatively well tolerated in the elderly, though rates of thrombocytopenia are substantial, and cognitive side effects may be seen. CBZ seems to be better tolerated than lithium in elderly patients with brain damage (Dubovsky 1994). Valproate is probably the mood stabilizer of choice for many elderly bipolar patients, though olanzapine and risperidone are increasingly being used as first-line treatments for geriatric mania (Jacobson et al. 2002).

Tables

Drug Class

TABLE 5–1. Selected mood stabilizers: preparations, usual daily doses, and putative therapeutic blood levels

Generic drug	Brand name(s)	Tablet/capsule strengths and other formulations	Usual adult total daily dose range[a]	Putative therapeutic blood level[b]
carbamazepine	Tegretol	100 mg (chewable), 200 mg Suspension: 100 mg/5 mL	400–1,200 mg	4–12 μg/mL
	Equetro[c]	100 mg, 200 mg, 300 mg (capsules)	400–1,000 mg (divided doses)	Approximately 5–9 μg/mL[d]
divalproex	Depakote Depakote Sprinkle Depakote-ER[e]	125 mg, 250 mg, 500 mg (tablets) 125 mg (capsules) 250 mg, 500 mg (tablets)	500–1,600 mg 500–1,600 mg 750–1,750 mg (single dose)	50–125 μg/mL
lamotrigine	Lamictal	25 mg, 100 mg, 150 mg, 200 mg (tablets) 2 mg, 5 mg, 25 mg (chewable dispersible tablets)	100–400 mg (without coadministration of valproic acid)	Levels not routinely monitored in bipolar disorder
lithium carbonate	Eskalith	150 mg, 300 mg, 600 mg (capsules)	600–1,500 mg (usually in divided doses)	0.4–1.4 mEq/L

TABLE 5–1. Selected mood stabilizers: preparations, usual daily doses, and putative therapeutic blood levels *(continued)*

Generic drug	Brand name(s)	Tablet/capsule strengths and other formulations	Usual adult total daily dose range[a]	Putative therapeutic blood level[b]
slow-release lithium carbonate	Lithobid	300 mg (slow-release tablets)	600–1,500 mg (usually as bid dosing)	
	Eskalith-CR	450 mg (controlled-release tablets)	450–1,350 mg (usually as bid dosing)	
lithium citrate (syrup)	—	8 mEq/5 mL	Each 5 mL = 300 mg lithium carbonate	
olanzapine[f]	Zyprexa	2.5 mg, 5 mg, 7.5 mg, 10 mg, 15 mg, 20 mg (tablets)	10–20 mg	Not well established in bipolar disorder
	Zydis	5 mg, 10 mg, 15 mg, 20 mg (dissolvable tablets)		
oxcarbazepine	Trileptal	150 mg, 300 mg, 600 mg (tablets)	600–1,800 mg (in divided doses)[g]	Not well established in bipolar disorder; in epilepsy, levels usually 10–35 μg/mL

TABLE 5–1. Selected mood stabilizers: preparations, usual daily doses, and putative therapeutic blood levels *(continued)*

Generic drug	Brand name(s)	Tablet/capsule strengths and other formulations	Usual adult total daily dose range[a]	Putative therapeutic blood level[b]
valproic acid	Depakene[h]	250 mg (capsules) Syrup: 250 mg/5mL	500–1,600 mg	Not well established in bipolar disorder

[a]The "usual" adult total daily dose does not necessarily reflect the full *dosage range,* which is generally broader.
[b]Therapeutic levels achieved in epilepsy not well validated in bipolar patients.
[c]Beaded extended-release formulation.
[d]In a study by Ketter et al. (2004a), there was no significant correlation between serum concentration and score on Young Mania Rating Scale, however.
[e]Extended-release (ER) formulation of divalproex has not been extensively studied in bipolar disorder. However, one study (Centorrino et al. 2003) found that dosage of the ER form needed to be about 20% higher than the dosage of standard divalproex in order to maintain comparable blood levels.
[f]Recently received U.S. Food and Drug Administration approval for use in bipolar maintenance. For information regarding other atypical antipsychotics, see Chapter 1 ("Introduction to Pharmacodynamics and Pharmacokinetics") and Chapter 3 ("Antipsychotics").
[g]About 30%–50% higher in dosing than carbamazepine.
[h]Rarely used in bipolar disorder because of poor gastrointestinal tolerance.
Source. Drug Facts and Comparisons 1995; Ghaemi 2003; Physicians' Desk Reference 2004; Post et al. 2003.

Indications

TABLE 5–2. Indications for lithium

Strength of database	Condition	Comments
Strong	Acute mania	Lithium seems most effective when acute mania is "classic" type, not mixed with depression, dysphoria, or irritability. (Valproate is more effective for mixed mania.)
	Prophylaxis of bipolar disorder	Lithium is definitely effective in prophylaxis, but as many as 50% of bipolar patients show inadequate long-term response to lithium monotherapy; lithium has well-documented efficacy in reducing suicide in bipolar disorder.
Moderate	Depressed phase of bipolar disorder	Lithium may be effective for the majority of depressed bipolar patients, but response is often partial; lithium averts risk of rapid cycling from antidepressant, though some depressed bipolar patients may require adjunctive antidepressant.
	Potentiation of anti-depressant response in unipolar and bipolar depression	Lithium potentiation of TCAs and perhaps SSRIs is successful in about 50% of cases, sometimes within 1–2 weeks (more likely to help in bipolar than unipolar depressive patients). Levels may need to be in usual "bipolar" range.
	Schizoaffective disorder	Overall response rate of lithium-treated schizoaffective patients is >70%; schizomanic patients respond better than do patients with depressed subtype.
	Impulsive aggression	Lithium has antiaggressive effects in wide range of psychiatric patients, including developmentally delayed/mentally retarded patients, prisoners with "rage outbursts," and self-injurious patients. However, patients with underlying brain damage may be prone to lithium toxicity (use lower doses?).

TABLE 5–2. Indications for lithium *(continued)*

Strength of database	Condition	Comments
Weak/Questionable	Schizophrenia	Lithium may improve some affective symptoms in schizophrenia, but rarely improves "core" features of the illness. However, a subset of psychotic patients with absence of negative features and schizophrenia spectrum disorders in family may be lithium-responsive.
	OCD (adjunct)	In OCD, addition of lithium to primary serotonergic agent appears to produce response in only a few patients; controlled data not supportive.
	BPD	Some BPD patients may show decreased impulsivity with lithium, but controlled studies are lacking.
	Alcoholism	Lithium for alcoholism has had mixed results (three positive, four negative outcome studies).

Note. BPD=borderline personality disorder; OCD=obsessive-compulsive disorder; SSRI=selective serotonin reuptake inhibitor; TCA=tricyclic antidepressant.

Source. Baldessarini et al. 2003; M.P. Freeman et al. 2004; Hester 1994; Lenox and Manji 1995; Pies 2002a; Pies and Popli 1995; Rifkin et al. 1972; Schexnayder et al. 1995.

TABLE 5–3. Preferred treatments of acute manic or mixed episodes in bipolar disorder

Clinical situation	Treatment
Choice of initial treatment modality for patients not yet in treatment for bipolar disorder[a]	
First-line pharmacological treatment for more severe mania or mixed episodes	Lithium or valproate, in combination with an antipsychotic (e.g., olanzapine, risperidone, quetiapine)[b]
First-line pharmacological treatment for less severely ill patients	Monotherapy with lithium, valproate, or an antipsychotic such as olanzapine[b] may be sufficient Short-term adjunctive treatment with a benzodiazepine may also be helpful
First-line pharmacological treatment for mixed episodes	Valproate may be preferred over lithium
Alternatives to lithium or valproate	Carbamazepine or oxcarbazepine
Patients already receiving maintenance treatment	
First-line intervention for patients who experience a "breakthrough" manic or mixed episode	Optimize current medication dosage Introduction or resumption of an antipsychotic may also be necessary
Management of severely ill or agitated patients	Short-term adjunctive treatment with a benzodiazepine may also be required
Patients who fail to respond after dosage is optimized	
First recommendation	Add lithium or valproate
Alternatives	Add carbamazepine or oxcarbazepine Change from one antipsychotic to another
Treatment of severely ill patients or patients with treatment-resistant illness	Clozapine may be especially effective for refractory illness, though controlled studies are lacking Consider electroconvulsive therapy (ECT) when appropriate
Treatment of patients experiencing mixed episodes or patients experiencing severe mania during pregnancy	ECT is a potential treatment (and may be treatment of choice during first trimester)

TABLE 5–3. Preferred treatments of acute manic or mixed episodes in bipolar disorder *(continued)*

Clinical situation	Treatment
Patients with features of psychosis	
Recommendation	An antipsychotic medication or ECT is virtually always required; antipsychotics may be useful even in nonpsychotic manic patients

[a]Antidepressants should be tapered or discontinued if possible. If psychosocial therapies are used, they should be in combination with pharmacotherapy.
[b]Atypical antipsychotics are preferred over typical antipsychotics because of their more benign side-effect profile. Ziprasidone and aripiprazole have antimanic effects but are less well studied than olanzapine, risperidone, and quetiapine.
Source. Modified and adapted from recommendations in American Psychiatric Association 2002.

TABLE 5–4. Preferred treatments of acute depressive episodes in bipolar disorder

Clinical situation	Treatment
Choice of initial treatment modality in patients not yet in treatment for bipolar disorder	
First-line pharmacological treatment for patients with bipolar depression	Monotherapy with lithium or lamotrigine Antidepressant monotherapy *not* recommended; however, olanzapine/fluoxetine combination (OFC; Symbyax) has FDA-approved labeling for bipolar depressive episodes
Alternative in treating more severely ill patients	Lithium and an antidepressant may be combined in some cases
Cases of life-threatening inanition (e.g., refusing food), suicidality, or psychosis; or, prominent catatonic features	Electroconvulsive therapy (ECT) is a reasonable alternative and may be treatment of choice
Severe (especially psychotic) depression during pregnancy	ECT is potential treatment, especially during first trimester (when risk of teratogenic effects of medications is increased); OFC could be considered if ECT not feasible
Concomitant psychosocial intervention	Interpersonal therapy and cognitive-behavioral therapy in combination with pharmacotherapy Psychodynamic psychotherapy with medication
Patients already receiving maintenance treatment[a]	
First-line approach for patients who experience a "breakthrough" depressive episode	Optimize dosage of maintenance medication
Patients who fail to respond after dosage is optimized[a]	
Next steps	Add lamotrigine Add bupropion or paroxetine
Alternative steps	Add newer antidepressants (other SSRIs or venlafaxine) or an MAOI
Management of patients with severe or treatment-resistant depression, or with psychotic or catatonic features	Consider ECT early in course

TABLE 5–4. Preferred treatments of acute depressive episodes in bipolar disorder *(continued)*

Clinical situation	Treatment
Patients with features of psychosis	
Recommendations	Adjunctive treatment with an antipsychotic medication is almost always required; ECT is reasonable alternative and may be used with antipsychotic

Note. FDA=U.S. Food and Drug Administration; MAOI=monoamine oxidase inhibitor; SSRI=selective serotonin reuptake inhibitor.

[a]Antidepressant-induced switch rates to hypomania/mania are probably lower in patients with bipolar II depression than in patients with bipolar I depression. Therefore, clinicians may elect using antidepressants earlier in the treatment of bipolar II patients.

Source. Modified and adapted from recommendations in American Psychiatric Association 2002; Fink 2003; Tohen et al. 2003.

TABLE 5–5. Preferred treatments of rapid cycling in bipolar disorder

Clinical situation	Treatment
Initial intervention	Identify and treat medical conditions such as hypothyroidism and drug or alcohol use Certain medications, particularly TCAs, may contribute to rapid cycling and should be tapered and discontinued if possible
Initial treatment	Include lithium or valproate
Alternative treatments	Lamotrigine, perhaps carbamazepine or oxcarbazepine Combinations of medications are required in many patients; thyroxine (T_4) may be useful; some evidence for nimodipine, other calcium channel blockers

Note. TCA=tricyclic antidepressant.

Source. Modified and adapted from recommendations in American Psychiatric Association 2002; Dunn et al. 1998.

TABLE 5–6. Preferred maintenance treatments in bipolar disorder

Clinical situation	Treatment
Choice of initial treatment modality following remission of acute episode (continuation phase treatment)	
Following manic episode; in bipolar II patients	Maintenance treatment is recommended
Treatment options[a]	Lithium or valproate
Alternative treatment options[a]	Lamotrigine, carbamazepine, or oxcarbazepine; ECT in patients who responded to it acutely; possibly olanzapine or other atypicals
Patients who have been treated with an antipsychotic agent during preceding acute episode	
Recommendations	Reassess need for antipsychotic treatment during maintenance phase
	Discontinue antipsychotic unless required for control of persistent psychosis
	Discontinue antipsychotic unless required for prophylaxis against recurrence
	However, maintenance therapy with atypical antipsychotic agents may be considered; olanzapine and aripiprazole now have FDA-approved labeling for maintenance treatment; depot risperidone could be considered for poorly compliant patients
Concomitant psychosocial intervention	Likely to benefit from psychotherapy (addressing illness management and interpersonal difficulties)
	Group psychotherapy
	Support groups. For dual-diagnosis patients (e.g., with comorbid alcohol abuse), parallel treatment (AA, 12-step programs) is critical
Patients who fail to respond or experience "breakthrough" mood episode	
Recommendations	Consider adding another maintenance medication
	Consider adding an atypical antipsychotic or an antidepressant
	Consider maintenance ECT for those who responded to ECT acutely

Note. ECT = electroconvulsive therapy; FDA = U.S. Food and Drug Administration.

[a]If one of these medications was used to achieve remission from the most recent depressive or manic episode, it should be continued.

Source. Modified and adapted from recommendations in Albanese and Pies 2004; American Psychiatric Association 2002.

Mechanisms of Action

TABLE 5–7. Mood stabilizer and anticonvulsant mechanisms of action

Agent	Putative mechanism of action
lithium	May reduce "excessive signaling" through the phosphatidylinositol (PI) system, at least during mania. Lithium is an inhibitor of GSK-3 activity, via competition with magnesium for a binding site on the enzyme. GSK-3 is critically involved in cellular signaling pathways and regulation of various transcription factors, as well as in "neuroprotection."
carbamazepine, oxcarbazepine topiramate (?) lamotrigine	Directly block presynaptic voltage-gated sodium channels, leading to reduced action potentials and reduced release of glutamate from presynaptic neuron; indirect augmentation of GABA?
valproate	Indirectly acts on voltage-gated sodium channels; indirect potentiation of GABA?
gabapentin pregabalin	Act on calcium channels by binding to α_2/δ subunits, normalizing excessive activation; reduced release of multiple neurotransmitters
tiagabine	Raises GABA levels; selective GABA reuptake inhibitor

Note. ?=evidence is preliminary. GABA=γ-aminobutyric acid; GSK-3=glycogen synthase kinase–3.

Source. El-Mallakh and Wyatt 1995; Gould et al. 2004; Stahl 2004.

Pharmacokinetics

TABLE 5–8. Pharmacokinetics of selected mood stabilizers

Chemical name	Half-life ($t_{1/2}$)[a]	Time to steady state[a]	Metabolism	Active metabolites
carbamazepine	15–50 hours initially; 8–20 hours chronically; approximately 6.5 hours for 10,11-epoxide metabolite	2–4 days initially; after first 2 weeks, because of autometabolism, more than a month may be required to reach stable level, assuming dose is increased	Hepatic microsomal oxidation (at least in part via CYP 3A4) Autoinduction present (leads to reduced blood levels)	10,11-Epoxide, which may be neurotoxic
divalproex	6–16 hours	1.5–3.5 days	Mainly hepatic, via several pathways: glucuronidation, mitochondrial B-oxidation, and P450 microsomal metabolism (2C9, 2C19)	Several active metabolites, including 2-propyl-4-pentanoic acid, which is hepatotoxic and teratogenic
lithium	20–27 hours	4–7 days	Renal excretion	—
olanzapine	21–54 hours	7–14 days	Hepatic CYP 1A2, CYP 2D6, and glucuronidation	—
oxcarbazepine	2.0–2.5 hours for parent compound; 9–11 hours for 10-hydroxy metabolite	±2 days for active metabolite	Mainly via noninducible cytosol enzyme, arylketone reductase; small portion of active metabolite goes through CYP 3A4 Autoinduction not present	10-Hydroxy metabolite may be active compound (does not produce epoxide, which may improve tolerability)

TABLE 5–8. Pharmacokinetics of selected mood stabilizers *(continued)*

Chemical name	Half-life ($t_{1/2}$)[a]	Time to steady state[a]	Metabolism	Active metabolites
lamotrigine	25–33 hours	7–10 days	Hepatic and extrahepatic, mainly via glucuronidation $t_{1/2}$ is increased if used concomitantly with valproic acid	—

Note. CYP = cytochrome P450.

[a]Values are only estimates derived from several studies.

Source. Cozza et al. 2003; DeVane 1994; Hellewell 2002; Janicak 1995; Ketter et al. 2004b; McElroy and Keck 1995; Physicians' Desk Reference 2004.

Main Side Effects

TABLE 5–9. Lithium side effects

Subjective side effects	% Patients reporting
Excessive thirst	35.9
Polyuria	30.4
Memory problems	28.2
Tremor	26.6
Weight gain	18.9
Drowsiness/Fatigue	12.4
Diarrhea	8.7

Source. Goodwin and Jamison 1990 (does not include placebo control data); Lenox and Manji 1995.

TABLE 5–10. Stages of lithium toxicity

Stage	Lithium level (mEq/L)	Clinical Picture
Early toxicity	1.2–1.5	Slight ataxia, dysarthria, lack of coordination
Mild toxicity	1.5–2.0	Listlessness, nausea, slurring of speech, diarrhea, coarse tremor
Moderate toxicity	2.0–2.5	Coarse tremor, confusion, delirium, pronounced ataxia
Severe toxicity	2.5–3.0 or greater	Stupor, spontaneous attacks of hyperextension of extremities, choreoathetosis, seizures, coma

Note: Recently, an "instant blood test" for lithium levels using a finger-stick sample of whole blood has been successfully field-tested. The test appears to have high reliability compared with standard methods (Glazer et al. 2004).
Source: Adapted from Janicak et al. 1993, p. 397.

TABLE 5–11. Five most common side effects of carbamazepine

Side effect	% Patients reporting
Dizziness	35
Drowsiness	29
Nausea	13
Skin reactions	12
Asthenia	11

Source. Sillanpaa 1981 (based on Ciba-Geigy data on patients taking carbamazepine for neuralgia, epilepsy, and other miscellaneous conditions).

TABLE 5–12. Management of common anticonvulsant mood stabilizer side effects (non-placebo-adjusted rates)

Agent	Side effects (average % patients reporting[a])	Management
carbamazepine	Neurological (e.g., ataxia, vertigo, diplopia, sedation, blurred vision) (36%)	Usually transient; reversible with dosage reduction; may be related to CBZ's metabolite CBZ-10,11-epoxide (not ordinarily measured by most laboratories)
	Leukopenia (10%)	Usually transient, benign granulocytopenia (not related to aplastic anemia); usually resolves spontaneously or with dosage reduction (aplastic anemia seen in about 1 in 575,000 cases)
	Rash (10%)	May respond to topical steroids; discontinue CBZ if rash accompanied by fever, bleeding, exfoliative skin lesions (Stevens-Johnson syndrome)
	Hyponatremia (5%)	If severe, may require discontinuation of CBZ; tetracyclines may be helpful (e.g., demeclocycline)
	Liver enzyme elevations (10%)	Usually benign; dose reduction helps Monitor clinical status to rule out malaise, vomiting, jaundice If levels of transaminases are three times normal, or if levels of alkaline phosphatase or bilirubin are elevated, hold CBZ, consider alternative agent Monitor LFTs periodically
	Thyroid dysfunction (8%)	Slight decrease in total or free T_4 or elevation of TSH levels, rarely of clinical significance; may be dose related Use thyroid supplement if necessary
	GI disturbances (10%)	Usually abate after the first few weeks of treatment; dosage reduction or multiple dosing schedule may help

TABLE 5–12. Management of common anticonvulsant mood stabilizer side effects (non-placebo-adjusted rates) *(continued)*

Agent	Side effects (average % patients reporting[a])	Management
lamotrigine (300 mg/day in adults with epilepsy)	Dizziness (31%) Diplopia (24%) Nausea (18%) Vomiting (11%) Blurred vision (11%) Ataxia (10%)	Dosage reduction and/or divided doses usually helpful Plasma levels not routinely obtained in bipolar disorder
	Benign rash (8%)	Any patient developing new-onset rash within first few months of treatment should be instructed to hold the next dose and immediately seek medical evaluation and/or treatment; see "Questions and Answers" section on side effects for details (risk of severe/life threatening rash is <1 in 1,000 in adults)
oxcarbazepine (2,400 mg/day monotherapy)	Headache (31%) Dizziness (28%) Nausea (22%) Fatigue (21%) Somnolence (19%) Vomiting (15%) Visual problem (14%) Diplopia (12%)	Dosage reduction and/or divided doses usually helpful Plasma levels are not usually obtained in bipolar disorder; in epilepsy, therapeutic range is roughly 10–35 μg/mL
	Hyponatremia (±2.5%)	Baseline serum Na^+, follow-up in 1–2 months; monitor as appropriate
valproate (divalproex)[b]	GI disturbances (e.g., anorexia, nausea, vomiting, diarrhea) (18%)	Related to onset of treatment (may be transient), dose, and plasma level; rarely a significant problem with plasma levels below 90 μg/mL; may be reduced with use of divalproex "sprinkles," addition of H_2 blocker (e.g., famotidine)
	Tremor (5%)	Dosage reduction or use of beta-blocker
	Hair loss/thinning (6%)	Usually transient; may respond to zinc/ selenium supplement

TABLE 5–12. Management of common anticonvulsant mood stabilizer side effects (non-placebo-adjusted rates) *(continued)*

Agent	Side effects (average % patients reporting[a])	Management
valproate (divalproex)[b] *(continued)*	Increased appetite, weight gain (5%)	Exercise and fat/sugar reduction occasionally helpful; but may be refractory
	Elevated liver functions (20%)	Usually benign, dose-related elevation of transaminase levels; not necessarily associated with hepatic dysfunction Monitor clinical status to rule out malaise, vomiting, jaundice If levels of transaminases are three times normal and/or if levels of bilirubin or alkaline phosphatase are elevated, hold valproate, consider alternative agent
	Platelet abnormalities	Thrombocytopenia may be seen in 13%–54% of patients, especially elderly patients; rarely, impairment of platelet activation Usually not clinically significant, but some patients may have substantial drop in platelet count and/or increased bleeding time Monitor platelet count periodically, especially in elderly patients Consider checking bleeding time if any signs indicate impaired hemostasis (e.g., petechiae)

Note. CBZ=carbamazepine; GI=gastrointestinal; LFT=liver function test; T_4=thyroxine; TSH=thyroid-stimulating hormone.

[a]Percentages of affected patients may vary considerably with population studied (epilepsy vs. bipolar disorder patients), dosing regimen, age of patient, etc.

[b]Published data regarding the percentage of side effects due to valproate monotherapy are rare. The figures above represent composite averages from several of the references cited in the source below, as well as the author's clinical experience.

Source. Calabrese et al. 1992; De Berardis et al. 2003; Janicak et al. 1993; Lenox and Manji 1995; Maxmen 1991; Physicians' Desk Reference 2004; Shelton and Calabrese 2004; Sillanpaa 1981; Trannel et al. 2001.

TABLE 5–13. Management of lithium side effects

Side effect	Specific symptoms	Clinical management
Gastrointestinal	Nausea, vomiting, anorexia, diarrhea, cramping; common at start of therapy, often transient	Reduce dose and/or slow rate of dose increase early in treatment; give lithium with meals Slow-release preparations can decrease nausea but increase diarrhea Lithium citrate syrup may help GI disturbances; if GI toxicity develops late in treatment, rule out toxicity.
Renal	Glomerular dysfunction is very rare at therapeutic doses (may occur in patients exposed to toxic blood levels) Renal tubular effects are fairly common (e.g., polyuria in about 60% of patients receiving long-term maintenance treatment) Nephrogenic diabetes insipidus (NDI) in about 10% of cases (>3 L/day urine output) Edema is usually not due to change in renal function and may resolve spontaneously	If creatinine level rises abruptly, hold lithium and check creatinine clearance; consider discontinuation of the lithium Some patients may experience less polydipsia/polyuria if most of the lithium dose is given at bedtime (reduce total dose by about 20%); some data suggest that every-other-day dosing schedule may be feasible Thiazide diuretics may help with polyuria but can increase lithium levels about 40% (must decrease lithium dose); thiazides also may reduce K^+; use of amiloride (K^+-sparing diuretic, 5–10 mg bid) may be preferable for treatment of polyuria and usually does not affect lithium or K^+ levels

TABLE 5–13. Management of lithium side effects *(continued)*

Side effect	Specific symptoms	Clinical management
Neurological/ Cognitive	Neurological side effects may be related to dose and/or peak plasma levels; include cognitive effects (slowing/ memory impairment), lethargy, weakness, postural tremor (7–16 Hz) Lithium may increase EPS in patients taking neuroleptics; rarely, lithium may reactivate NMS, cause pseudotumor cerebri	*Always rule out lithium toxicity with new-onset neurological symptoms* Dosage reduction or increasing interdose interval may help For tremor, reduce caffeine, stimulant, tricyclic use Beta-blockers (e.g., atenolol 50 mg bid) may help with tremor (must *monitor pulse* to avert bradycardia) Use lower lithium levels in dementia or brain-injured patients, some elderly patients
Endocrine	Hypothyroidism develops in about 20% of patients treated chronically. Rarely, elevation of parathyroid hormone and serum calcium levels; usually not clinically significant, but could lead to osteoporosis	Check baseline TFTs and follow-up every 6 months; if TSH level is elevated, consider adding T_4; hypothyroidism is not a reason to discontinue lithium, but different agent could be considered Baseline calcium, phosphorus levels with one follow-up after 6 months of lithium may be prudent
Cardiac	T-wave flattening/inversion, sinoatrial node dysfunction; bradycardia; rare ventricular premature contractions	Obtain baseline ECG for patients over age 50 or with history of cardiac symptoms, concomitant use of beta-blockers or calcium channel blockers Check K^+ if T-wave flattening present (usually not due to low serum K^+ levels) Monitor pulse periodically; avoid coprescription of other drugs that cause bradyarrhythmias

TABLE 5–13. Management of lithium side effects *(continued)*

Side effect	Specific symptoms	Clinical management
Dermatological	Acne, worsening of psoriasis; pruritis, hair loss Dermatological side effects not clearly dose-related	Anti-acne regimens may help; consider alternative mood stabilizer Check TFTs if hair loss is present (rule out hypothyroidism)
Weight gain	Lithium may have insulin-like effect on carbohydrate metabolism; increased intake of liquids may promote weight gain	Begin comprehensive weight management program (increase exercise, avoid fats); avoid sugary drinks Consider use of orlistat, if appropriate Avoid sibutramine (Meridia) since it may induce mood elevation or psychosis If clinically feasible, changing to lamotrigine, carbamazepine, or oxcarbazepine may help (weight gain associated with valproate) Adjunctive topiramate may help reduce weight but carries other risks Caution patients against using diuretics to reduce weight (may elevate serum lithium levels)

Note. ECG=electrocardiogram; EPS=extrapyramidal side effects; GI=gastrointestinal; NMS=neuroleptic malignant syndrome; T4=thyroxine; TFT=thyroid function test; TSH=thyroid-stimulating hormone.

Source. Anghelescu et al. 2000; Arana and Hyman 1991; Shader 1994; Taflinski and Chojnacka 2000; Wang et al. 2003.

TABLE 5–14. Potential risk factors for antidepressant-induced mania (AIM) or cycling

Personal history	Numerous antidepressant trials, substance abuse history, early age at first treatment for mood disorder
Family history	Strongly positive for bipolar disorder
Response to previous antidepressant trials	Documented AIM, increased cycling, dysphoric reaction (e.g., feeling "wired," restless, irritable, poor sleep, but not always meeting DSM-IV criteria for hypomania)
Demographic factors	Female; possibly bipolar II disorder
Medical factors	Hypothyroidism (TSH > 5–8 mU/L)
Nature of antidepressant	Possibly TCAs have greater risk than newer agents (SSRIs, bupropion), but little randomized controlled evidence available

Note. SSRI = selective serotonin reuptake inhibitor; TCA = tricyclic antidepressant; TSH = thyroid-stimulating hormone.
Source. Altshuler et al. 1995; Goldberg and Whiteside 2002; Yildiz and Sachs 2003; and author's clinical experience.

Drug–Drug Interactions

TABLE 5–15. Drug–drug interactions with lithium

Agent added to lithium	Potential interaction	Clinical management
ACE inhibitors (enalapril, captopril, lisinopril)	Increased lithium serum levels due to decreased clearance	Monitor lithium levels during treatment with an ACE inhibitor
Acetazolamide	Decreased lithium level due to increased renal excretion	Monitor lithium level closely with this combination
Calcium channel blockers (verapamil, diltiazem)	Increased risk of cardiac and/or neurotoxicity (ataxia, tremors, nausea, vomiting, diarrhea, tinnitus)	Avoid combination if possible
Carbamazepine	Increased neurotoxic effect despite therapeutic lithium and CBZ levels (mechanism unknown)	Usually this combination is well tolerated; toxicity may be more likely in patients with medical illness, previous history of lithium neurotoxicity; monitor carefully for clinical signs/symptoms when this combination is used
COX-2 inhibitors (celecoxib, rofecoxib [removed from U.S. market in 2004], valdecoxib)	Increased lithium serum levels due to decreased clearance	Monitor lithium levels during and after discontinuation of COX-2 inhibitors

TABLE 5–15. Drug–drug interactions with lithium *(continued)*

Agent added to lithium	Potential interaction	Clinical management
Fluoxetine, fluvoxamine, other SSRIs	Increased serum lithium levels and/or lithium toxicity occasionally reported; tremor common; neurotoxicity may progress to ataxia, serotonin syndrome, confusion Fluvoxamine may provoke hyperpyrexia, seizures when combined with lithium, perhaps as part of serotonin syndrome	Consider lithium dose reduction, change to different SSRI, or change to nonserotonergic antidepressant (e.g., bupropion)
Haloperidol, other antipsychotics	Reported increased neurotoxic effects, despite therapeutic lithium levels; similar to NMS (confusion, rigidity)	Not clear that haloperidol is more likely than other neuroleptics to interact in this way with lithium; any antipsychotic may increase EPS associated with lithium, and vice versa; dosage reduction of one or both agents indicated
Methyldopa	Increased lithium level or increased lithium toxicity without change in level	Avoid combination
Metronidazole	Increased lithium level due to decreased renal clearance	Monitor lithium levels closely during treatment

TABLE 5–15. Drug–drug interactions with lithium *(continued)*

Agent added to lithium	Potential interaction	Clinical management
NSAIDs	Increased lithium level, perhaps due to NSAID effect on renal prostaglandin synthesis	Monitor lithium levels closely and use sulindac if NSAID must be used; consider aspirin instead
Theophylline	Decreased lithium level due to increased renal excretion	Monitor lithium level closely with this combination
Thiazide diuretics	Increased serum lithium level due to decreased renal lithium clearance; possible lithium toxicity	50% reduction in lithium dose indicated with use of hydrochlorothiazide 50 mg qd; consider use of furosemide instead
TCAs	A few reports of combination of lithium and TCA (amitriptyline, imipramine, ? others) leading to increased likelihood of seizures, tremor, ? cardiac toxicity	Usually this combination is well tolerated and may be good strategy for refractory unipolar depression Monitor for signs and symptoms of neurotoxicity and consider reduced lithium dose if neurotoxicity is present ECG is prudent with this combination

Note. ACE=angiotensin-converting enzyme; CBZ=carbamazepine; COX-2=cyclooxygenase-2; ECG=electrocardiogram; EPS=extrapyramidal side effects; NMS=neuroleptic malignant syndrome; NSAID=nonsteroidal anti-inflammatory drug; SSRI=selective serotonin reuptake inhibitor; TCA=tricyclic antidepressant.

Source. Brodie and Dichter 1996; Ciraulo et al. 1995; Drug Facts and Comparisons 1995; Ketter et al. 1995a, 1995b; Krishnan et al. 1996; Popli et al. 1995; Venkatakrishnan et al. 2003.

TABLE 5–16. Drug–drug interactions with carbamazepine (CBZ)

Agent added to CBZ	Potential interaction	Clinical management
Anticoagulants	Possibly increased metabolism of anticoagulants; this may reduce their effects	Adjustment of warfarin (Coumadin) dose may be necessary when CBZ is coadministered (or dose is changed or drug is discontinued)
Aripiprazole	Increased clearance of aripiprazole through hepatic induction	Manufacturer recommends doubling the dose of aripiprazole; clinical monitoring is recommended
Bupropion	Possibly decreased plasma levels of bupropion with greatly increased levels of hydroxy-bupropion; this may lead to toxicity in some patients	If bupropion is used with CBZ, obtain plasma level of both bupropion and its metabolite; watch for signs of confusion, psychosis secondary to very high hydroxybupropion levels
Calcium channel blockers	Increased CBZ levels and neurotoxicity, probably due to inhibition of CYP 3A4 system; added cardiac effects	Seems to occur with use of verapamil or diltiazem, but not nifedipine, which is calcium channel blocker of choice in this context
Cimetidine	Transient increase in CBZ levels, with possible increase in CBZ side effects during first 3–5 days of treatment	When possible, use ranitidine, famotidine, or other antacid in patients taking CBZ

TABLE 5–16. Drug–drug interactions with carbamazepine (CBZ) *(continued)*

Agent added to CBZ	Potential interaction	Clinical management
Clozapine, haloperidol (? other antipsychotics)	Induced metabolism of clozapine and haloperidol, which reduces levels of both agents; reduction of haloperidol may be clinically significant in some cases (reduction of antipsychotic effect in some, but not all, cases) Theoretically, increased risk of agranulocytosis when CBZ is used with clozapine	Monitor clinical response when CBZ and antipsychotic are coprescribed Monitor clozapine or other antipsychotic levels; consider dosage increase when CBZ is coadministered; if CBZ is discontinued, may need to *reduce* antipsychotic dose Consider switch to *oxcarbazepine* if clinically appropriate, but oxcarbazepine may induce CYP 3A4, inhibit 2C9
Isoniazid (INH)	Increased CBZ level and toxicity, and possible increased risk of INH-induced hepatotoxicity	Monitor CBZ levels, LFTs carefully with this combination
Lamotrigine	Increased clearance, reduced blood levels of lamotrigine through induction of glucuronidation; *possibly* increased production of neurotoxic CBZ-epoxide metabolite (conflicting reports)	Dose of lamotrigine may need to be increased Oxcarbazepine might be alternative but can reduce lamotrigine levels by about 30%
Macrolide antibiotics (erythromycin, clarithromycin, troleandomycin)	CBZ toxicity, probably due to inhibition of CYP 3A4 system by macrolides	May be more likely with larger doses of macrolides; if possible, use different type of antibiotic; monitor CBZ levels and clinical signs of weakness, lethargy, ataxia, etc. Use azithromycin or dirithromycin (less 3A4 inhibition)

TABLE 5–16. Drug–drug interactions with carbamazepine (CBZ) *(continued)*

Agent added to CBZ	Potential interaction	Clinical management
Oral contraceptives	Effectiveness of oral contraceptives reduced in presence of CBZ, via induction of metabolism; unwanted pregnancy possible	Breakthrough bleeding may be warning of interaction; avoid CBZ in patients taking oral contraceptives or Norplant
Phenobarbital, primidone	Reduced CBZ levels, via enhanced hepatic metabolism; apparently no loss of seizure control	Monitor CBZ levels
	Possibly increased levels of phenobarbital (a metabolite of primidone)	
Phenytoin	Reduced CBZ levels, via enhanced hepatic metabolism of CBZ; effect of CBZ on phenytoin highly variable	Monitor CBZ and phenytoin levels
SSRIs	Studies inconsistent, but possible impairment of CBZ metabolism by fluoxetine and perhaps other SSRIs (e.g., fluvoxamine), leading to CBZ toxicity and/or serotonin syndrome	Monitor CBZ levels closely when SSRI (especially fluoxetine or fluvoxamine) is used concomitantly; in theory, nefazodone may also increase CBZ levels via inhibition of CYP 3A4
TCAs	Additive sedation, cardiac conduction effects; high doses of CBZ associated with anticholinergic side effects, which may be additive	Use cautious dosing; check ECG; monitor for dry mouth, urinary retention, tachycardia

TABLE 5–16. Drug–drug interactions with carbamazepine (CBZ) *(continued)*

Agent added to CBZ	Potential interaction	Clinical management
Valproate	Increased ratio of CBZ epoxide to CBZ via inhibition of epoxide hydroxylase (possible neurotoxicity) Valproate may cause displacement of CBZ from plasma binding proteins CBZ *reduces* valproate levels but *increases* levels of 2-propyl-4-pentanoic acid metabolite, which is hepatotoxic and teratogenic	If CBZ and valproate are used together, monitor levels of both closely; obtain level of CBZ epoxide if possible and closely monitor patient for signs of neurotoxicity; check LFTs more frequently than with either agent alone

Note. CBZ=carbamazepine; CYP=cytochrome P450; ECG=electrocardiogram; LFT=liver function test; SSRI=selective serotonin reuptake inhibitor; TCA=tricyclic antidepressant.

Source. Brodie and Dichter 1996; Ciraulo et al. 1995; Drug Facts and Comparisons 1995; Ketter et al. 1995a, 1995b; Krishnan et al. 1996; Physicians' Desk Reference 2004; Popli et al. 1995; Sandson 2003.

TABLE 5–17. Drug–drug interactions with valproate

Agent added to valproate	Potential interaction	Clinical management
Aspirin, naproxen	Aspirin and naproxen may displace valproate from its binding sites on plasma proteins, but this effect is of doubtful clinical significance; however, aspirin also *inhibits valproate metabolism* Some clinical evidence suggests aspirin/valproate toxicity	Use nonaspirin pain relievers, if possible, with valproate; or reduce valproate dose if aspirin is required
Bupropion	Bupropion concentration unaffected, but increased hydroxybupropion level	Consider reduction of bupropion dose if signs of toxicity develop
Carbamazepine	CBZ *reduces* valproate levels but *increases* levels of 2-propyl-4-pentanoic acid metabolite, which is hepatotoxic and teratogenic	May need to monitor LFTs more closely; adjust one or both anticonvulsant doses and follow levels periodically
Chlorpromazine (? other antipsychotics)	Increased valproate levels due to competitive inhibition of metabolism	Monitor valproate levels closely when valproate and phenothiazines are used concomitantly; haloperidol may not have this effect on valproate
Cimetidine	Increased valproate levels due to decreased clearance	Use ranitidine or famotidine with valproate
Fluoxetine	Increased valproate levels via inhibition of hepatic metabolism	Monitor valproate levels and adjust dose

TABLE 5–17. Drug–drug interactions with valproate *(continued)*

Agent added to valproate	Potential interaction	Clinical management
Lamotrigine	Modest decrease in valproate levels (±25%) after addition of lamotrigine in healthy volunteers; no change in valproate steady-state levels in clinical trials; however, *lamotrigine levels will rise in presence of valproate* (see Table 5–18)	Addition of valproate to lamotrigine not usually recommended in routine cases If lamotrigine must be added to valproate in adults, titrate slowly with low lamotrigine doses (e.g., 25 mg qod for first 2 weeks; then 25 mg qd for 2 weeks; then increase dosage by 25–50 mg/day every 1–2 weeks to target dosage of 100–400 mg/day in one or two divided doses); monitor closely for rash
Magnesium/ aluminum hydroxide antacids	Increased valproate levels	Adjust dosage of valproate if side effects occur
Phenobarbital	Increased phenobarbital levels	Reduce phenobarbital dose
Topiramate	Valproate and topiramate may slightly decrease each other's levels	Monitor valproate blood levels

Note. CBZ = carbamazepine; LFT = liver function test.

Source. Ciraulo and Slattery 1995; Drug Facts and Comparisons 1995; Physicians' Desk Reference 2004; Shelton and Calabrese 2004; Venkatakrishnan et al. 2003.

TABLE 5–18. Drug–drug interactions with lamotrigine

Agent added to lamotrigine	Potential interaction	Clinical management
Carbamazepine/ Oxcarbazepine	Decreased lamotrigine levels with CBZ, less so with oxcarbazepine; *possibly* increased production of neurotoxic CBZ-epoxide metabolite (conflicting reports); some reports of toxicity when lamotrigine is added to CBZ, probably due to pharmacodynamic interaction	Carefully monitor combined use of CBZ and lamotrigine, using lower than usual doses of one or both agents Toxicity more likely when lamotrigine is added to CBZ if initial CBZ level > 8 mg/L; reduction of CBZ dose usually resolves toxicity Oxcarbazepine plus lamotrigine may be safe (based on anecdotal reports)
Oral contraceptives	Decreased lamotrigine levels; conversely, increased lamotrigine levels with discontinuation of oral contraceptive	Adjust lamotrigine dosage accordingly
Phenytoin, phenobarbital, primidone	Decreased lamotrigine levels	Adjust lamotrigine dosage accordingly
Sertraline (? other SSRIs)	Inhibition of glucuronidation may increase lamotrigine levels substantially	Adjust lamotrigine dosage accordingly
Topiramate	No major pharmacokinetic interactions	Watch for pharmacodynamic interactions (e.g., increased sedation, cognitive problems)

TABLE 5–18. Drug–drug interactions with lamotrigine *(continued)*

Agent added to lamotrigine	Potential interaction	Clinical management
Valproate	Addition of adjunctive valproate leads to increased lamotrigine $t_{1/2}$ (from ±25 to 70 hours) and blood levels, due to valproate's inhibition of glucuronidation; may lead to neurotoxicity, increased incidence of Stevens-Johnson syndrome	Slower titration of lamotrigine dose is necessary; monitor more closely for any complaint of rash

Note. CBZ=carbamazepine; SSRI=selective serotonin reuptake inhibitor.
Source. Besag et al. 1998; Doose et al. 2003; Kaufman and Gerner 1998; Physicians' Desk Reference 2004; Sandson 2003; Shelton and Calabrese 2004.

Potentiating Maneuvers

TABLE 5–19. Augmenting strategies in treating patients with bipolar disorder

Combination strategy	Efficacy/Clinical experience	Comments
Lithium + CBZ	Number of major mood episodes, hospitalization, and “cumulative affective morbidity” may be reduced after CBZ augmentation of lithium	Lithium/CBZ combination generally well tolerated Reduction of lithium dose sometimes facilitated by combined treatment; tremor, polyuria, and weight gain may thereby decrease Complaints during combined treatment include sexual dysfunction, decreased energy, hypersomnia CBZ may lead to reduction in TSH levels, perhaps reflecting a shift in favor of free (versus protein-bound) thyroxine (T_4)

TABLE 5–19. Augmenting strategies in treating patients with bipolar disorder *(continued)*

Combination strategy	Efficacy/Clinical experience	Comments
Lithium + divalproex	Expert consensus guidelines (Sachs et al. 2000) list divalproex as the "preferred mood stabilizer to add," when a manic patient has failed to respond fully to initial lithium treatment; however, few controlled studies of efficacy of lithium/divalproex combinations for any phase of bipolar disorder Preliminary evidence suggests that combination of lithium and divalproex is effective for patients not responding to monotherapy with either agent In rapidly cycling patients, combination of lithium and divalproex is associated with acute and continuation antimanic efficacy (85% of patients) and antidepressant efficacy (60% of patients); however, only 50% of patients experience bimodal mood stabilization; most rapidly cycling patients with poor response are depressed	Overall tolerability of the lithium/divalproex combination is usually good Most common adverse effects of combined treatment are GI distress, tremor, cognitive impairment, and alopecia; these appear to occur more frequently than with lithium alone; alopecia possibly improves with zinc/selenium treatment, but few controlled data are available

TABLE 5–19. Augmenting strategies in treating patients with bipolar disorder *(continued)*

Combination strategy	Efficacy/Clinical experience	Comments
Lithium + lamotrigine	Almost no controlled studies of this combination Few of the "add-on" studies break down the results according to subjects who were treated with a combination of lamotrigine and lithium, as opposed to lamotrigine and *other* mood stabilizers Lamotrigine may be effective in treating patients with either no response or only partial response to other agents used to treat bipolar disorder. Expert consensus guidelines (Sachs et al. 2000) endorse a combination of lamotrigine and lithium in selected bipolar patients; that is, for those experiencing depressive breakthrough after a prolonged remission, lamotrigine is a "preferred strategy" for patients already taking high doses of lithium	Administration of lamotrigine with lithium does not cause clinically significant changes in the pharmacokinetics of lithium Combination is well tolerated in most patients; however, dose-related cognitive side effects may occur in some patients, particularly when other medications besides lithium and lamotrigine are being used; reducing the dose of lamotrigine, lithium, or both may help

TABLE 5–19. Augmenting strategies in treating patients with bipolar disorder *(continued)*

Combination strategy	Efficacy/Clinical experience	Comments
Lithium + topiramate	Few studies of the risks and benefits of combined lithium/topiramate therapy; open studies suggest possible antimanic or anticycling effects (not antidepressant) *Note:* Antimanic effects of topiramate monotherapy have not been confirmed in controlled studies	Dosage range of topiramate in bipolar illness is roughly 50–600 mg/day Topiramate has numerous side effects (e.g., tremor, paresthesia) Both pharmacodynamic and pharmacokinetic side effects may be increased with this combination When topiramate is used as an add-on (e.g., with lithium), use conservative topiramate dosing Overly rapid increases in topiramate dosage may lead to neuropsychiatric complications, via topiramate's blockade of AMPA-type glutamate receptors

TABLE 5–19. Augmenting strategies in treating patients with bipolar disorder *(continued)*

Combination strategy	Efficacy/Clinical experience	Comments
Lithium + T_4	Few controlled studies Small, open studies suggest adjunctive T_4 may decrease cycling frequency and severity in rapid cyclers who are unresponsive to lithium alone Some clinicians aim for free T_4 150% of normal	T_4 is used at dosages ranging from 0.1 to 0.3 mg/day, usually as an adjunct to ongoing treatment with lithium or with lithium plus another mood stabilizer Some clinicians "titrate to mood stability" Do not use in patients with underlying cardiac arrhythmia Note use of T_4 in *augmentation* differs from its use in *replacement* treatment in cases of primary or lithium-induced hypothyroidism Perform periodic check of thyroid functions with long-term lithium treatment
CBZ + valproate	May result in sustained prophylactic response in patients who are poorly responsive to CBZ or valproate alone	May be well tolerated; however, valproate inhibits epoxide hydrolase, potentially leading to increased plasma levels of CBZ epoxide and potential neurotoxicity CBZ leads to reduced valproate blood levels

TABLE 5–19. Augmenting strategies in treating patients with bipolar disorder *(continued)*

Combination strategy	Efficacy/Clinical experience	Comments
Valproate, lithium, other mood stabilizers + gabapentin	No controlled evidence supports use of gabapentin as primary mood stabilizer; however, some clinical experience suggests that adjunctive gabapentin may sometimes be useful in bipolar patients with comorbid anxiety, insomnia; some *open* data suggest that adjunctive gabapentin may reduce hypomanic and depressive symptoms Gabapentin may be of more benefit to younger patients with shorter duration of illness	Gabapentin dosage begins at 300–600 mg/day; effective range seems to be 500–3,600 mg/day in divided doses. Gabapentin does not have significant interactions with valproate or other anticonvulsants Combination generally well tolerated, but side effects may include somnolence, dizziness, ataxia, fatigue, nystagmus

Note. AMPA = α-amino-3-hydroxy-5-methylisoxazole-4-propionic acid; CBZ = carbamazepine; GI = gastrointestinal; TSH = thyroid-stimulating hormone.

Source. Altshuler et al. 1999; Bauer and Whybrow 1991; Bochetta et al. 1997; Calabrese et al. 2001; Chengappa et al. 1999, 2001; Fogelson and Sternbach 1997; Frye et al. 2000; McElroy et al. 2000; Obrocea et al. 2002; Pies 2002b; Post et al. 2001; Sachs et al. 2000; Solomon et al. 1997; Sporn and Sachs 1997; Zerjav-Lacombe and Tabarsi 2001.

Use in Special Populations

TABLE 5–20. Use of mood stabilizers in special populations

Population	Special concerns
Women of child-bearing age, pregnant women	Risk of Ebstein's anomaly in infants exposed to lithium in first trimester Exposure to CBZ, valproate is linked to craniofacial defects, spinal cord malformations; if CBZ or valproate must be used during pregnancy, supplemental folate is recommended Teratogenesis risk appears lower with oxcarbazepine, lamotrigine; folate supplementation still recommended Olanzapine appears relatively unlikely to cause teratogenic effects, obstetrical complications
Children, adolescents	Very few controlled studies of mood stabilizers in younger populations Lithium appears to be safe and effective, with side effects similar to those in adults; psychosis may reduce response to lithium in adolescents Valproate and valproate/lithium combinations appear effective in pediatric bipolar populations, but few controlled studies are available Valproate can cause hepatotoxicity in children under age 3 CBZ may be less effective than valproate in younger cohorts, but few controlled studies are available Few data for oxcarbazepine are available Limited experience with lamotrigine in pediatric bipolar patients; some evidence of adjunctive benefit in refractory bipolar depression; higher risk of serious rash with lamotrigine in pediatric populations (up to 1%)

TABLE 5–20. Use of mood stabilizers in special populations *(continued)*

Population	Special concerns
Elderly, medically or neurologically ill persons	Elderly brain more sensitive to drugs Lithium $t_{1/2}\beta$ increased in elderly persons (especially those with renal dysfunction), and neurotoxicity may occur at lower plasma levels; dementia/poststroke patients are especially susceptible to lithium neurotoxicity, even when the lithium is at a therapeutic blood level CBZ may be more likely to produce neurotoxicity in older populations No controlled data on oxcarbazepine in elderly bipolar patients Valproate may be effective at lower dosage/plasma levels than in younger populations, especially in dementia patients; some reports of skeletal muscle weakness with valproate in the elderly (may interfere with walking, etc.); thrombocytopenia in the elderly is common with valproate; valproate may be useful in aggressive, disinhibited dementia patients Limited data for lamotrigine are available in elderly bipolar patients; lamotrigine clearance is reduced by about a third in the elderly Olanzapine is generally safe in the elderly, albeit with some reports of higher rates of laxative use and urinary retention compared with risperidone

Note. CBZ=carbamazepine; $t_{1/2}\beta$=elimination half-life.

Source. Dubovsky 1994; Dulcan et al. 1995; Jacobson et al. 2002; Jeste et al. 2003; Martin et al. 2003; Newport et al. 2004; Wagner 2004.

Questions and Answers

Indications

Q. What are the mood stabilizers of choice in "mixed" or dysphoric mania?

A. There is a reasonably strong consensus that for mixed bipolar episodes, divalproex is somewhat more effective than lithium (T.W. Freeman et al. 1992; Keck et al. 1996). Thus, the American Psychiatric Association (APA) (2002) guideline lists lithium as a first-line agent for essentially every type and phase of bipolar disorder, but notes that for "mixed" manic episodes, valproate "may be preferred over lithium." Similarly, the Texas Medication Algorithm (Suppes et al. 2002) favors either divalproex or olanzapine over lithium for mixed or dysphoric mania/hypomania. Nevertheless, further controlled studies, naturalistic trials, and long-term maintenance-phase studies are needed in order to corroborate the apparent differences in treatment outcome in treating mixed mania with anticonvulsant mood stabilizers versus lithium (Boland and Keller 1999). Indeed, some naturalistic studies (e.g., Tondo et al. 2001) suggest that lithium may be effective in mixed bipolar patients.

Q. What is the role of newer atypical antipsychotics in the management of mania?

A. As discussed in Chapter 3 ("Antipsychotics"), atypical antipsychotics are playing an increasingly important role in the early management of mania. For example, in the 2000 Texas Medication Algorithm (Suppes et al. 2002), the treatment of first choice for euphoric mania was lithium, divalproex, or olanzapine. Five atypical agents—olanzapine, risperidone, quetiapine, aripiprazole, and ziprasidone—already have U.S. Food and Drug Administration (FDA)–approved labeling for use in mania. In light of newer data demonstrating antimanic effects for ziprasidone and aripiprazole, the updated Texas Medication Algorithm is likely to include a broader array of atypical antipsychotics for use in mania and to recommend their use in the first stage of management (Shivakumar and Suppes 2004).

Q. Can atypical antipsychotics sometimes exacerbate mania or agitation?

A. Despite occasional case reports of atypical antipsychotic–related mania or agitation (e.g., John et al. 1998; London 1998), there is little evidence from the controlled outcome literature that this is a common problem. When this phenomenon does occur, it seems to be associated with atypical antipsychotic *monotherapy,* rather than with the combination of atypical antipsychotics and "classical" mood stabilizers, such as lithium (F. K. Goodwin and Ghaemi 2001). Nonetheless, a recent report of hypomania associated with ziprasidone (Brieger 2004) in a schizoaffective patient taking concomitant valproate, and a report of worsening agitation associated with aripiprazole in two patients with chronic schizophrenia (DeQuardo 2004), suggest that such untoward reactions to atypical antipsychotics can occasionally occur. In some cases, this may be a dose-related phenomenon (John et al. 1998).

Q. What are the mood stabilizers of choice for treating rapid-cycling bipolar patients?

A. Several studies have suggested that lithium and carbamazepine (CBZ) are not as effective as divalproex in the treatment of rapid-cycling bipolar disorder (Dilsaver et al. 1993; Okuma 1993). Similarly, Calabrese et al. (1996) concluded that the presence of rapid cycling appeared to be a predictor of nonresponse to lithium and possibly to CBZ.

Not all the evidence supports this conclusion, however (Gelenberg and Pies 2003). The largest of the retrospective/naturalistic studies examined 360 bipolar I and II patients with predominantly mixed, psychotic, and rapid-cycling features (Tondo et al. 2001). Overall, lithium was found to be effective over the course of 1 year, even in those bipolar patients with these supposedly refractory subtypes. Episode frequency and "time ill" were both reduced. These same researchers reported earlier, in this same group of patients (N=360), that overall morbidity was *not* greater in rapid-cycling bipolar patients treated with lithium than in non–rapid-cycling patients (Baldessarini et al. 2000). Specifically, the proportion of time in mania or depression and psychiatric hospitalization rates were not greater in the rapid-cycling patients treated with lithium versus non–rapid-cycling patients. Indeed, with respect to rapid cycling, the APA guideline specifies that the initial treatment may be either lithium or valproate (American Psychiatric Association 2002). There is also some evidence pointing to the effectiveness of lamotrigine in treating rapid-cycling bipolar disorder, particularly in patients with bipolar II disorder (Calabrese et al. 2000). In light of these and other data, the APA guideline considers lamotrigine to be an "alternative" agent in the treatment of rapid-cycling bipolar disorder (American Psychiatric Association 2002).

Q. What is the role of mood stabilizers versus antidepressants in the treatment of patients with bipolar disorder, particularly during the depressed phase of bipolar illness?

A. Bipolar depression represents a dilemma for psychiatrists, and the use of antidepressants for this condition remains controversial (Altshuler et al. 2003; Gelenberg and Pies 2003; F.K. Goodwin and Ghaemi 2001). On the one hand, the development of an effective agent that does not worsen cycling or induce a "switch" into mania remains a major unmet need. On the other hand, so too does development of an effective treatment for the depressed phases of bipolar disorder, which often predominate in many patients (Ketter and Calabrese 2002). In a recent 1-year prospective study, Altshuler's group found that the risk of depressive relapse in bipolar illness was increased when antidepressants were discontinued soon after remission (Altshuler et al. 2003). Furthermore, the risk of *manic* relapse was not significantly associated with continuing use of antidepressants. However, this study had some significant limitations. Aside from lacking blinding or randomization, the study followed only those bipolar patients *who had been successfully treated* with an antidepressant. Experienced clinicians know that not all bipolar patients have such a good response to antidepressants. Furthermore, the antidepressant was an *adjunctive* treatment, used concomitantly with a mood stabilizer. Thus, this study does not demonstrate that antidepressants—either as monotherapy or as adjunctive treatment—are either safe or necessary in the maintenance treatment of all bipolar patients.

Some bipolar patients may be at especially high risk for antidepressant-induced mania or worsened cycling (see Table 5–14); in such patients, antidepressants should be used only with extreme caution, if at all, in the author's view. However, an emerging consensus suggests that a small but vulnerable subgroup of bipolar patients may need adjunctive maintenance antidepressant treatment in order to avoid depressive relapse and recurrence (Altshuler et al. 2003; Post et al. 2003). Nevertheless, most recent guidelines urge caution in the use of antidepressants and advise against antidepressant monotherapy (American Psychiatric Association 2002; Shivakumar and Suppes 2004).

To be sure, "classical" mood stabilizers leave much to be desired in the treatment of bipolar depression. Thus, there is a clinical consensus that divalproex is only modestly effective in the treatment of acute bipolar depression (West et al. 1998). Lithium's effects in bipolar depression are generally modest to moderate and quite variable. For example, Strakowski and colleagues (2000) found a relatively wide range of responses to lithium in bipolar depression, with rates varying from 44% to 100%. They noted that the patients in these studies (*N*= 160) had an overall response rate of 72%, although in many cases the response was only partial. But this is hardly support for the commonly held belief—encountered in the author's experience as a teacher and consultant—that lithium "doesn't work" in the depressed phase of bipolar disorder (Pies 2002b). On the contrary, F.K. Goodwin and Jamison (1990) noted significant antidepressant effects in six of the seven studies they reviewed with a 4-week or longer treatment period. A recent meta-analysis of randomized controlled trials (Geddes et al. 2004) found that lithium has robust protective effects against manic relapse and a more modest effect on depressive relapse (the average risk of relapse in the placebo group was 32%, vs. 25% in the lithium group). Still, the authors characterized this as a "moderate beneficial effect" against depressive relapse, noting that some patients will probably be protected by lithium against both manic and depressive relapses.

Recently, the FDA approved the anticonvulsant lamotrigine for "the maintenance treatment of adults with bipolar I disorder to delay the time to occurrence of mood episodes (depression, mania, hypomania, mixed episodes) in patients treated for acute mood episodes with standard therapy" (R.A. Leadbetter, GlaxoSmithKline "Dear Doctor" letter, June 2003). The data on which this approval was based (Bowden et al. 2003) suggest that lamotrigine has more robust effects in bipolar depression than in mania, hypomania, or mixed episodes. In controlled studies of bipolar I patients, there seems to be a low rate (about 2%) of switching and/or hypomania with lamotrigine (Bowden et al. 2003), notwithstanding one report of apparent lamotrigine-related hypomania in a patient who had also been taking bupropion (Margolese et al. 2003).

In summary: When clinically feasible, minimize or avoid antidepressant use in bipolar patients; instead, optimize use of classical mood stabilizers and perhaps atypical antipsychotics (F.K. Goodwin and Ghaemi 2001). Avoidance of antidepressant use seems especially appropriate in patients with rapid, ultrarapid, or continuous cycling, for whom an increased risk of manic "switching" seems more likely (Post et al. 2003). One recent naturalistic study also found that females may be particularly at risk for antidepressant-induced mania—that is, there was a significant association between *rapid cycling* and *antidepressant use prior to first episode of mania/hypomania* for women, but not for men (Yildiz and Sachs 2003). If a bipolar patient who has done well taking a combination of mood stabilizer(s) and an antidepressant clearly decompensates without the antidepressant, it may be reasonable to include the antidepressant in the maintenance regimen. Alternatively, lamotrigine might be used in lieu of the antidepressant.

Q. What is the role of the new combination treatment (olanzapine–fluoxetine) in the treatment of bipolar depression?

A. The FDA's approval of olanzapine–fluoxetine combination (OFC; Symbyax) was based on findings from a double-blind, 8-week, randomized, placebo-controlled trial in bipolar I depressed patients (Tohen et al. 2003). Patients were randomly assigned to receive placebo ($n=377$), olanzapine 5–20 mg/day ($n=370$), or OFC (as separately administered olanzapine, up to 12 mg/day, plus fluoxetine, up to 50 mg/day) ($n=86$). Using Montgomery-Åsberg Depression Rating Scale (MADRS) scores, the study found that the OFC group showed statistically greater improvement than the olanzapine (monotherapy) group or the placebo group. There were no statistically significant differences in rates of mania among the three groups over the 8-week study period. Common side effects with OFC included weight gain, drowsiness, and occasional orthostatic hypotension associated with dizziness. Rosenblatt and Rosenblatt (2004), in critically reviewing this study, argued the following:

1. The study "more plausibly corroborates antidepressant effects of fluoxetine than…superior antidepressant effects…of coadministering fluoxetine and olanzapine…," and the antidepressant effects of olanzapine monotherapy were modest.
2. The study had a short duration and a high dropout rate, and lacked a fluoxetine monotherapy arm.
3. The study found significant rates of weight gain with olanzapine-treated patients, and high rates of orthostatic hypotension with OFC treatment.

It should also be noted that 8 weeks is a rather brief period in the overall "life history" of a patient with bipolar disorder; hence, claims about manic "switch" rates in this study should be taken with a large grain of salt.

The use of a combination agent (i.e., two drugs in a single capsule) may increase "compliance" in some patients who dislike taking several medications; on the other hand, the fixed dosages of such combination agents may limit flexibility in dosing. Symbyax does not have FDA-approved labeling for use in elderly patients with dementia. Finally, it is not clear whether OFC is effective in the long-term treatment of bipolar patients with predominantly depressed features.

Q. If an antidepressant must be used in treating a patient with bipolar disorder, which agent is preferred?

A. There is a good deal of "received wisdom" and clinical lore on this issue but far less in the way of randomized controlled studies. Most clinical guidelines recommend the use of a selective serotonin reuptake inhibitor (SSRI) or sustained-release bupropion (Shivakumar and Suppes 2004). However, to the author's knowledge, there has never been a randomized, prospective, "head-to-head" comparative study of "manic switch" rates with any of these agents. In one small double-blind study of bipolar depressed patients (Sachs et al. 1994), switch rates into mania or hypomania were statistically lower with bupropion than with the tricyclic antidepressant (TCA) desipramine (11% vs. 50%). In contrast, Fogelson and colleagues (1992) observed incipient mania in 6 of the 11 patients whom they treated with bupropion; however, nearly all had a previous history of manias induced by other antidepressants. Although paroxetine is sometimes cited as the "preferred" SSRI for bipolar depression, there are no prospective, randomized, "head-to-head" trials comparing paroxetine with other SSRIs vis-à-vis switch rates in bipolar disorder. Furthermore, lifetime naturalistic data from the Cornell Bipolar Disorders Research Clinic cohort indicate no significant differences across antidepressant classes with regard to the prevalence of antidepressant-induced manias. Across all classes studied, there was an overall mania induction rate of 16%, ranging from as low as 10% to 15% with TCAs or SSRIs to as high as 25% with venlafaxine (Goldberg and Whiteside 2002). Finally, although some open data (not based on assessment with mania rating scales) support the use of an SSRI as *monotherapy* in bipolar II patients (e.g., Amsterdam et al. 1998), there are currently no professional guidelines that recommend antidepressant monotherapy in bipolar depression (American Psychiatric Association 2002; Shivakumar and Suppes 2004).

Q. Can mood stabilizers prevent a bipolar patient from "switching" into mania while taking an antidepressant?

A. This seems to be a widely held assumption among clinicians, though the supporting evidence is meager (Bowden and Goldberg 2003). For example, Altshuler et al. (1995) found that the majority of patients who had probable antidepressant-induced mania were concurrently taking a mood stabilizer during the switch; hence, evidence of a "protective" effect was lacking. Similarly, in a double-blind comparison of bupropion or desipramine added to lithium, valproate, lithium–valproate combination, or CBZ for bipolar depression, manic inductions occurred in 3 of 10 patients taking desipramine (Sachs et al. 1994). Over the course of a 1-year continuation phase, a total of 5 of 10 patients taking desipramine had a manic or hypomanic episode, versus 1 of 9 bupropion-treated patients. These included 3 of 8 taking lithium (37.5%), 1 of 4 taking valproate alone (25%), 1 of 2 taking lithium plus valproate (50%), and none taking CBZ. The treatment subgroups in this study were too small to permit statistical analysis of differences among mood stabilizers; however, the results do not seem to show a robust protective effect of mood stabilizers (Bowden and Goldberg 2003). Similarly, Goldberg and Whiteside (2002) observed no significant differences in rates of manic or hypomanic inductions across antidepressant classes in either the presence or absence of concurrent therapy with lithium or divalproex. On the other hand, a small (*N*=44) naturalistic study of antidepressant-induced mania (Henry et al. 2001) found that patients taking concomitant anticonvulsant medications did not differ in their switch rate from those not taking a mood stabilizer. However, those taking concomitant lithium had a lower rate of antidepressant-induced mania. Finally, the whole notion of antidepressant-induced "switching" is fraught with controversy, since it is difficult to discriminate a patient's "natural" manic periods from those induced by external causes (see Bowden and Goldberg 2003 for a comprehensive review).

Q. What factors differentially predict response to lithium, valproate, and CBZ in the treatment of bipolar disorder?

A. High likelihood of response to lithium is predicted by the presence of a milder manic episode; one with "pure" manic symptoms (e.g., elation and grandiosity without a mix of depressive features); prior good response to lithium; and a history of fewer manic episodes. Some data suggest that the episode sequence of mania, followed by depression, followed by euthymia (M-D-Eu) responds better to lithium than does the pattern of depression–mania–euthymia (D-M-Eu) (Bowden 1995b; Grof et al. 1993). A history of many previous mood episodes (manic and depressed) also appears to predict a diminished response to lithium, compared with divalproex, in acute mania (Swann et al. 2000). Patients with complicated types of mania (e.g., secondary to substance abuse, underlying brain pathology) and "mixed" manic states generally have poorer responses to lithium (Bowden 1995b). Valproate seems to be a "broader spectrum" mood stabilizer, in that mixed mania responds as well to divalproex as does pure mania and responds better to divalproex than to lithium. (Although valproate is often said to be superior to lithium for the treatment of rapid-cycling bipolar disorder, the evidence for this is somewhat mixed.) Bipolar disorder is highly comorbid with alcohol and substance abuse (Albanese and Pies 2004). Goldberg and colleagues (1999) found a lower response to lithium than to CBZ or divalproex in comorbid substance abusers. Similarly, Albanese et al. (2000), in treating 20 substance-abusing mood disorder patients with divalproex, found that divalproex was efficacious for the mood disorder and safe when used as monotherapy or in combination with other psychiatric medications.

Predictors of response to CBZ and oxcarbazepine are less clear, though CBZ appears to be more effective than lithium in treating secondary mania and may be useful in patients who have not responded to lithium (Bowden 1995b). The data on CBZ in mixed and rapid-cycling bipolar disorder are contradictory (Bowden 1995b). Although both CBZ and (in small and underpowered studies) oxcarbazepine have shown benefits in acute mania (Emrich 1990; Ketter et al. 1998), there are few controlled studies of either agent in patients with mixed bipolar states. In part, this may be a consequence of the declining use of CBZ in American psychiatry, as divalproex and other anticonvulsants have gained favor.

Q. What evidence is there that oxcarbazepine actually works in bipolar disorder?

A. The controlled evidence is limited mostly to older, European studies of acute manic patients (e.g., Emrich 1990; Ketter et al. 2004b), for whom oxcarbazepine was as effective as haloperidol and lithium. However, in a comprehensive review, Hellewell (2002) cited some uncontrolled evidence for oxcarbazepine's usefulness in bipolar depression, as well as (less convincing) evidence for its benefits in maintenance treatment of bipolar disorder. Recently, Ghaemi (2003) performed a chart review (*N*=42) of naturalistic treatment with oxcarbazepine as monotherapy or adjunctive therapy. Overall, oxcarbazepine appeared effective in about half of patients with bipolar disorder and was well tolerated, with sedation being the most common side effect. The type of bipolar disorder (e.g., mixed, type I, type II) did not differentially predict response. Thus, the role of oxcarbazepine in treating bipolar disorder is still not clear, though it is considered a treatment option in two expert guidelines (e.g., American Psychiatric Association 2002; Suppes et al. 2002). In the author's experience, oxcarbazepine is useful mainly in patients who would otherwise be good candidates for CBZ treatment but who experience side effects or drug–drug interactions with that agent (Gelenberg and Pies 2003).

Q. What are the risks of stopping lithium therapy in bipolar patients?

A. Withdrawing lithium from stable bipolar patients taking long-term lithium is associated with a high risk of early recurrence; increased mortality from suicide; and probably a "rebound" treatment-refractory state (Faedda et al. 1993; G.M. Goodwin 1994; Osser 1996; Suppes et al. 1991). Rapid discontinuation produces the worst outcome, with a 50% relapse rate (within 6 months) and increased risk of suicide (Baldessarini et al. 1999). Post et al. (2001) described the phenomenon of "lithium discontinuation–induced treatment resistance"—a condition that may be associated with extreme difficulty in reacquiring adequate response, despite new pharmacotherapy trials. More gradual tapering of lithium improves 6-month outcome, but not relapse rate over a 5-year period. Some data suggest that relapse rates for bipolar patients who have their lithium discontinued may be worse than those for patients never treated with lithium (G.M. Goodwin 1994). Thus, lithium treatment may not be prudent if there is a very high probability the patient will discontinue it within the first year or two. On the other hand, given the clear antisuicidal benefits of lithium, the clinician should make every reasonable effort to maintain a lithium-responsive patient on this agent, even in the face of some significant side effects (Pies 2002b).

Q. What is the role of lithium in the management of psychosis?

A. The answer may depend on the nature of the psychotic disturbance. Hirschowitz et al. (1980) found that patients with DSM-III (American Psychiatric Association 1980) schizophreniform disorder and those with so-called good prognosis schizophrenia (essentially, those with significant recovery from previous psychotic episodes) tend to be lithium-responsive. The authors hypothesized that such patients may have "lithium-responsive affective disorders masquerading phenomenologically as schizophrenic-like illnesses" (p. 919). Schexnayder et al. (1995) examined a group of 66 psychotic patients treated with lithium alone. Lithium responders showed fewer negative symptoms of schizophrenia (e.g., apathy, withdrawal) and lacked a family history of "schizophrenic spectrum" disorders (defined as schizophrenia, schizoaffective disorder, schizophreniform disorder, or schizotypal personality disorder). (Note that the earlier study by Hirschowitz et al. [1980]) looked at schizophreniform disorder but did not "lump it in" with these other conditions.)

Q. In what psychiatric conditions (besides bipolar disorder) is lithium useful?

A. Lithium has been found useful as an adjunctive agent (i.e., added to a primary antidepressant) in treating both unipolar and bipolar depression. Some data suggest that lithium augmentation in unipolar depression represents a viable alternative to changing the primary agent (Lenox and Manji 1995). Many studies of lithium augmentation suffer from retrospective analysis, uncontrolled design, or inadequate dose/duration of treatment (Nierenberg et al. 2003; O'Reardon 2004). Furthermore, one recent placebo-controlled trial (Nierenberg et al. 2003) found lithium augmentation of nortriptyline ineffective in patients with multiple antidepressant failures. Nevertheless, in their review of placebo-controlled studies of lithium augmentation in refractory depression, Price et al. (2001) concluded that 7 of 10 trials (total *N*=226) showed a positive effect. Some data suggest a preferential effect of lithium augmentation in bipolar depression, whereas other data show no difference. In unipolar depression, response to adjunctive lithium may be evident within 1–2 weeks; however, a 3- to 4-week trial is recommended. Sometimes response to lithium augmentation may be seen at relatively low dosages of lithium (e.g., 300–600 mg/day), but many patients will require higher dosages and plasma levels in the usual therapeutic range (0.5–0.9 mEq/L) (Price et al. 2001). Pope et al. (1988) found lithium useful when added to fluoxetine in five patients with treatment-refractory depression, and clinical experience has tended to support the view that lithium may augment response to SSRIs in some patients. However, confirmatory controlled data are lacking.

Lithium has also been found useful in treating schizoaffective disorder, though this category has been defined in various ways over the years. After reviewing virtually the entire literature on schizoaffective disorder as of 1988, Levitt and Tsuang (1988) concluded that the most helpful therapeutic maneuver is to divide the disorder by "polarity"—that is, whether the patient shows "schizomanic" or "schizodepressive" features. These authors noted several studies showing that schizomanic patients respond to lithium. In schizodepressive patients, the benefits of lithium are less clear. Lithium has not been found particularly useful in schizophrenia, but there may be a lithium-responsive subset of psychotic (nonbipolar) patients. Schexnayder et al. (1995) examined a group of 66 psychotic patients who were diagnosed with schizophrenia or schizophreniform disorder. These patients were then treated with lithium alone. Lithium responders and nonresponders did not differ according to DSM-III or RDC (Research Diagnostic Criteria) diagnoses or number of "positive" schizophrenic symptoms. However, the lithium responders showed a paucity of negative symptoms and an absence of "familial schizophrenic spectrum disorders." This "spectrum" was defined as including schizophrenia, schizophreniform disorder, schizotypal personality disorder, and schizoaffective disorder. One could argue that inclusion of schizoaffective disorder in this spectrum begs the question of schizoaffective disorder's "true nature"; nevertheless, the results of the study support the clinical impression that lithium response is not robust in psychotic patients with marked emotional withdrawal, blunted affect, and a family history more suggestive of schizophrenia than of affective illness. The Schexnayder and colleagues study does suggest that a paucity of negative symptoms and lack of a family history of schizophrenia-like illness may predict good response to lithium in psychotic patients. Other possible indications for lithium include impulsive aggression, borderline personality disorder, and alcoholism. However, with the exception of impulsive aggression, the data for use in the other conditions mentioned are relatively weak.

Q. Besides their use in bipolar disorder, what other indications exist for valproate, CBZ, and lamotrigine?

A. With respect to "off-label" uses (nonapproved by the FDA), valproate has been found variably effective in the treatment of acute major depression; impulsive/aggressive behavior in dementia patients; panic disorder; posttraumatic stress disorder (PTSD); and borderline personality disorder (Bowden 2004). (Valproate is also FDA-approved for use in migraine prophylaxis.) Recently, adjunctive divalproex was found useful in a 4-week, randomized, double-blind study of 242 patients with schizophrenia being treated with risperidone or olanzapine (Casey et al. 2003). Addition of divalproex led to greater improvement in the PANSS (Positive and Negative Syndrome Scale) scores from day 3 through day 21, but not at day 28. CBZ has also been used for impulsive/aggressive disorders, borderline personality disorder, various anxiety states, alcohol or sedative-hypnotic withdrawal, and trigeminal neuralgia (Keck et al. 1992a; Klein et al. 1986). It appears that the use of valproate in panic disorder is better substantiated than the use of CBZ; conversely, the use of CBZ in the treatment of "behavioral dyscontrol" appears to be better supported than the use of valproate (Keck et al. 1992a). However, most of the data supporting use of valproate and CBZ in treating patients with nonbipolar psychiatric disorders are derived from open studies and case reports.

Lamotrigine is currently being investigated for use in a variety of neuropsychiatric conditions, including PTSD, borderline personality disorder, depersonalization disorder, cocaine abuse, schizoaffective disorder, and refractory schizophrenia (Shelton and Calabrese 2004). However, it is too early to recommend its use for these conditions.

Q. How useful are calcium channel blockers in treating bipolar disorder? What are the potential risks?

A. Initial enthusiasm about calcium channel blockers as antimanic agents (Dubovsky et al. 1986) was reflected as recently as the mid-1990s; for example, one textbook stated that "available data support the use of verapamil for both the short-term and maintenance treatment of bipolar I disorder," adding that verapamil "should be considered a fourth-line drug," following trials with standard mood stabilizers (Kaplan et al. 1994, p. 923). More recent reviews have been more cautious. Gelenberg (1997), in his review of the use of verapamil in treating mania, discussed the work of Walton et al. (1996). In this study, acutely manic patients were randomly assigned to treatment with either verapamil 230–360 mg/day or lithium 500–1,000 mg/day (mean serum level = 0.51 mmol/L). Over the 28 days of the study, patients treated with lithium, but not those treated with verapamil, showed significant improvement on all rating scales. However, Dunn et al. (1998), in their review, found evidence from small studies that dihydropyridine L-type calcium channel blockers may have mood-stabilizing properties. Furthermore, Goodnick (1995) reported that nimodipine (up to 60 mg tid) was effective as the sole agent in the treatment of two patients with rapid-cycling bipolar disorder, with the effectiveness evident at 5- to 12-month follow-up (see also subsection "Potentiating Maneuvers" later in this section). Gelenberg (1997) concluded, on the basis of these and other studies, that verapamil "might still be considered (alone or as an adjunct) for occasional patients unresponsive to or intolerant of more standard treatments. Certainly, lithium divalproex, and carbamazepine, alone or in combination, should be considered first…" (p. 7). The more recent Texas Medication Algorithm Project (Suppes et al. 2002; Shivakumar and Suppes 2004) does not include calcium channel blockers in the algorithm for treatment of mania. The APA revised "Practice Guideline for the Treatment of Patients With Bipolar Disorder" (American Psychiatric Association 2002) notes that randomized controlled trials have provided little support for use of calcium channel blockers in the treatment of mania and mixed episodes.

Verapamil is usually administered at dosages ranging from 120 to 480 mg/day, in divided doses, in the treatment of mania (Arana and Hyman 1991; Dubovsky 1995). Constipation, vertigo, headache, cardiac conduction problems, and hypotension have been reported with verapamil (Arana and Hyman 1991). Drug–drug interactions may occur when calcium channel blockers are coprescribed with lithium or CBZ (see subsection "Drug-Drug Interactions" in the "Overview" section of this chapter).

Q. What is the role of newer anticonvulsants in bipolar disorder, including topiramate, zonisamide, levetiracetam, and tiagabine?

A. The role of these agents remains uncertain (see Wang et al. 2003 for review). Although topiramate (Topamax) 175–200 mg/day has shown promise in open studies of bipolar disorder (Marcotte 1998), results of controlled trials have been disappointing. Topiramate is sometimes used as an "add on" in bipolar patients, owing to its weight-reducing properties. (Weight loss may be 2–6 kg in some patients.) This effect may be useful in some bipolar patients who would not otherwise take their mood stabilizers. However, topiramate is not especially "user friendly," and it may be associated with numerous side effects. Dose-related adverse events in placebo-controlled add-on trials (200 mg/day) included tremor (about 7% placebo-adjusted rate); nervousness (about 6%); impaired concentration/attention (about 6%); confusion (about 4%); and weight decrease (about 2%) (Physicians' Desk Reference 2004). Two recent "Dear Doctor" letters (July 2003 and December 2003) from the manufacturer noted that 1) oligohydrosis (i.e., decreased sweating) and hyperthermia may rarely occur (about 35 cases per million), mainly in children, and usually in a hot environment; and 2) decreased serum bicarbonate and/or metabolic acidosis may occur in as many as two-thirds of patients, with severely reduced bicarbonate in 3%–11% of patients. High dosages (>400 mg/day) of topiramate may be associated with paresthesias, weight gain, constipation, and nausea (all in more than 10% of patients). Concomitant use with other carbonic anhydrase inhibitors, such as acetazolamide, may increase risk of renal stone formation and should be avoided. Given these side effects and the paucity of positive controlled data in bipolar disorder, the routine use of topiramate in bipolar disorder appears unwarranted.

Zonisamide (Zonegran), a sulfonamide derivative with γ-aminobutyric acid (GABA)–ergic and antiglutamatergic effects, showed some antimanic effects in one open study (Kanba et al. 1994); however, it is premature at this time to recommend its use in bipolar disorder. Indeed, recent reports of zonisamide-related visual hallucinations (Akman et al. 2003) and mood disturbances (depression and mania) in patients with epilepsy (Osawa et al. 2004) raise further concerns. Similarly, the data remain scanty regarding the use of levetiracetam in bipolar disorder, although open, "add on" studies in manic patients look promising (Wang et al. 2003). Tiagabine (Gabitril), a GABA receptor reuptake inhibitor, has shown inconsistent effects in mania and may have numerous side effects.

In short: Topiramate, zonisamide, levetiracetam, and tiagabine have an uncertain role in the routine management of bipolar disorder. However, these agents might be considered in extremely refractory cases that are unresponsive to agents with established efficacy.

Q. What about omega-3 fatty acids (OFAs) as adjunctive treatment in bipolar disorder?

A. Adjunctive OFAs showed some efficacy in one double-blind study of bipolar patients, in which depressive symptoms, mood cycling, and relapse rates were decreased (Stoll et al. 1999). However, Altshuler (2004) has recently commented on an unpublished Stanley Network study in which rapid-cycling or depressed bipolar patients were treated with either OFAs or placebo in addition to their existing (suboptimal) medication regimen. Adjunctive OFA treatment was no better than placebo for either rapid cycling or depression. Thus, while promising and apparently very benign, OFAs remain an experimental treatment in bipolar disorder.

Mechanisms of Action

Q. What are the postulated mechanisms of action (MOAs) of lithium in bipolar disorder (manic-depressive illness)?

A. The exact mechanism is not known, though the answer may be intimately related to the mechanisms underlying bipolar disorder itself. Lithium has a plethora of effects on neurotransmitters, intracellular "secondary messenger" systems, and even gene expression (Lenox and Manji 1995). Lithium's antimanic action may be related, in part, to its ability to reduce both pre- and postsynaptic dopamine receptor function, and perhaps dopamine formation as well. Its antidepressant action may be related to enhanced presynaptic serotonergic activity, among other mechanisms. Interest has also focused on lithium's potent inhibition of the intracellular enzyme *inositol monophosphatase* (IMPase), leading to reduced production of free *inositol*—the substrate that "fuels" intracellular and intercellular signaling (Lenox and Manji 1995). Interestingly, this property does *not* seem to be shared with CBZ or valproate, suggesting that IMPase inhibition is not a necessary property for mood stabilization (Vadnal and Parthasarathy 1995). A review by Stoll and Severus

(1996) also suggests that lithium may reduce "excessive signaling" through the phosphatidylinositol (PI) system, at least during mania. Models of bipolar illness, and a hypothesis focusing on abnormalities in the Na, K–ATPase system (sodium, potassium–activated adenosine triphosphatase pump), were reviewed by El-Mallakh and Wyatt (1995). More recently, Gould and colleagues (2004) reviewed the role of the enzyme glycogen synthase kinase–3 (GSK-3) in lithium's MOA. GSK-3 is critically involved in cellular signaling pathways and in regulation of various transcription factors, as well as in "neuroprotection"—for example, inhibition of GSK appears to decrease programmed neuronal death (apoptosis). Lithium is an inhibitor of GSK-3 activity, via competition with magnesium for a binding site on the enzyme (Gould et al. 2004).

Q. What is the MOA of valproate in treating psychiatric illnesses?

A. Valproate's MOA is not known. Valproate inhibits breakdown of GABA and may also enhance neuronal sensitivity to GABA (McElroy and Keck 1995). Valproate may exert its antiseizure effects via these effects on GABA and/or via direct neuronal effects on sodium and potassium exchange (e.g., reducing sodium influx). Valproate appears to have modest antiglutamatergic effects (Wang et al. 2003). It is not known which, if any, of these mechanisms is involved in valproate's effects on mania, depression, and anxiety. In the rat, valproate has *regional* effects on norepinephrine (NE)—that is, it *increases* NE in the hippocampus but *decreases* it in the hypothalamus (Baf et al. 1994). It is tempting to speculate that such regional modulation might allow valproate to have both antimanic and antidepressive effects in humans, although the latter effects are modest. Other studies in the rat suggest that valproate does not have significant effects on serotonin$_{1A}$ (5-HT$_{1A}$), serotonin$_2$ (5-HT$_2$), or β-adrenergic receptor number (Khaitan et al. 1994). Nor does valproate appear to have any significant effect on myoinositol monophosphatase (cf. lithium; see beginning of this subsection) (Vadnal and Parthasarathy 1995). Valproate may decrease dopamine turnover (McElroy and Keck 1995), possibly accounting for its modest antipsychotic effects.

Q. What are the MOAs of CBZ and lamotrigine in treating psychiatric illness?

A. As with valproate, the MOAs of CBZ and lamotrigine are not precisely known. CBZ's antiseizure effects are probably mediated via inactivation of sodium channels, with consequent reduction of sodium influx into the neuron. The antimanic and mood-stabilizing properties of CBZ have not yet been linked to a specific biochemical mechanism (McElroy and Keck 1995), though CBZ has effects on numerous neurotransmitters. In theory, CBZ's acute effects in mania may relate to its enhancement of GABA and its reduction of glutamate activity (Wang et al. 2003). Subchronic treatment with CBZ may decrease NE and dopamine turnover, which might have implications for CBZ's antimanic properties. Unlike lithium, which inhibits IMPase, CBZ seems to *stimulate* this system in bovine brain preparations (Vadnal and Parthasarathy 1995).

Lamotrigine demonstrates antiglutamatergic effects via presynaptic sodium channel blockade and, to some extent, calcium channel blockade (Shelton and Calabrese 2004). These effects apparently lead to *decreased glutamate release*. Most likely, it has other MOAs. In contrast to some anticonvulsants (e.g., tiagabine), lamotrigine has an "activating" profile, perhaps associated with its antidepressant effects in bipolar disorder (Wang et al. 2003). Thus, lamotrigine may "stabilize from below" (Ketter and Calabrese 2002). Lamotrigine inhibits glutamate release secondary to ischemia and other conditions of abnormal neuronal activation, thus acting as a neuroprotective agent (Shelton and Calabrese 2004).

Q. Doesn't the effect of anticonvulsants on "kindling" have something to do with their mood-stabilizing effects?

A. The term *kindling* originally referred to a process whereby, in effect, it becomes progressively easier to "set off" neuronal firing. In technical terms, repeated *subthreshold* stimuli progressively increase the responsivity of some brain regions until, eventually, a seizure occurs. Over time, application of even a *single* subthreshold stimulus can evoke a seizure (Ayd 1995). Kindling occurs most readily in limbic regions and may be pharmacologically induced by substances like metrazol or cocaine. This process may explain why alcohol withdrawal symptoms recur more readily with repeated episodes of drinking (Ayd

1995). Kindling is associated with induction of *transcription factors* under the regulation of *immediate early genes,* such as c-fos. This induction process may in turn regulate neurotransmitter metabolism and neuronal receptor production. Post (1993) adduced evidence showing that cycle acceleration in bipolar patients may be related to so-called kindling phenomena—namely, that "with sufficient numbers of episodes, the illness may, as in the kindling model, become progressively more 'well grooved' or autonomous" (p. 88). The anticonvulsants CBZ and valproate appear to have antikindling properties in animal models of amygdala kindling and may reduce affective cycling via a similar mechanism. The kindling model predicts tolerance (declining clinical effect at the same dose) to anticonvulsants and some degree of cross-tolerance between CBZ and valproate, but it is not clear that this occurs in clinical practice. If such tolerance did develop in bipolar patients, theory would predict that *brief interruption* of anticonvulsant treatment might restore responsivity in patients with loss of efficacy (Post 1993). To the author's knowledge, this hypothesis has not been tested in controlled clinical studies.

Q. Does response to one mood stabilizer predict response to another?

A. The short answer seems to be no, as might be expected from the differing mechanisms of action of these agents. Although previous response to lithium strongly predicts lithium response for the index episode of mania, response to divalproex is *not* related to previous lithium response (i.e., patients with poor lithium response often do quite well with valproate [Bowden et al. 1994]). The relationship between lithium and CBZ response is less clear, but some lithium nonresponders do respond to CBZ. Post (1993) cited "many individual cases" of patients who respond to one anticonvulsant but not another, as well as cases in which patients do not respond to either agent alone but do respond well to a combination of CBZ and valproate (Keck et al. 1992b). This combination, however, may produce complex pharmacokinetic interactions (see subsection "Drug–Drug Interactions" later in this "Questions and Answers" section).

Pharmacokinetics

Q. How does the "autometabolism" of CBZ affect dosing strategy? Does autometabolism also apply to oxcarbazepine?

A. Because CBZ induces its own metabolism when given chronically, its $t_{1/2}\beta$ ranges from 15–50 hours initially but 8–20 hours chronically. In practical terms, this means that unless the dosage is adjusted to "keep up" with dropping plasma levels, the patient may eventually fail to respond to CBZ. CBZ is usually started at a dosage of 200–600 mg/day in divided doses, with increases of about 100–200 mg every 3–5 days as tolerated. This rate may need to be slowed in patients who develop significant side effects (e.g., sedation, dizziness). A typical daily dose after 2 weeks would be about 1,000 mg, but there is wide variability among patients. Clinical response and adverse effects are more important in dosing than the plasma level, though generally one aims for a level of about 5–12 μg/mL. (Keep in mind that toxicity due to the 10,11-epoxide metabolite will not be evident from routine plasma levels of CBZ.) Plasma levels should be monitored every 5–7 days for the first 3 weeks or so. By this time, autometabolism may be starting (Gerner and Stanton 1992), although this is sometimes not evident until weeks 4–8 of treatment (Bowden 1995b). Depending on the individual patient, upward adjustment of CBZ dosage will soon become necessary, sometimes requiring *twice the dose* arrived at during the first 2–3 weeks of treatment (Potter and Ketter 1993). As the $t_{1/2}$ of CBZ drops, the time to steady state after each dosage change will also drop, since steady state is reached after four to five half-lives. Plasma levels should generally be obtained at each new "steady state" level. If we assume a $t_{1/2}$ (after 6 weeks) of about 15 hours, each new steady state would be reached after about 68 hours, or roughly 3 days (four to five half-lives). *Thus, in theory, if the dosage is still being increased 6 weeks into treatment (in order to "keep up" with autometabolism), levels should be checked roughly every 3 days.* In clinical practice, weekly levels are probably adequate for most patients during this "transitional" phase. Once two or three stable levels have been obtained—presumably reflecting maximum autometabolism—plasma levels are usually obtained once every 1–3 months, depending on several variables. If the patient requires a dosage change or is prescribed a medication that may affect CBZ metabolism (see subsection "Drug–Drug Interactions" later in this "Questions and Answers" section), more frequent checks may be necessary. As always, remember that it is the patient, not laboratory values, that is being treated. Autometabolism is not seen with oxcarbazepine (Wang et al. 2003)—a feature that simplifies dosing considerably.

Q. Does the daily dosing schedule of lithium affect the plasma level and/or therapeutic efficacy (e.g., bid vs. qd)?

A. The basic answer is no. The steady-state concentration ("plasma level") of a drug with first-order kinetics (cf. nonlinear pharmacokinetics; see Chapter 1, "Introduction to Pharmacodynamics and Pharmacokinetics") is chiefly determined by the *total* dose given during a 24-hour period and the rate of the drug's clearance (typically via hepatic and renal elimination). So long as the *total* dose and rate of clearance remain constant during a given time period of administration, the concentration at steady state (C_{SS}) will not be affected by the daily dosing schedule. This may be seen if we plug arbitrary values into the following equation (Magliozzi and Tupin 1988):

$$C_{ss} = \frac{D}{t \times CL}$$

Where *D* is the fixed dose, *t* is the dosing interval per day (e.g., every 4 hours, 8 hours, 24 hours), and *CL* is the systemic clearance. Let's compare the values for C_{SS} if the total daily dose of lithium (1,200 mg) is given according to two different schedules: as a single daily dose versus four doses of 300 mg each (every 6 hours). Let's assume an arbitrary clearance of 20. The equations now look like this:

$$(1) \quad C_{ss} = \frac{1200}{24 \times 20}$$

$$(2) \quad C_{ss} = \frac{300}{6 \times 20}$$

The C_{SS} in *both* cases is 2.5. However, although the C_{SS} does not differ in these two scenarios, there will be a difference in the *peak* plasma levels achieved during a 24-hour period, as well as a difference in the "delta" (fluctuation) between *peaks and troughs.* In effect, a more frequent dosing schedule results in a lower peak plasma level and a "smoother" plasma level curve (i.e., less interdose fluctuation). This can often lead to fewer side effects for many patients, including some taking lithium. On the other hand, there may be advantages to a single daily dose of lithium for some patients (see subsection "Main Side Effects" later in this "Questions and Answers" section). The equation above assumes, of course, that *clearance is constant.* In actuality, the renal clearance of lithium is *slightly less during sleep,* and this leads to somewhat higher than predicted plasma levels if the same total dose is given "all at night" instead of, say, as three daily doses.

Q. How are the various preparations of valproate absorbed and eliminated? What are "therapeutic" levels with divalproex in treating patients with bipolar disorder?

A. Valproate is available in five oral preparations: valproic acid (Depakene and others); sodium valproate (Depakene syrup); divalproex sodium (Depakote, an enteric-coated, delayed-release tablet); divalproex sodium extended-release (Depakote ER); and divalproex sodium sprinkle capsules (Depakote Sprinkle capsules) that can be pulled apart and sprinkled on food (McElroy and Keck 1995; Physicians' Desk Reference 2004). In the management of psychiatric disorders, it is primarily formulations of *divalproex sodium* that are utilized. Regular divalproex sodium tablets reach peak serum concentrations within 3–8 hours. The $t_{1/2}\beta$ of divalproex is about 11 hours, and steady state is reached within about 2 days. With Depakote ER, peak serum valproate concentrations are reached within 4–17 hours. Experience in patients with epilepsy suggests that the extended-release formulation should be administered once daily, with the dose about *15% higher* than the total daily dose of regular Depakote (Physicians' Desk Reference 2004); a similar approach has been employed in treating bipolar disorder (Centorrino et al. 2003). A valproate *loading-dose strategy* has also been found to be rapidly effective, with divalproex given in divided doses of 20–30 mg/kg per day (Keck et al. 1993; Post et al. 2003). Therapeutic levels of divalproex in bipolar disorder are generally in the range of 50 to 125 μg/mL and are reached more rapidly with a loading-dose strategy (Post et al. 2003). Severely manic patients may sometimes require even higher divalproex blood levels, as tolerated (R. Dunn, M.D., personal communication, June 20, 2004). The sprinkle formulation of valproate has an *earlier onset* of absorption but a *slower rate* of absorption than the tablets and produces a somewhat *lower peak plasma level* (McElroy and Keck 1995; Wilder 1992). (It is probably these characteristics that result in fewer gastrointestinal (GI) side effects with the sprinkles.)

Valproate metabolism is quite complex (Wilder 1992), mediated via two hepatic pathways (one mitochondrial, one via the microsomal P450 route), as well as via glucuronidation (Cozza et al. 2003). Numerous metabolites are produced, at least one of which appears to be hepatotoxic (see next subsection, "Main Side Effects" in this "Questions and Answers" section). Valproate's $t_{1/2}\beta$ is roughly 5–20 hours. Some data indicate a mild "autoinduction" of valproate beta-oxidative metabolism, but not glucuronidation, with chronic use (McLaughlin et al. 2000); however, it is not clear that this feature leads to significant decreases in valproate blood levels for most patients. As the plasma concentration of valproate increases, clearance also increases, owing to saturation of protein binding sites and the resultant increased availability of unbound valproate. Transient side effects may be more frequent at higher serum concentrations, and the laboratory levels may be less useful for purposes of monitoring. Their lack of usefulness in monitoring is probably due to rapid shifts in concentrations of unbound valproate as plasma proteins become saturated (McElroy and Keck 1995).

Main Side Effects

Q. What are the advantages and disadvantages of giving lithium as a single daily or "at bedtime" dose?

A. There are some data showing that patients who take lithium as a single daily dose have less *glomerular* pathology than those who receive multiple doses (Hetmar et al. 1987; Plenge et al. 1982); however, these studies did not control for total dosage, since patients receiving the multiple-dose regimen received a higher total daily dose. In a study in which total lithium dosage was kept the same in both the once-daily and multiple-dose groups, 24-hour urine volume fell significantly after 12 days of single-dose treatment (Perry et al. 1981). Furthermore, patients who take lithium in a single dose at bedtime are *less likely to develop polyuria* than are patients who take lithium in multiple daily doses (Bowen et al. 1991). Severe polyuria, of course, can lead to dehydration and consequent lithium toxicity. Since plasma levels of lithium may increase by about 20% on a "single-dose hs" regimen (owing, in part, to decreased nocturnal clearance), total daily dose may need to be decreased when converting a patient from a multiple-dose to a single-dose hs regimen. Some patients who are given their entire lithium dose as bedtime may awaken with GI side effects (diarrhea, nausea), probably owing to higher (though briefer) peak plasma levels. Patients with lithium -induced tremor may sometimes benefit from having all or most of their total dose given at bedtime.

Q. What side effects of lithium are most likely to produce noncompliance?

A. When patients are asked this question, the most frequent answer involves *cognitive side effects,* such as mental confusion, poor concentration, memory problems, and mental slowness (F.K. Goodwin and Jamison 1990; Lenox and Manji 1995). Lithium may exert some of these cognitive effects via its action on protein kinase C (PKC), with consequent effects on neurotransmission (Lenox and Manji 1995). However, not all studies of neuropsychiatric function have demonstrated cognitive impairment from lithium, and in some patients, gradual tolerance to cognitive side effects may develop. (Dosage reduction or multiple dosing may also help.) Many patients also complain of significant weight gain from lithium and may refuse to take it for that reason.

Q. What is the acute management of lithium toxicity?

A. Lithium toxicity may exist even within the so-called therapeutic range of roughly 0.5–1.4 mEq/L. Symptoms may include nausea, tremor, muscle fasciculations, twitching, rigidity, hyperreflexia, fever, confusion, and coma. For patients with mild to moderate signs of toxicity, normal renal function, and levels less than 2.0 mEq/L, a period of observation and monitoring of vital signs, coupled with substantial dosage reduction, may be all that is necessary (Janicak et al. 1993)—for example, reducing the lithium dose by 75% for 24 hours, resuming at one-half the usual dose for an additional 24 hours, and then resuming the usual dose. A repeat lithium serum level determination is appropriate after 3–4 days. (This period—just less than four times the $t_{1/2}$ of lithium, and hence slightly sooner than the expected new steady-state lithium level—is chosen in order to err on the side of caution.) Since lithium may cause bradyarrhythmias, an electrocardiogram (ECG) should be considered for patients with pulse rates below 55. For more severe toxicity (levels above

2.5 mEq/L), *forced saline diuresis* is indicated. *Hemodialysis* may be necessary in some cases; however, recent concerns have been raised regarding *too rapid a correction* of "hyperlithemia" (Schou 1996; Swartz and Jones 1996). Since rapid diminution of intraneuronal lithium leads to replacement by sodium, the brain may be subject to massive electrolyte shifts when lithium toxicity is corrected too rapidly, with these shifts possibly leading to increased risk of seizures and delirium (Swartz and Jones 1996).

Q. Can lithium withdrawal lead to mania in some patients with unipolar depression?

A. On the basis of two cases, Hoaken and Hoaken (1996) suggested that *discontinuation of lithium augmentation* may induce hypomanic or manic symptoms in apparently *unipolar* depressed patients. Both patients had a history of recurrent depression without known hypomanic/manic episodes; both had lithium added to their ongoing TCA treatment. Their lithium was stopped over periods of 5–14 days. The authors speculated that "some patients with mood disorder have only depressive episodes until lithium, used as monotherapy…or as an antidepressant augmentating agent, is withdrawn, causing a temporary destabilization and the eruption of hypomania or mania" (p. 48). Such an effect would be consistent with the so-called permissive hypothesis of serotonergic function, which holds that both mania and depression are characterized by low central serotonergic function (Mendels and Frazer 1975). In this view, lithium acts to stabilize serotonergic systems and—when withdrawn—can cause an excursion into either depression or mania. More recent theories of lithium action, however, might suggest different mechanisms. For example, if lithium acts (in mania) to inhibit excessive signaling through the PI system (Stoll and Severus 1996), it is theoretically possible that sudden discontinuation of lithium might lead to some form of "rebound" hyperactivity in the PI system—though this must remain speculation at this time. When lithium augmentation is discontinued in patients with recurrent unipolar depression, it may be prudent to do so very gradually, over a period of 1–2 months.

Q. What is the best approach to new-onset rash with lamotrigine use?

A. Most rashes seen with lamotrigine prove to be benign, and controlled outcome data find a rate of serious lamotrigine-related rash comparable to that of placebo (Shelton and Calabrese 2004). Nevertheless, rash is the side effect that most often complicates treatment, and it is a source of anxiety for both patients and clinicians. Furthermore, it is incumbent upon physicians to recognize and prevent the (very rare) occurrence of severe or life-threatening rash, such as that of Stevens-Johnson syndrome. The clinician should be able to recognize the hallmarks of serious and life-threatening rashes, such as when the patient shows one or more of the following:

- Confluent areas of erythema
- Facial edema
- Skin pain
- Blisters or epidermal detachment
- Positive Nikolsky's sign (easy separation of outer layer of epidermis from basal layer, with thumb pressure)
- Mucous membrane erosions
- Fever
- Enlarged lymph nodes
- Arthralgias or arthritis
- Shortness of breath, wheezing, laryngeal edema
- Elevated eosinophil count (>1,000)
- Abnormal liver function tests (LFTs)

In contrast, most benign rashes lack these features, and are typically maculopapular in appearance. Nevertheless, some rashes that appear "benign" may evolve into more serious ones. Thus, patients taking lamotrigine should be instructed to report *any* new rash immediately to the psychiatrist or other physician and to *hold the next dose of lamotrigine.* The patient should not resume taking lamotrigine until he or she has been assessed by an appropriate medical professional—ideally, a dermatologist, though this is not always feasible. Patients who develop a serious lamotrigine-related rash should generally not be "rechallenged" with this agent (Shelton and Calabrese 2004).

Q. What is the treatment approach to CBZ- or oxcarbazepine-induced hyponatremia?

A. CBZ has been implicated in causing a state of hyponatremia and water intoxication that resembles the syndrome of inappropriate antidiuretic hormone (SIADH) (Lahr 1985). Oxcarbazepine is also associated with hyponatremia in about 2.5%–20% of patients. Usually, this hyponatremia is not clinically significant, but serum sodium may drop below 125 mmol/L in about 2% of cases (Ketter et al. 2004b; Reinstein et al. 2002). Since hyponatremia of <125 mEq/L may lead to anorexia, vomiting, confusion, and coma, recognition and treatment of this condition is important, particularly in the elderly. Successful treatment of CBZ-induced hyponatremia has been reported with use of either of two tetracyclic antibiotics, demeclocycline or doxycycline (Boutros et al. 1995). Doxycycline (100 mg bid) has the advantages of not being dependent on renal excretion and of having a longer $t_{1/2}$ than demeclocycline. Similar strategies with oxcarbazepine have not yet been reported; hence, periodic monitoring (baseline and follow-up serum sodium) is the main recommendation at this time. Rapid overcorrection of hyponatremia may lead to *central pontine myelinolysis.*

Q. Are there advantages to the new extended-release form of CBZ (Equetro), compared with the regular formulation of CBZ and other anticonvulsant mood stabilizers?

A. Extended-release CBZ (ERC) recently received FDA-approval for use in acute manic and mixed episodes of bipolar disorder (Table 5-1). In one open-label evaluation of ERC (Ketter et al. 2004a), the drug was generally well-tolerated, with side effects typical of carbamazepine (e.g., headache, dizziness, and rash). Significant weight gain was not noted (as is also the case with the standard formulation of this drug), certainly an advantage vis-à-vis several other mood stabilizers. One study of patients with partial onset–seizures who converted from immediate- to extended-release carbamazepine (A.D. Miller et al. 2004) found reduced neuropsychiatric side effects and improved tolerability with ERC; however, such comparative studies in bipolar patients are lacking. Further controlled study will be needed to determine the relative advantages of ERC versus other mood stabilizers, in the management of bipolar patients.

Q. What is the risk of hepatotoxicity with valproate and CBZ, and how is hepatotoxicity managed?

A. Divalproex does have a black box warning regarding the risk of serious hepatic dysfunction (Physicians' Desk Reference 2004). Although neither valproate nor CBZ is highly hepatotoxic, both may cause alterations in LFTs that may (often unnecessarily) alarm clinicians. Baseline LFTs are indicated, with periodic follow-ups, depending on subsequent LFT values *and the patient's clinical status.* Valproate (divalproex) has been associated with fatal hepatotoxicity in about 1 in 49,000 cases, almost entirely in patients under the age of 2 years who were receiving multiple anticonvulsants (Janicak 1995) or who had medical/neurological abnormalities besides epilepsy (Bowden 2004). Fatal hepatotoxicity is idiosyncratic and *not* related to dose. In contrast, transient alterations in levels of liver enzymes (particularly transaminases) do occur in a dose-related fashion with valproate but are not generally suggestive of impending hepatic toxicity. Unless the levels of transaminases reach three times normal values; *or* alkaline phosphatase or bilirubin values have risen from baseline (which may suggest an obstructive process); *or*—perhaps most important—the patient shows *clinical evidence of hepatotoxicity* (malaise, fever, anorexia, vomiting, easy bruising, jaundice), there is no need to discontinue the valproate. Dosage reduction and the passage of time may suffice. Janicak (1995) recommends baseline LFTs, a single follow-up during the first few weeks of valproate treatment, then a repeat of LFTs every 6–12 months, under ordinary circumstances. However, the patient's clinical status appears to be a better predictor of incipient hepatic dysfunction than any single laboratory finding (Konig et al. 1998). With CBZ, elevation of LFTs occurs in 5%–15% of patients (McElroy and Keck 1995) and is usually a benign dose-related finding. Dosage reduction, or brief interruption of CBZ treatment followed by rechallenge at a lower dose, often suffices.

Q. What is the management of valproate-induced hair loss or thinning?

A. Hair loss from valproate is usually transient; new hair tends to be more curly than it was prior to medication use. Interruption of valproate treatment is rarely necessary, and multivitamins containing selenium (25 μg/day) and zinc (50 mg/day) are said to be useful in preventing or stabilizing this hair loss

(Potter and Ketter 1993). However, there appears to be virtually no controlled evidence supporting this often-repeated advice.

Drug–Drug Interactions

Q. How does one safely use a combination of valproate and CBZ in patients with refractory bipolar disorder?

A. As noted earlier, addition of valproate to CBZ may lead to an increased ratio of CBZ epoxide to CBZ via inhibition of epoxide hydroxylase, which, in theory, could lead to neurotoxicity in some patients. Also, in theory, valproate may cause displacement of CBZ from plasma binding proteins, thereby producing a transient increase in CBZ effects. Conversely, CBZ *reduces* valproate levels but *increases* levels of valproate's 2-propyl-4-pentanoic acid metabolite, which is hepatotoxic and teratogenic. Given these concerns, it is reassuring that clinical experience is generally positive regarding CBZ–valproate combination therapy in bipolar patients (Tohen et al. 1994). In a study by Tohen and colleagues (1994), all 12 bipolar patients given this combination showed moderate to marked response; only 2 patients had minor side effects (mild drowsiness). (In contrast, none of the 4 schizoaffective patients responded to this combination. Patients with "organic" brain syndromes fared less well on the CBZ–valproate combination, showing adverse effects such as slurred speech and oversedation.) In this study—which was based on a review of pharmacy records, not prospective monitoring—patients received an average dosage of 1,500 mg/day of valproate and 1,200 mg/day of CBZ. In the 7 cases in which CBZ was added to valproate, the valproate level declined (as predicted). However, in the cases in which valproate was added to CBZ, there was no change in CBZ blood levels. It should be noted that *metabolite levels* were not reported (and are rarely obtained in clinical practice). While Tohen et al. did conclude that the CBZ–valproate combination is "usually well tolerated," they advised reduction in CBZ dosage to avoid potential toxicity. Furthermore, if CBZ and valproate are used together, monitor levels of both closely; obtain levels of the CBZ epoxide if possible, and closely monitor the patient for signs of neurotoxicity. LFTs should be checked more frequently than with either agent alone. This combination does not seem as useful or safe in patients with schizoaffective disorder and in brain-damaged patients. Keep in mind that in some patients maintained on this combination, discontinuation of CBZ may lead to increased valproate levels (Jann et al. 1988). Finally, consider using oxcarbazepine instead of CBZ, since oxcarbazepine does not generate the epoxide metabolite.

Q. How does valproate interact with anticonvulsants other than CBZ?

A. Valproate may reduce elimination and/or raise plasma levels of *ethosuximide, lamotrigine,* and *phenobarbital,* with this effect sometimes leading to significant toxicity (Ciraulo and Slattery 1995). Interactions between valproate and *phenytoin* are quite variable and usually not of clinical significance. *Felbamate* may inhibit metabolism of valproate, an effect that can possibly lead to toxicity (Ciraulo and Slattery 1995). There is little published information on the interaction between valproate and oxcarbazepine. The interaction between valproate and lamotrigine may increase the risk of serious rash.

Q. Can CBZ be used safely with monoamine oxidase inhibitors (MAOIs) in treating patients with refractory unipolar or bipolar depression?

A. The structural similarities between CBZ and TCAs have led some clinicians to warn against the CBZ–MAOI combination. Theoretical concerns include the development of hypertensive and hyperpyrexic states, postural hypotension, muscle twitching, convulsions, delirium, and coma (Ketter et al. 1995b). Moreover, some data suggest that phenelzine (Nardil) and tranylcypromine (Parnate) could inhibit hepatic metabolism of CBZ. Nevertheless, in a small (N=10) double-blind study in which MAOIs were added to CBZ, no major adverse reactions occurred (Ketter et al. 1995b). Furthermore, 4 of the 10 patients (7 bipolar, 3 unipolar depressed inpatients) improved substantially on the CBZ–MAOI combination. These 4 patients' illness had previously been refractory to either agent alone. Responder polarity was not discussed, but responders and nonresponders did not differ significantly in polarity of illness. CBZ pharmacokinetics did not seem to be altered in this study.

Q. What precautions are indicated when a patient is taking concomitant lithium and nonsteroidal anti-inflammatory drugs (NSAIDs)?

A. Several NSAIDs can increase serum lithium levels; they do so apparently by decreasing renal blood flow. Thus, *ibuprofen, indomethacin, diclofenac,* and *ketorolac* can significantly increase serum lithium levels, with this effect potentially leading to toxicity (Ayd 1995; Sarid-Segal et al. 1995). It appears that *sulindac, aspirin,* and *acetaminophen* do *not* significantly raise serum lithium levels (Ayd 1995; Ragheb 1990) and may be the analgesics of choice for patients taking lithium. Recently, several COX-2 (cyclooxygenase-2) inhibitors (rofecoxib [now off U.S. market] and *celecoxib*) have been found to increase serum lithium levels, perhaps by increasing tubular reabsorption of lithium (Phelan et al. 2003).

Q. What is the basis for, and management of, *neurotoxicity* associated with combined lithium and neuroleptic use? What about increased risk of extrapyramidal side effects (EPS)?

A. The degree to which lithium and antipsychotics interact to cause neurotoxicity is still debated. The original report of W.J. Cohen and Cohen (1974) implicated the combination of lithium and haloperidol in four cases of irreversible neurotoxicity; however, subsequent reviews have seriously impugned both the basis and the likelihood of this putative interaction (see Goff and Baldessarini 1995 for discussion). Still, given lithium's ability to *reduce both pre- and postsynaptic dopaminergic function* (Lenox and Manji 1995), a pharmacodynamic interaction with antipsychotics is plausible. This interaction may manifest as frank neurotoxicity (e.g., confusion, disorientation, ataxia) or as increased EPS (Ayd 1995; Ghadirian et al. 1996) in a susceptible subgroup of patients. However, some cases of apparent lithium/neuroleptic neurotoxicity may actually be cases of neuroleptic malignant syndrome (NMS); interestingly, lithium itself may be a precipitant of NMS (Susman and Addonizio 1987). It is not clear that any particular neuroleptic is especially likely to interact adversely with lithium, though most cases have involved haloperidol—probably because haloperidol is so frequently used. The best management strategy entails 1) using low initial and maintenance doses of the neuroleptic when it is combined with lithium; 2) carefully monitoring mental status and vital signs after one agent is added to the other; 3) avoiding *simultaneous* prescription of lithium and neuroleptic (i.e., starting both drugs at precisely the same time, thus obfuscating which agent is causing adverse effects), and 4) decreasing the dose of neuroleptic if signs of neurotoxicity appear in this context (F. Miller and Menninger 1987). The management of NMS is discussed in Chapter 3 ("Antipsychotics").

Q. Can angiotensin-converting enzyme (ACE) inhibitors (for hypertension) be used safely with lithium?

A. ACE inhibitors such as *captopril, enalapril,* and *lisinopril* are often used in the treatment of hypertension and congestive heart failure. Many elderly bipolar patients may be prescribed lithium and an ACE inhibitor. A study by DasGupta and colleagues (1992) found that, overall, enalapril did not significantly affect steady-state lithium levels in 9 healthy volunteers, who were tested over 10 days. In contrast, a larger study (Finley et al. 1996) of 20 hypertensive patients previously stabilized with lithium therapy showed that after initiation of an ACE inhibitor, the steady-state lithium concentration increased by about 36%. Four patients presented with signs suggesting lithium toxicity (i.e., increased tremor, ataxia, confusion). The increased lithium levels (and decreased lithium clearance) were correlated with increasing age. The authors concluded that elderly patients should generally not be treated with lithium plus an ACE inhibitor. An alternative approach in such cases would be to use a reduced dose of lithium, with frequent monitoring of clinical state and serum lithium levels.

Q. Are there any significant interactions between lithium and valproate?

A. There are no clinically significant *pharmacokinetic* interactions when these two agents are used together, though divalproex (Depakote) levels may be slightly increased by the lithium carbonate preparation. This increase may be due to neutralization of gastric acid by the carbonate form of lithium (Granneman et al. 1996). GI side effects do not appear to be significantly increased by this combination versus lithium alone.

Q. What drug–drug interactions may be seen with topiramate?

A. Topiramate may increase phenytoin (Dilantin) levels, whereas phenytoin may substantially decrease topiramate levels. Topiramate has little effect on CBZ levels, but CBZ (and phenytoin) may substantially decrease topiramate levels (Cozza et al. 2003). Topiramate may also decrease estrogen concentration, and this may reduce efficacy of oral contraceptives (Wang et al. 2003). Valproate and topiramate may slightly decrease each other's levels. It appears that there are no significant pharmacokinetic interactions between topiramate and lamotrigine (Doose et al. 2003), though pharmacodynamic interactions cannot be ruled out. Concomitant use of topiramate with other carbonic anhydrase inhibitors, such as acetazolamide, may increase risk of renal stone formation.

Potentiating Maneuvers

Q. If a nonpsychotic bipolar patient is unresponsive to lithium alone, what might be the best "first move" in terms of potentiation?

A. That depends on the "target symptoms" that are not responding (see Tables 5–3 through 5–5). If a patient shows primarily *depressive* symptoms, it may be worthwhile *raising the lithium level* prior to adding any augmenting agent (e.g., from 0.8 to 1.2 mEq/L) (Srisurapanont et al. 1995). Alternatively, lamotrigine could be added (American Psychiatric Association 2002). The APA guideline on treatment of bipolar disorder also notes that bupropion or paroxetine may be used adjunctively in this situation, though several experts in treating bipolar disorder prefer to avoid the use of antidepressants until other options (e.g., addition of an atypical antipsychotic) have been tried (F. K. Goodwin and Ghaemi 2001). The new combination agent Symbyax (olanzapine/fluoxetine) might be useful when added to lithium; however, this strategy has not been tested in controlled studies. If a patient shows primarily *manic* symptoms refractory to lithium, adding one of the anticonvulsant mood stabilizers (divalproex, oxcarbazepine) is often useful, with the likely exception of lamotrigine. Divalproex is preferable if there is a "mixed" presentation (mania with irritable or depressive features). Short-term adjunctive treatment with a benzodiazepine may also be helpful for refractory mania. Adding olanzapine, risperidone, or another atypical antipsychotic would also be reasonable. For patients with rapid-cycling bipolar disorder, the "antimanic" strategies just described may be helpful. Adding thyroxine (T_4) to lithium may reduce rapid cycling (Bauer and Whybrow 1991), as may the calcium channel blocker nimodipine (Goodnick 1995; Pazzaglia et al. 1993; see below). However, neither of these strategies (i.e., T_4, nimodipine) has been well validated in large, double-blind, randomized controlled trials.

Q. What are the guidelines for use of thyroxine in rapid-cycling bipolar patients?

A. The benefits of T_4 (usually as an adjunctive agent) have not been documented in large-scale, controlled studies of rapid-cyclers. Nevertheless, T_4 was deemed a useful treatment in such patients by one expert consensus panel for bipolar disorder (Kahn et al. 1996). T_4 is used in doses ranging from 0.1 to 0.3 mg/day, usually as an adjunct to ongoing treatment with lithium or with lithium plus another mood stabilizer (Bauer and Whybrow 1991). Behavioral response often occurs before complete suppression of thyroid-stimulating hormone (TSH) and appears to be a function of increased T_4 levels rather than triiodothyronine (T_3) levels (Bauer and Whybrow 1991). Although rapid cycling is associated with clinical or subclinical hypothyroidism, euthyroid rapid-cyclers may also respond to this T_4 augmentation strategy (Bauer and Whybrow 1991).

Q. How is T_4 tolerated in rapid-cycling bipolar patients?

A. On the basis of reports on a fairly small number of patients, T_4 is usually tolerated well (Bauer and Whybrow 1991), though, in the author's experience, some patients will complain of excessive perspiration, mild excitation, or mild, transient tachycardia. (These side effects are usually responsive to dosage reduction.) Patients with atrial or "fast" cardiac arrhythmias are not good candidates for T_4 augmentation. There have been concerns about bone demineralization in pre- and postmenopausal women receiving long-term T_4 therapy, but the evidence for such an effect is equivocal (Fujiyama et al. 1995; Marcocci et al. 1994). Nevertheless, with T_4 augmentation, the clinician should avoid TSH levels < 0.35 mIU, since long-term suppression of TSH may be associated with osteoporosis (Kahn et al. 1996).

Q. What is the role of calcium channel blockers (CCBs) as adjunctive agents in treating bipolar disorder?

A. Dubovsky (1995) noted that "clinical experience suggests that combining a CCB with another antimanic drug may be helpful for some treatment-refractory patients, but this approach...has not been studied formally" (p. 385). Verapamil has been used as an adjunct to lithium in a few patients unresponsive to lithium alone (Brotman et al. 1986), but large, controlled studies are lacking. Lenzi and colleagues (1995) used verapamil in combination with chlorpromazine in treating 15 female inpatients with acute mania and found that the combination produced global improvement in manic symptoms in most of the patients (see Gelenberg 1997). Calcium channel blockers such as verapamil appear to be most useful for manic patients who are responsive to lithium but cannot tolerate it; indeed, acutely manic patients who do *not* respond to lithium seem less responsive to verapamil (Dubovsky 1995). Calcium channel blocker/lithium interactions include neurotoxicity, parkinsonism, and cardiac slowing (Dubovsky 1995). The usefulness of calcium channel blockers in depression has not been clearly established, and these agents have the potential to exacerbate depression. However, Goodnick (1995) found nimodipine (up to 60 mg tid) effective as the sole agent in the treatment of two patients with rapid-cycling bipolar disorder, even after 5–12 month follow-up. Pazzaglia and colleagues (1993) found nimodipine superior to placebo in a crossover study of rapid-cycling bipolar patients. Larger-scale and better-controlled studies are needed before the role of calcium channel blockers in bipolar disorder is securely established. (See subsection "Indications" in this "Questions and Answers" section for further discussion.)

Q. What is the role of pramipexole in treating bipolar depression?

A. Pramipexole, a dopamine D_2/D_3 receptor agonist, has shown preliminary evidence of benefit as an adjunctive treatment in refractory bipolar depression. In a double-blind, placebo-controlled study of bipolar I and II patients (N=22) conducted by Goldberg et al. 2004, the addition of pramipexole (mean maximum dosage = 1.7 mg/day) to existing mood stabilizers proved safe and effective, compared with placebo. Eight of 12 patients taking pramipexole improved, versus 2 of 10 patients taking placebo. However, one patient developed mania and psychosis while taking pramipexole, despite receiving concomitant divalproex, and some patients experienced nausea and sedation. Overall, this pilot study suggests that larger, randomized controlled trials are indicated, but that the risk of "switching" or induction of mania cannot be ruled out with pramipexole.

Use in Special Populations

Q. What are the teratogenic risks of various mood stabilizers during pregnancy?

A. Early, retrospective data gathered by the International Register of Lithium Babies suggested a rate of Ebstein's anomaly approximately 500 times higher in infants exposed to lithium during the first trimester than in the general population. But these data were gathered from *physicians' reports,* a method that often leads to overestimation of adverse outcomes. As L. S. Cohen (1992) noted, more recent studies point to a *28-fold increase* in the risk of Ebstein's anomaly due to first-trimester lithium exposure—roughly 1 in 700 lithium-exposed infants versus 1 in 20,000 in the general population. In a review of the available data, Altshuler and colleagues (1995) concluded that Ebstein's anomaly following first-trimester exposure to lithium is roughly 10–20 times the rate in the general population. Thus, while the risk is not insignificant, it is considerably less than once feared. Furthermore, *the risk of untreated bipolar illness must also be considered;* for example, abrupt discontinuation of lithium will typically lead to relapse of mania or major depression and occasionally to lithium "resistance" upon restarting treatment. Recent studies have linked first-trimester maternal exposure to CBZ with higher-than-expected rates of fetal craniofacial defects, fingernail hypoplasia, developmental delay, and spina bifida. There is also a 1% rate of spina bifida in infants exposed to the anticonvulsant mood stabilizer valproate (divalproex; Depakote); minor dysmorphic syndromes have also been reported with this agent (McElroy and Keck 1995). The risk with these agents is clearly much higher than the risk of Ebstein's anomaly induced by lithium, and most clinicians now regard lithium as safer than anticonvulsants in bipolar patients in the first trimester of pregnancy (Chaudron and Pies 2003). Folic acid and multivitamins with trace metals (e.g., selenium) may decrease risk in pregnant patients who must take CBZ or valproate (McElroy and Keck 1995). Oxcarbazepine has not been rigorously studied in pregnancy, but preliminary data suggest it is relatively free of major teratogenic effects; however, folic acid supplementation is still recommended in women of childbearing age who are taking oxcarbazepine (Newport et al. 2004).

Q. How is lithium use adjusted for use in the pregnant patient?

A. If lithium is prescribed during pregnancy, it is best to minimize or eliminate its use during the first trimester, when organogenesis is proceeding. However, abrupt discontinuation of lithium should be avoided whenever possible, owing to the high risk of bipolar relapse (Viguera et al. 2000). For pregnant women who have been treated with lithium during the first trimester, a fetal echocardiogram between the sixteenth and eighteenth week of gestation is recommended. Since renal clearance of lithium increases during pregnancy and returns to baseline after delivery, dosage and serum levels may need careful adjustment during these periods. Serum lithium levels usually *decrease* as pregnancy progresses, and this necessitates dosage *increases.* Adjusting the dosage is best achieved using divided doses and aiming for the lowest effective level. With the massive fluid loss (and consequent decrease in plasma volume) associated with delivery, maternal lithium levels may rise dramatically. For this reason—as well as to avert lithium toxicity in the neonate—lithium dosage should be decreased by about 50% prior to delivery. Lithium toxicity in the neonate may appear as flaccidity, lethargy, or poor sucking reflex and may occur at serum levels lower than that of the mother. Transient neonatal hypothyroidism has also been reported (L.J. Miller 1994). Antipsychotics or bilateral electroconvulsive therapy (ECT) may be preferable to lithium for the severely disturbed bipolar patient in the first trimester. Since some manic patients may worsen with unilateral ECT—perhaps due to suboptimal stimulus dosage—bilateral ECT is generally the method of choice in pregnant manic patients (L.J. Miller 1994; Milstein et al. 1987; Pies 1995a; Weiner and Coffey 1988; Zornberg and Pope 1993). However, given the increased cognitive side effects from bilateral ECT, the choice must be individualized and made a part of the informed-consent process (see Abrams 1996 for discussion).

Q. Is the postpartum period one of "high risk" for female bipolar patients, and does mood-stabilizing medication help reduce this risk?

A. The link between bipolar disorder and heightened risk of postpartum mood disorder is well established. One study suggested that the risk of postpartum relapse is around 50% in manic-depressive women (Reich and Winokur 1970). Women with bipolar disorder have up to a 100-fold higher risk than women without a history of psychiatric illness of developing a puerperal psychosis (Chaudron and Pies 2003; Pariser 1993). These episodes are often life-threatening and virtually always require hospitalization (Viguera et al. 2000) for the safety of both mother and child. Whereas the need for vigorous medical treatment is clear in such cases, the optimal choice of medication remains unclear. In a study of mood stabilizer prophylaxis in postpartum bipolar patients (L.S. Cohen et al. 1995), only 1 of 14 patients who received a mood stabilizer postpartum demonstrated recurrent mood disturbance in the first 3 months postpartum. Of the 13 women who did not receive mood stabilizers in the acute postpartum period, 8 experienced manic or depressive relapse within the first 3 months postpartum. The authors concluded that "women with bipolar disorder appear to benefit from puerperal prophylaxis with mood stabilizers" (L.S. Cohen et al. 1995, p. 1641). Burt and Hendrick (1997) recommended that mood stabilizers be started immediately in postpartum psychosis and noted that antipsychotics are often required. There is, as yet, no consensus regarding which mood stabilizer (lithium, divalproex, among others) is the drug of first choice in the acute management of postpartum psychosis. Burt and Hendrick (1997) cautioned that antidepressants may precipitate a protracted and complicated course with rapid cycling in this population. ECT may be an important treatment alternative in many cases of postpartum psychosis, although medicolegal issues often complicate implementation.

Q. What mood stabilizers are indicated for children and adolescents with bipolar disorder, and what special considerations apply?

A. Historically, lithium has been the most commonly prescribed mood stabilizer in younger bipolar populations, although valproate has become increasingly accepted (Dulcan et al. 1995). CBZ is also used in this population, though much of the literature on this agent relates to the treatment of aggression in younger patients (Dulcan et al. 1995). There have been very few controlled studies of any of the mood stabilizers in children and adolescents; however, clinical experience suggests that lithium is usually well tolerated in this population, with the most common side effects being tremor, weight gain, polyuria, polydipsia, polyphagia, and accentuation of preexisting enuresis (Dulcan et al. 1995; Weller et al. 1986). Lithium does not appear to affect growth in children, but its cognitive side effects have not been well studied.

One study of brain-to-serum lithium ratio (Moore et al. 2002) found that while serum and brain lithium concentrations were positively correlated, younger subjects had *lower brain-to-serum concentration ratios* than adults. This suggests that some children and adolescents may need higher maintenance serum lithium concentrations than adults to ensure that brain lithium concentrations reach therapeutic levels. Valproate—and valproate–lithium combinations—appear effective in pediatric bipolar populations, but there are few controlled studies (Wagner 2004). As in adult populations, valproate may produce GI side effects. Valproate can cause hepatotoxicity in children less than 3 years of age, but this event is very rare in children older than 10 years (Dulcan et al. 1995). Even more rare in this population are cases of (potentially fatal) valproate-induced pancreatitis (Trimble 1990). CBZ appears to be eliminated more rapidly in children than in adults, with a $t_{1/2}$ of around 9 hours (subject to autoinduction). The usual total daily dose range of CBZ is 10–50 mg/kg, but there is not a good correlation between weight-based dosage and plasma level. The most common CBZ-related side effects in younger populations include drowsiness, nausea, rash, diplopia, nystagmus, and dose-related leukopenia (Dulcan et al. 1995). There are virtually no published data on use of oxcarbazepine in younger cohorts with bipolar disorder (Wagner 2004). There is also very limited published information on lamotrigine use in pediatric bipolar patients (Wagner 2004). One open trial (Kusumakar and Yatham 1997) found adjunctive lamotrigine useful in a small group of adolescents (*N*=16) with treatment-refractory bipolar depression. However, given the relatively higher risk of serious rash with lamotrigine in pediatric populations (up to 1%), the role for lamotrigine may be more limited in younger patients.

Q. What concerns arise when mood stabilizers are used in elderly patients or dementia patients?

A. As a general rule, elderly patients and dementia patients tend to be more sensitive to both pharmacokinetic and pharmacodynamic factors than do younger patients (Jacobson et al. 2002). Adverse drug reactions may occur in the elderly even at so-called therapeutic plasma levels of mood stabilizers, particularly lithium, whose concentration in the brain may not be accurately reflected in the plasma level. Despite clinical lore, it has not been established in randomized controlled studies that lithium's *therapeutic effects* occur at lower levels in the elderly (Dubovsky 1994). However, to minimize neurocognitive side effects in older patients, it is often necessary to begin at lower doses and to use more gradual dosing increments than in younger patients. Lithium $t_{1/2}\beta$ may be increased (from 24 hours in younger patients to about 40 hours in some elderly patients), resulting in both a longer time to reach steady state (Dubovsky 1994) and a longer "washout" period when the lithium is discontinued. In a retrospective study of 114 elderly outpatients maintained on lithium, Holroyd and Rabins (1994) found that side effects were correlated with higher mean serum lithium levels; however, delirium—which was the most common side effect (19.3% of patients)—occurred at serum lithium levels ranging from 0.3 to 1.5 mmol/L. In this sample, tremor occurred in 20% of patients and hypothyroidism occurred in 18%. Hypothyroidism was more prevalent than in some other studies and may reflect the long-term usage of lithium in this population. Nevertheless, few patients in this elderly population had side effects so serious that discontinuation of the lithium was necessary. Lithium distribution in the brain can be nonuniform (Sansone and Ziegler 1985), and patients with underlying brain damage may show selective "take-up" of lithium in damaged regions of the brain. This may lead to focal neurological side effects (e.g., unilateral tremor) or to generalized neurotoxicity and impaired mentation.

The anticonvulsant mood stabilizers have not been systematically studied in large populations of elderly or dementia patients. While valproate seems generally well tolerated, lower initial dosage may be necessary in the elderly so as to avoid side effects. Some geriatric psychiatrists have observed skeletal muscle (especially truncal) weakness in valproate-treated patients (Jacobson et al. 2002). Valproate has been found useful in the management of aggressive, disinhibited behavior in dementia patients; however, valproate blood levels may need to be lower (roughly 30–50 μg/mL) in dementia than in bipolar disorder (Jacobson et al. 2002). CBZ may also be useful in agitated dementia patients but may be more likely than valproate to produce neurotoxicity, perhaps via accumulation of its 10,11-epoxide metabolite. Again, dosage and plasma levels should probably be kept in the lower therapeutic ranges in elderly and dementia patient populations, with slow increases and frequent monitoring of mental status.

There is still limited experience with lamotrigine in treating elderly bipolar and dementia patients. Robillard and Conn (2002) studied the effectiveness of adding lamotrigine to the treatment regimens of five female geriatric inpatients (average age=71.5) with bipolar depression (four with rapid cycling, one with mixed features). Lamotrigine was started at 25 mg hs, with weekly incremental increases of 12.5 mg daily until a total daily dose of either 75 mg or 100 mg was obtained. Three of the 5 patients had remission of symptoms, as judged by clinical interview and reduction of their Hamilton Rating Scale for Depression score by 50%. Lamotrigine was well tolerated, and none of the patients developed a rash. One patient developed coarse hand tremor that improved with lamotrigine dose reduction. The authors concluded that lamotrigine in conjunction with lithium and valproate may be effective in treating geriatric patients with bipolar depression; however, given the small number of patients in this study and the study's uncontrolled design, more research is necessary before this combination is recommended.

Vignettes/Puzzlers

Q. A 70-year-old man with bipolar disorder is admitted to the inpatient unit in the depressed phase of his illness. However, he has some "mixed" features of irritability and aggressive behaviors. He has been maintained for several years on a regimen of lithium 300 mg bid (level at admission = 0.86 mEq/L) and nortriptyline 35 mg/day (level = 78 ng/mL). Attempts over the years to discontinue nortriptyline inevitably led to recurrent depressive bouts. The patient had been prescribed valproate briefly, but he experienced intolerable nausea and diarrhea, even though the enteric coated form (divalproex) and the Sprinkle formulation were used. At the time of admission, all laboratory studies, ECG, and physical exam results are within normal limits. The patient is started on CBZ 100 mg hs, with increases in dosage as tolerated to a total of 600 mg/day. Plasma CBZ level after 10 days is 7 μg/mL (therapeutic = 4–12 μg/mL). The patient's mood symptoms improve significantly, but he complains of feeling "spacey" and "dizzy." A nurse notes one episode in which the patient fell backward onto his bed, with transient loss of consciousness. A repeat ECG is markedly abnormal. What is the most likely problem and its cause?

A. CBZ has a tricyclic-like structure and shares with the TCAs their quinidine-like properties. CBZ can cause atrioventricular conduction abnormalities, and, as in this case, such conduction abnormalities may be more likely when another quinidine-like agent (e.g., nortriptyline) is used simultaneously. Such problems can occur even at therapeutic CBZ levels. The patient's repeat ECG most likely showed the presence of second- or third-degree atrioventricular block, with its attendant interruption of cerebrovascular circulation leading to cardiac syncope (Stokes-Adams attack). CBZ has been known to produce intermittent total atrioventricular block and asystole, sometimes requiring insertion of a demand pacemaker (Boesen et al. 1983; Ladefoged and Mogelvang 1982).

Q. A 60-year-old woman with a history of panic disorder has been maintained on alprazolam 0.5 mg tid with good control of her anxiety. She suddenly develops severe, unilateral, lancinating facial pain, diagnosed as trigeminal neuralgia (*tic douloureux*), and is prescribed CBZ 200 mg bid. She reports significant pain relief after 4 days but also complains of increased anxiety. Five days later, she experiences two severe panic attacks. What is the most likely explanation?

A. CBZ may increase clearance of both clonazepam and alprazolam, decreasing plasma levels of the latter by as much as 50% (Arana et al. 1988). Patients taking CBZ with a benzodiazepine may require increased dosage of the latter.

Q. A 26-year-old woman with bipolar disorder begins taking oxcarbazepine (with dosage adjusted up to 1,500 mg/day) for recent onset of manic symptoms. She has been intolerant of divalproex, lithium, and olanzapine. Her medication regimen includes occasional (prn) use of loratadine (10 mg tabs) for "allergic symptoms" and use of oral contraceptives. Her manic symptoms are under good control, and she appears to be tolerating the medication well for the first 4 months of use. She then reports nausea and vomiting upon awakening for several mornings in a row. What condition must be immediately ruled out?

A. *Pregnancy* must be ruled out. Oxcarbazepine—though perhaps not as strong an inducer of cytochrome enzymes as CBZ—may increase clearance of estrogen/progesterone agents via induction of cytochrome P450 (CYP) 3A4 (Cozza et al. 2003), thus reducing the effectiveness of oral contraceptives. The prn use of loratadine was probably not relevant in this case.

Q. A 30-year-old woman with unipolar major depression has been maintained on fluoxetine 40 mg/day. When her depression suddenly worsens, her psychiatrist adds lithium 300 mg tid as an augmenting agent. After 1 week, her lithium level has reached 0.8 mEq/L (therapeutic level = 0.5–1.4 mEq/L). At the same time, the woman complains of diarrhea, muscle twitching, shivering, and confusion. Her temperature is 100.4°F. Blood cultures, chest X ray, and urinalysis are all negative. What is the most likely diagnosis?

A. This is probably a case of *serotonin syndrome* (see Chapter 2, "Antidepressants), brought on by a pharmacodynamic interaction between fluoxetine and lithium (Muly et al. 1993; Sternbach 1991). Other case reports suggest that fluoxetine—and perhaps other SSRIs—may increase neurotoxicity in patients taking lithium, sometimes (but not always) elevating plasma lithium levels. The mechanism of action underlying this putative adverse interaction is not known (Sarid-Segal et al. 1995; Venkatakrishnan et al. 2003). Furthermore, one observational drug utilization study using a matched cohort control design (Bauer et al. 1996) found no evidence of major adverse reactions to the combination of lithium and fluoxetine.

Q. A 23-year-old man with refractory bipolar disorder has had his illness poorly controlled with a combination of lithium 300 mg tid (level = 0.9 mEq/L, therapeutic level = 0.5–1.4 mEq/L) and CBZ 400 mg bid (level = 11 μg/mL, therapeutic level = 4–15 μg/mL). His psychiatrist adds valproate 250 mg bid and increases the dosage up to a total of 1,000 mg/day. A valproate level after 1 week is 78 μg/mL (therapeutic level = 50–125 μg/mL). Although the patient's mania is reduced, he shows marked drowsiness, ataxia, and vertigo. A repeat CBZ level is 12 μg/mL. What is the likely cause of the patient's new problems?

A. Valproate inhibits the enzyme epoxide hydrolase, and this leads to increased plasma levels of *CBZ epoxide*—a potentially neurotoxic metabolite. This increase may occur even when levels of the parent compound (CBZ) are within the putative therapeutic range (Ciraulo and Slattery 1995; Sovner 1988).

Q. **A 24-year-old female bipolar patient is started on CBZ 200 mg tid, with good effect after 1 week. Her baseline total white blood cell (WBC) count is 5,200 cells/μL (i.e., 5.2×10^3 cells/μL; normal range = 4–11) with 65% neutrophils (normal = 50%–70%). After 1 week, her total WBC is 4.0, with 60% neutrophils. Is this likely to represent the beginning of an aplastic anemia?**

A. No. Transient, benign leukopenia—usually involving primarily the granulocyte fraction—is seen in about 10%–12% of patients taking CBZ (McElroy and Keck 1995). This reaction does not predispose to infection, nor is it related to serious blood dyscrasias, such as aplastic anemia. The latter occurs in only around 1 in 575,000 cases, usually after 2–3 months of treatment (Ayd 1995; McElroy and Keck 1995).

Q. **A 20-year-old male college student has recently been diagnosed as having bipolar I disorder. He is initially seen in the manic phase and is begun on lithium 300 mg tid (plasma level = 0.9 mEq/L). Because he experiences significant cognitive "slowing" while taking the lithium, he increases his caffeine intake from his usual two cups of caffeinated coffee per day to four cups per day. One week later, he suffers another manic episode. What is the most likely explanation, other than spontaneous cycling?**

A. Caffeine (and related methylxanthines) can increase lithium excretion, sometimes dropping blood levels below the minimum therapeutic range (Ayd 1995). It is also possible, in this case, that the increased caffeine acted directly (i.e., via a pharmacodynamic effect) by increasing neuronal sensitivity to catecholamines, thereby increasing the likelihood of mania.

Q. **A 40-year-old woman with bipolar II disorder has been taking lithium 300 mg tid for the depressed phase of her illness (blood level = 0.7 mEq/L). Because her depression has responded only partially, lamotrigine (up to 100 mg/day) is added to her regimen. She appears to tolerate this combination well for the first 2 weeks of treatment. After 15 days, however, she develops a rash on her legs, sore throat, general malaise, conjunctivitis, and a temperature of 103°F. Intra-oral ruptured bullae and "target" lesions of the skin are observed on the patient's hands and feet. What is the most likely diagnosis?**

A. Most likely, this represents a case of Stevens-Johnson syndrome, a potentially lethal form of erythema multiforme. This syndrome is probably a hypersensitivity reaction due to various drugs, including barbiturates, meprobamate, fluoxetine, CBZ, and—very rarely—lamotrigine. If current dosing guidelines are followed, the incidence of severe rash with lamotrigine appears to be no greater than about 1% (1/100) in pediatric patients (ages <16 years) and 0.3% (3/1000) in adults (Messenheimer et al. 2000). Recent analysis of controlled studies suggests even lower rates in adults (Shelton and Calabrese 2004).

Q. A 35-year-old woman with schizoaffective disorder has been successfully treated with clozapine 450 mg/day and lamotrigine 200 mg/day. Unfortunately, the patient develops a rash that is attributed to the lamotrigine, and this agent is discontinued. Divalproex 750 mg/day is started, and the dosage is titrated to a plasma level of 75 μg/mL. Within 3 weeks after the discontinuation of the lamotrigine, the patient begins complaining of new and unusual auditory hallucinations, despite therapeutic levels of clozapine (355 ng/mL). What pharmacodynamic and/or pharmacokinetic effects can explain this sequence of events?

A. Lamotrigine has been shown to antagonize the psychoactive ("psychotogenic") effects of the dissociative anesthetic agent ketamine. This effect is most likely due to lamotrigine's antagonism at the glutamate receptor. Furthermore, this medication has demonstrated pharmacodynamic synergism in patients with treatment-resistant schizophrenia who are being treated with clozapine. It is possible that this patient was benefiting from lamotrigine because of its direct pharmacodynamic (antipsychotic) effects (Tiihonen et al. 2003); hence, discontinuation of lamotrigine may have led to psychotic relapse. Theoretically, pharmacokinetic factors may also have contributed to this event. One report suggests that lamotrigine may elevate serum clozapine levels, owing to competitive inhibition of glucuronidation (Cozza et al. 2003; Kossen et al. 2001). Discontinuation of the lamotrigine may have led to "deinhibition" of this metabolic pathway, with a resultant drop in serum clozapine levels. Even though the clozapine levels may have been within the putative therapeutic range of 350 ng/mL or higher (Marder and Wirshing 2004), this particular patient might have required higher clozapine levels for control of psychotic symptoms. The effect of *divalproex* on clozapine has been equivocal, with case reports of both increased or decreased clozapine levels (Cozza et al. 2003).

Q. A hospitalized 17-year-old woman with bipolar disorder has been receiving divalproex 750 mg bid for the past 18 months. She has tolerated the medication well, except for a gain of 8 pounds. Despite therapeutic valproate levels, symptoms of irritability, insomnia, and racing thoughts are still present. Olanzapine is considered as adjunctive treatment, but both the patient and her family are concerned about the risk of further weight gain with olanzapine. Therefore, topiramate is started at a dose of 50 mg qd, and the dose is increased to 150 mg over the next week. After about 2 weeks at this dose, the patient is found confused and ataxic. After a sudden fall, she is difficult to awake and is transferred to the ICU. All labs are normal (including "liver functions") except for her serum ammonia level, which is twice the upper limits of normal. What factors might have led to this outcome?

A. Valproic acid and its derivatives can cause *hyperammonemic encephalopathy,* particularly in patients with underlying urea cycle disorders (Physicians' Desk Reference 2004). Though this patient had been taking divalproex for a long time, a new drug was added to the regimen. Topiramate, which is not FDA-approved for bipolar disorder or weight loss, is an inhibitor of *carbonic anhydrase* and cerebral *glutamine synthetase.* Normally, the production of these enzymes is responsible for decreasing ammonia levels. Therefore, the addition of topiramate may have enhanced the hyperammonemic effects of valproic acid through additional mechanisms (Hamer et al. 2000).

References

Abrams R: ECT stimulus parameters as determinants of seizure quality. Psychiatr Ann 26:701–704, 1996

Akman CI, Goodkin HP, Rogers DP, et al: Visual hallucinations associated with zonisamide. Pharmacotherapy 23:93–96, 2003

Albanese MJ, Pies R: The bipolar patient with comorbid substance use disorder: recognition and management. CNS Drugs 18:585–596, 2004

Albanese MJ, Clodfelter RC Jr, Khantzian EJ: Divalproex sodium in substance abusers with mood disorder. J Clin Psychiatry 61:916–921, 2000

Altshuler LL: Bipolar depression revisited: review and recent findings (interview). Currents in Affective Illness 23:5–10, 2004

Altshuler LL, Post RM, Leverich GS, et al: Antidepressant-induced mania and cycle acceleration: a controversy revisited. Am J Psychiatry 152:1130–1138, 1995

Altshuler LL, Keck PE Jr, McElroy SL, et al: Gabapentin in the acute treatment of refractory bipolar disorder. Bipolar Disord 1:61–65, 1999

Altshuler LL, Suppes T, Black D, et al: Impact of antidepressant discontinuation after acute bipolar depression remission on rates of depressive relapse at 1-year follow-up. Am J Psychiatry 160:1252–1262, 2003

American Psychiatric Association: Diagnostic and Statistical Manual of Mental Disorders, 3rd Edition. Washington, DC, American Psychiatric Association, 1980

American Psychiatric Association: Diagnostic and Statistical Manual of Mental Disorders, 4th Edition. Washington, DC, American Psychiatric Association, 1994

American Psychiatric Association: Practice guideline for the treatment of patients with bipolar disorder (revision). Am J Psychiatry 159:1–50, 2002

Amsterdam JD, Garcia-Espana F, Fawcett J, et al. Efficacy and safety of fluoxetine in treating bipolar II major depressive episode. J Clin Psychopharmacol 18:435–440, 1998

Andrews DG, Schweitzer I, Marshall N: The comparative side effects of lithium, carbamazepine and combined lithium-carbamazepine in patients treated for affective disorders. Hum Psychopharmacol 5:41–45, 1990

Anghelescu I, Klawe C, Benkert O: Orlistat in the treatment of psychopharmacologically induced weight gain. J Clin Psychopharmacol 20:716–717, 2000

Arana GW, Hyman SE: Handbook of Psychiatric Drug Therapy, 2nd Edition. Boston, MA, Little, Brown, 1991

Arana GW, Epstein S, Molloy M, et al: Carbamazepine-induced reduction of plasma alprazolam concentrations: a clinical case report. J Clin Psychiatry 49:448–449, 1988

Ayd FJ: Lexicon of Psychiatry, Neurology, and the Neurosciences. Baltimore, MD, Williams & Wilkins, 1995

Baf MH, Subhash MN, Lakshmana KM, et al: Sodium valproate induced alterations in monoamine levels in different regions of the rat brain. Neurochem Int 24:67–72, 1994

Baldessarini RJ, Tondo L, Viguera AC: Discontinuing lithium maintenance treatment in bipolar disorders: risks and implications. Bipolar Disord 1:17–24, 1999

Baldessarini RJ, Tondo L, Floris G, et al: Effects of rapid cycling on response to lithium maintenance treatment in 360 bipolar I and II disorder patients. J Affect Disord 61:13–22, 2000

Baldessarini RJ, Tondo L, Hennen J: Lithium treatment and suicide risk in major affective disorders: update and new findings. J Clin Psychiatry 64 (suppl 5):44–52, 2003

Bauer MS, Mitchner L: What is a "mood stabilizer"? An evidence-based response. Am J Psychiatry 161:3–18, 2004

Bauer MS, Whybrow PC: Rapid cycling bipolar disorder: clinical features, treatment, and etiology, in Refractory Depression. Edited by Amsterdam JD. New York, Raven, 1991, pp 191–208

Bauer M, Linden M, Schaaf B, et al: Adverse events and tolerability of the combination of fluoxetine/lithium compared with fluoxetine. J Clin Psychopharmacol 16:130–134, 1996

Besag FM, Berry DJ, Pool F, et al: Carbamazepine toxicity with lamotrigine: pharmacokinetic or pharmacodynamic interaction? Epilepsia 39:183–187, 1998

Bochetta A, Chillotti C, Severino G, et al: Carbamazepine augmentation in lithium-refractory bipolar patients: a prospective study on long-term prophylactic effectiveness. J Clin Psychopharmacol 17:92–96, 1997

Boesen F, Andersen EB, Jensen EK, et al: Cardiac conduction disturbances during carbamazepine therapy. Acta Neurol Scand 68:49–52, 1983

Boland RJ, Keller MB: Mixed-state bipolar disorders: outcome data from the NIMH Collaborative Program on the Psychobiology of Depression, in Bipolar Disorders: Clinical Course and Outcome. Edited by Goldberg JF, Harrow M. Washington, DC, American Psychiatric Press, 1999, pp 115–128

Boutros NN, Guerra BM, Votolato NA, et al: Carbamazepine-induced hyponatremia resolved with doxycycline. J Clin Psychiatry 56:377–378, 1995

Bowden CL: Predictors of response to divalproex and lithium. J Clin Psychiatry 56 (suppl 3):25–30, 1995a

Bowden CL: Treatment of bipolar disorder, in The American Psychiatric Press Textbook of Psychopharmacology. Edited by Schatzberg AF, Nemeroff CB. Washington, DC, American Psychiatric Press, 1995b, pp 603–614

Bowden CL: Valproate, in The American Psychiatric Publishing Textbook of Psychopharmacology, 3rd Edition. Edited by Schatzberg AF, Nemeroff CB. Washington, DC, American Psychiatric Publishing, 2004, pp 567–579.

Bowden CL, Goldberg JF: Switching and Destabilization in Bipolar Disorder. CME Program Monograph. Boston, MA, Boston University School of Medicine, 2003

Bowden CL, Brugger AM, Swann AC, et al: Efficacy of divalproex vs lithium and placebo in the treatment of mania. JAMA 271:918–924, 1994

Bowden CL, Calabrese JR, Sachs G, et al: A placebo-controlled 18-month trial of lamotrigine and lithium maintenance treatment in recently manic or hypomanic patients with bipolar I disorder. Arch Gen Psychiatry 60:392–400, 2003

Bowen RC, Grof P, Grof E: Less frequent lithium administration and lower urine volume. Am J Psychiatry 148:189–192, 1991

Bradwejn J, Shriqui C, Koszycki D, et al: Double-blind comparison of the effects of clonazepam and lorazepam in acute mania. J Clin Psychopharmacol 10:403–408, 1990

Brieger P: Hypomanic episodes after receiving ziprasidone: an unintended "on-off-on" course of treatment. J Clin Psychiatry 65:132–135, 2004

Brodie MJ, Dichter MA: Antiepileptic drugs. N Engl J Med 334:168–175, 1996

Brotman AW, Farhadi AM, Gelenberg AJ, et al: Verapamil treatment of acute mania. J Clin Psychiatry 47:136–138, 1986

Burt VK, Hendrick VC: Postpartum psychiatric disorders, in Concise Guide to Women's Mental Health. Washington, DC, American Psychiatric Press, 1997, pp 63–77

Calabrese JR, Markowitz PJ, Kimmel SE, et al: Spectrum of efficacy of valproate in 78 rapidly cycling bipolar patients. J Clin Psychopharmacol 12 (suppl):53S–56S, 1992

Calabrese JR, Fatemi SH, Kujawa M, et al: Predictors of response to mood stabilizers. J Clin Psychopharmacol 16 (2, suppl 1):24S–31S, 1996

Calabrese JR, Suppes T, Bowden CL, et al: A double-blind, placebo-controlled, prophylaxis study of lamotrigine in rapid-cycling bipolar disorder. Lamictal 614 Study Group. J Clin Psychiatry 61:841–850, 2000

Calabrese JR, Shelton MD, Bowden CL, et al: Bipolar rapid cycling: focus on depression as its hallmark. J Clin Psychiatry 62 (suppl 14):34–41, 2001

Casey DE, Daniel DG, Wassef AA, et al: Effect of divalproex combined with olanzapine or risperidone in patients with an acute exacerbation of schizophrenia. Neuropsychopharmacology 28:182–192, 2003

Centorrino F, Kelleher JP, Berry JM, et al: Pilot comparison of extended-release and standard preparations of divalproex sodium in patients with bipolar and schizoaffective disorder. Am J Psychiatry 160:1348–1350, 2003

Chaudron LH, Pies RW: The relationship between postpartum psychosis and bipolar disorder: a review. J Clin Psychiatry 64:1284–1292, 2003

Chengappa KN, Rathore D, Levine J, et al: Topiramate as add-on treatment for patients with bipolar mania. Bipolar Disord 1:42–53, 1999

Chengappa KNR, Gershon S, Levine J: The evolving role of topiramate among other mood stabilizers in the management of bipolar disorder. Bipolar Disord 3:215–232, 2001

Ciraulo DA, Slattery M: Anticonvulsants, in Drug Interactions in Psychiatry, 2nd Edition. Edited by Ciraulo DA, Shader RI, Greenblatt DJ, et al. Baltimore, MD, Williams & Wilkins, 1995, pp 249–310

Ciraulo DA, Shader RI, Greenblatt DJ, et al: Drug Interactions in Psychiatry, 2nd Edition. Baltimore, MD, Williams & Wilkins, 1995

Cohen LS: Interview. Currents in Affective Illness, September 1992

Cohen LS, Sichel DA, Robertson LM, et al: Postpartum prophylaxis for women with bipolar disorder. Am J Psychiatry 152:1641–1645, 1995

Cohen WJ, Cohen NJ: Lithium carbonate, haloperidol, and irreversible brain damage. JAMA 230:1283–1287, 1974

Cozza KL, Armstrong SC, Oesterheld JR: Concise Guide to Drug Interaction Principles for Medical Practice: Cytochrome P450s, UGTs, P-Glycoproteins, 2nd Edition. Washington, DC, American Psychiatric Publishing, 2003

DasGupta K, Jefferson JW, Kobak KA, et al: The effect of enalapril on serum lithium levels in healthy men. J Clin Psychiatry 53:398–400, 1992

De Berardis D, Campanella V, Matera F, et al: Thrombocytopenia during valproic acid treatment in young patients with new-onset bipolar disorder. J Clin Psychopharmacol 23:451–458, 2003

DeQuardo JR: Worsened agitation with aripiprazole: adverse effect of dopamine partial agonism? J Clin Psychiatry 65:132–133, 2004

DeVane CL: Pharmacogenetics and drug metabolism of newer antidepressant agents. J Clin Psychiatry 55 (12, suppl):38–45, 1994

Dilsaver SC, Swann AC, Shoaib AM, et al: The manic syndrome: factors which may predict a patient's response to lithium, carbamazepine and valproate. J Psychiatry Neurosci 18:61–66, 1993

Doose DR, Brodie MJ, Wilson EA, et al: Topiramate and lamotrigine pharmacokinetics during repetitive monotherapy and combination therapy in epilepsy patients. Epilepsia 44:917–922, 2003

Drug Facts and Comparisons. St Louis, MO, Facts & Comparisons, 1995

Dubovsky SL: Geriatric neuropsychopharmacology, in The American Psychiatric Press Textbook of Geriatric Neuropsychiatry. Edited by Coffey CE, Cummings JL. Washington, DC, American Psychiatric Press, 1994, pp 595–631

Dubovsky SL: Calcium channel antagonists as novel agents for manic-depressive disorder, in The American Psychiatric Press Textbook of Psychopharmacology. Edited by Schatzberg AF, Nemeroff CB. Washington, DC, American Psychiatric Press, 1995, pp 377–388

Dubovsky SL, Franks RD, Allen S, et al: Calcium antagonists in mania: a double-blind study of verapamil. Psychiatry Res 18:309–312, 1986

Dulcan MK, Bregman JD, Weller EB, et al: Treatment of childhood and adolescent disorders, in The American Psychiatric Press Textbook of Psychopharmacology. Edited by Schatzberg AF, Nemeroff CB. Washington, DC, American Psychiatric Press, 1995, pp 669–706

Dunn RT, Frye MS, Kimbrell TA, et al: The efficacy and use of anticonvulsants in mood disorders. Clin Neuropharmacol 21:215–235, 1998

El-Mallakh RS, Wyatt RJ: The Na,K-ATPase hypothesis for bipolar illness. Biol Psychiatry 37:235–244, 1995

Emrich HM: Studies with oxcarbazepine (Trileptal) in acute mania, in Carbamazepine and Oxcarbazepine in Psychiatry. Edited by Emrich HM, Schiwy W, Silverstone T. London, Clinical Neuroscience Publishers, 1990, pp 83–88

Faedda GL, Tondo L, Baldessarini RJ: Outcome after rapid vs gradual discontinuation of lithium treatment in bipolar disorders. Arch Gen Psychiatry 50:448–455, 1993

Fink M: Separating psychotic depression from nonpsychotic depression is essential to effective treatment. J Affect Disord 76:1–3, 2003

Finley PR, O'Brien JG, Coleman RW: Lithium and angiotensin-converting enzyme inhibitors: evaluation of a potential interaction. J Clin Psychopharmacol 16:68–71, 1996

Fogelson DL, Sternbach H: Lamotrigine treatment of rapid cycling bipolar disorder. J Clin Psychiatry 58:271–273, 1997

Fogelson DL, Bystritsky A, Pasnau R: Bupropion in the treatment of bipolar disorders: the same old story? J Clin Psychiatry 53:443–446, 1992

Freeman MP, Wiegand C, Gelenberg AJ: Lithium, in The American Psychiatric Publishing Textbook of Psychopharmacology, 3rd Edition. Edited by Schatzberg AF, Nemeroff CB. Washington, DC, American Psychiatric Publishing, 2004, pp 547–565

Freeman TW, Clothier JL, Pazzaglia P, et al: A double-blind comparison of valproate and lithium in the treatment of acute mania. Am J Psychiatry 149:108–111, 1992

Frye MA, Ketter TA, Kimbrell TA, et al: A placebo-controlled study of lamotrigine and gabapentin monotherapy in refractory mood disorders. J Clin Psychopharmacol 20:607–614, 2000

Fujiyama K, Kiriyama T, Ito M, et al: Suppressive doses of thyroxine do not accelerate age-related bone loss in late postmenopausal women. Thyroid 5:13–17, 1995

Geddes JR, Burgess S, Hawton K, et al: Long-term lithium therapy for bipolar disorder: systematic review and meta-analysis of randomized controlled trials. Am J Psychiatry 161:217–222, 2004

Gelenberg AJ: Verapamil for mania? Biological Therapies in Psychiatry Newsletter 20:6–7, 1997

Gelenberg A, Pies R: Matching the bipolar patient and the mood stabilizer. Ann Clin Psychiatry 15:203–216, 2003

Gerner RH, Stanton A: Algorithm for patient management of acute manic states: lithium, valproate, or carbamazepine? J Clin Psychopharmacol 12 (suppl):57S-63S, 1992

Ghadirian A-M, Annable L, Belanger M-C, et al: A cross-sectional study of parkinsonism and tardive dyskinesia in lithium-treated affective disordered patients. J Clin Psychiatry 57:22–28, 1996

Ghaemi SN: Mood Disorders. Philadelphia, PA, Lippincott Williams & Wilkins, 2003

Ghaemi SN, Boiman EE, Goodwin FK: Diagnosing bipolar disorder and the effect of antidepressants: a naturalistic study. J Clin Psychiatry 61:804–808, 2000

Glazer WM, Sonnenberg JG, Reinstein MJ, et al: A novel, point-of-care test for lithium levels: description and reliability. J Clin Psychiatry 65:652–655, 2004

Goff DC, Baldessarini RJ: Antipsychotics, in Drug Interactions in Psychiatry, 2nd Edition. Edited by Ciraulo DA, Shader RI, Greenblatt DJ, et al. Baltimore, MD, Williams & Wilkins, 1995, pp 129–174

Goldberg JF, Whiteside JE: The association between substance abuse and antidepressant-induced mania in bipolar disorder: a preliminary study. J Clin Psychiatry 63:791–795, 2002

Goldberg JF, Garno JL, Leon AC, et al: A history of substance abuse complicates remission from acute mania in bipolar disorder. J Clin Psychiatry 60:733–740, 1999

Goldberg JF, Burdick KE, Endick CJ: Preliminary randomized, double-blind, placebo-controlled trial of pramipexole added to mood stabilizers for treatment-resistant bipolar depression. Am J Psychiatry 161:564–566, 2004

Goodnick P: Nimodipine treatment of rapid cycling bipolar disorder (letter). J Clin Psychiatry 56:330, 1995

Goodwin FK, Ghaemi SN: The difficult-to-treat patient with bipolar disorder, in The Difficult-to-Treat Psychiatric Patient. Edited by Dewan MJ, Pies RW. Washington, DC, American Psychiatric Publishing, 2001, pp 7–39

Goodwin FK, Jamison KR: Manic-Depressive Illness, New York, Oxford University Press, 1990

Goodwin GM: Recurrence of mania after lithium withdrawal: implications for the use of lithium in the treatment of bipolar affective disorder. Br J Psychiatry 164:149–152, 1994

Gould TD, Zarate CA, Manji HK: Glycogen synthase kinase–3: a target for novel bipolar disorder treatments. J Clin Psychiatry 65:10–21, 2004

Granneman GR, Schneck DW, Cavanaugh JH, et al: Pharmacokinetic interactions and side effects resulting from concomitant administration of lithium and divalproex sodium. J Clin Psychiatry 57:204–206, 1996

Grof P, Alda M, Grof E, et al: The challenge of predicting response to stabilising lithium treatment: the importance of patient selection. Br J Psychiatry 21 (suppl):16–19, 1993

Hamer HM, Knake S, Schomburg U, et al: Valproate-induced hyperammonemic encephalopathy in the presence of topiramate. Neurology 54:230–232, 2000

Hellewell JS: Oxcarbazepine (Trileptal) in the treatment of bipolar disorders: a review of efficacy and tolerability. J Affect Disord 72 (suppl 1):S23–S34, 2002

Henry C, Sorbara F, Lacoste J, et al: Antidepressant-induced mania in bipolar patients: identification of risk factors. J Clin Psychiatry 62:249–255, 2001

Hester RK: Outcome research: alcoholism, in The American Psychiatric Press Textbook of Substance Abuse Treatment. Edited by Galanter M, Kleber HD. Washington, DC, American Psychiatric Press, 1994, pp 35–44

Hetmar O, Brun C, Clemmensen L, et al: Lithium: long-term effects on the kidney, II: structural changes. J Psychiatry Res 21:279–288, 1987

Hirschowitz J, Casper R, Garver DL, et al: Lithium response in good prognosis schizophrenia. Am J Psychiatry 137:916–920, 1980

Hoaken PCS, Hoaken P: Undue mood elevation in unipolar patients following cessation of lithium augmentation treatment: implications for the understanding of mood disorders. Can J Psychiatry 41:46–48, 1996

Holroyd S, Rabins PV: A retrospective chart review of lithium side effects in a geriatric outpatient population. Am J Geriatr Psychiatry 4:346–351, 1994

Jacobson SA, Pies RW, Greenblatt DJ: Handbook of Geriatric Psychopharmacology. Washington, DC, American Psychiatric Publishing, 2002

Janicak PG, Davis JM, Preskorn SH, et al: Principles and Practice of Psychopharmacotherapy. Baltimore, MD, Williams & Wilkins, 1993

Janicak PG (ed): Advances in the pharmacotherapy of bipolar disorder. Principles and Practice of Psychopharmacotherapy, Vol 1, Update. Baltimore, MD, Williams & Wilkins, 1995, pp 1–20

Janicak PG, Davis JM, Preskorn SH, et al: Principles and Practice of Psychopharmacotherapy. Baltimore, MD, Williams & Wilkins, 1993

Jann MW, Fidone GS, Israel MK, et al: Increased valproate serum concentrations upon carbamazepine cessation. Epilepsia 29:578–581, 1988

Jeste DV, Barak Y, Mahusoodanan S, et al: International multisite double-blind trial of the atypical antipsychotics risperidone and olanzapine in 175 elderly patients with chronic schizophrenia. Am J Geriatr Psychiatry 11:638–647, 2003

John V, Rapp M, Pies R: Aggression, agitation and mania with olanzapine (letter). Can J Psychiatry 43:1054, 1998

Kahn DA, Carpenter D, Docherty JP, et al (eds): The Expert Consensus Guidelines for treatment of bipolar disorder. J Clin Psychiatry 57 (suppl 12A):41, 1996

Kanba S, Yagi G, Kamijima K, et al: The first open study of zonisamide, a novel anticonvulsant, shows efficacy in mania. Prog Neuropsychopharmacol Biol Psychiatry 18:7–15, 1994

Kaplan HI, Sadock BJ, Grebb JA (eds): Synopsis of Psychiatry, 7th Edition. Baltimore, MD, Williams & Wilkins, 1994, pp 918–925

Kaufman KR, Gerner R: Lamotrigine toxicity secondary to sertraline. Seizure 7:163–165, 1998

Keck PE Jr, McElroy SL, Friedman LM: Valproate and carbamazepine in the treatment of panic and posttraumatic stress disorders, withdrawal states, and behavioral dyscontrol syndromes. J Clin Psychopharmacol 12 (suppl):36S–41S, 1992a

Keck PE Jr, McElroy SL, Vuckovic A, et al: Combined valproate and carbamazepine treatment of bipolar disorder. J Neuropsychiatry Clin Neurosci 4:319–322, 1992b

Keck PE Jr, McElroy SL, Tugrul KC, et al: Valproate oral loading in the treatment of acute mania. J Clin Psychiatry 54:305–308, 1993

Keck PE Jr, Nabulsi AA, Taylor JL, et al: A pharmacoeconomic model of divalproex vs lithium in the acute and prophylactic treatment of bipolar I disorder. J Clin Psychiatry 57:213–222, 1996

Ketter TA, Calabrese JR: Stabilization of mood from below versus above baseline in bipolar disorder: a new nomenclature. J Clin Psychiatry 63:146–151, 2002

Ketter TA, Jenkins JB, Schroeder DH, et al: Carbamazepine but not valproate induces bupropion metabolism. J Clin Psychopharmacol 15:327–333, 1995a

Ketter TA, Post RM, Parekh PI, et al: Addition of monoamine oxidase inhibitors to carbamazepine: preliminary evidence of safety and antidepressant efficacy in treatment-resistant depression. J Clin Psychiatry 56:471–475, 1995b

Ketter TA, Post RM, Denicoff K: Carbamazepine, in Mania: Clinical and Research Perspectives. Edited by Goodnick PJ. Washington, DC, American Psychiatric Press, 1998, pp 263–300

Ketter TA, Kalali AH, Weisler RH [SPD417 Study Group]: A 6-month, multicenter, open-label evaluation of beaded, extended-release carbamazepine capsule monotherapy in bipolar disorder patients with manic or mixed episodes. J Clin Psychiatry 65:668-673, 2004a

Ketter TA, Wang PW, Post RM: Carbamazepine and oxcarbazepine, in The American Psychiatric Publishing Textbook of Psychopharmacology, 3rd Edition. Edited by Schatzberg AF, Nemeroff CB. Washington, DC, American Psychiatric Publishing, 2004b, pp 581–606

Khaitan L, Calabrese JR, Stockmeier CA: Effects of chronic treatment with valproate on serotonin-1A receptor binding and function. Psychopharmacology (Berl) 113:539–542, 1994

Klein E, Uhde TW, Post RM: Preliminary evidence for the utility of carbamazepine in alprazolam withdrawal. Am J Psychiatry 143:235–236, 1986

Konig SA, Elger CE, Vassella F, et al: Recommendations for blood studies and clinical monitoring in early detection of valproate-associated liver failure: results of a consensus conference 9 May–11 May 1997 in Berlin. Nervenarzt 69:835–840, 1998

Kossen M, Selten JP, Kahn RS: Elevated clozapine plasma level with lamotrigine (letter). Am J Psychiatry 158:1930, 2001

Krishnan KRR; Steffans DC, Doraiswamy PM: Psychotropic drug interactions. Primary Psychiatry 3:21–45, 1996

Kusumakar V, Yatham LN: An open study of lamotrigine in refractory bipolar depression. Psychiatry Res 72:145–148, 1997

Ladefoged SD, Mogelvang JC: Total atrioventricular block with syncope complicating carbamazepine therapy. Acta Med Scand 212:185–186, 1982

Lahr MB: Hyponatremia during carbamazepine therapy. Clin Pharmacol Ther 37:693–696, 1985

Lenox RH, Manji HK: Lithium, in The American Psychiatric Press Textbook of Psychopharmacology. Edited by Schatzberg AF, Nemeroff CB. Washington, DC, American Psychiatric Press, 1995, pp 303–349

Lenzi A, Marazziti D, Raffaelli S, et al: Effectiveness of the combination of verapamil and chlorpromazine in the treatment of severe manic or mixed patients. Prog Neuropsychopharmacol Biol Psychiatry 19:519–528, 1995

Levitt JJ, Tsuang MT: The heterogeneity of schizoaffective disorder: implications for treatment. Am J Psychiatry 145:926–936, 1988

London J: Mania associated with olanzapine (letter). J Am Acad Child Adolesc Psychiatry 37:997–1008, 1998

Magliozzi JR, Tupin JP: Glossary of pharmacological terms, in Handbook of Clinical Psychopharmacology. Edited by Tupin JP, Shader RI, Harnett DS. Northvale, NJ, Jason Aronson, 1988, pp 455–465

Maidment ID: Gabapentin treatment for bipolar disorders. Ann Pharmacother 35:1264–1269, 2001

Marcocci C, Golia F, Bruno-Bossio G, et al: Carefully monitored levothyroxine suppressive therapy is not associated with bone loss in premenopausal women. J Clin Endocrinol Metab 78:818–823, 1994

Marcotte D. Use of topiramate, a new antiepileptic as a mood stabilizer. J Affect Disord 50:245–251, 1998

Marder SR, Wirshing DA: Clozapine, in The American Psychiatric Publishing Textbook of Psychopharmacology, 3rd Edition. Edited by Schatzberg AF, Nemeroff CB. Washington, DC, American Psychiatric Publishing, 2004, pp 443–456

Margolese HC, Beauclair L, Szkrumelak N, et al: Hypomania induced by adjunctive lamotrigine. Am J Psychiatry 160:183–184, 2003

Martin H, Slyk MP, Deymann S, et al: Safety profile assessment of risperidone and olanzapine in long-term care patients with dementia. J Am Med Dir Assoc 4:183–188, 2003

Mattson RH, Cramer JA, Collins JF, et al: A comparison of valproate with carbamazepine for the treatment of complex partial seizures and secondarily generalized tonic-clonic seizures in adults. N Engl J Med 327:765–771, 1992

Maxmen JS: Psychotropic Drugs: Fast Facts. New York, WW Norton, 1991

McElroy SL, Keck PE: Antiepileptic drugs, in The American Psychiatric Press Textbook of Psychopharmacology. Edited by Schatzberg AF, Nemeroff CB. Washington, DC, American Psychiatric Press, 1995, pp 351–375

McElroy SL, Suppes T, Keck PE Jr, et al: Open-label adjunctive topiramate in the treatment of bipolar disorders. Biol Psychiatry 47:1025–1033, 2000

McLaughlin DB, Andrews JA, Hooper WD, et al: Apparent autoinduction of valproate beta-oxidation in humans. Br J Clin Pharmacol 49:409–415, 2000

Mendels J, Frazer A: Reduced central serotonergic activity in mania: implications for the relationship between depression and mania. Br J Psychiatry 126:241–248, 1975

Messenheimer JA, Giorgi L, Risner ME: The tolerability of lamotrigine in children. Drug Saf 22:303–312, 2000

Miller AD, Krauss GL, Hanzeh FM: Improved CNS tolerability following conversion from immediate- to extended release carbamazepine. Acta Neurol Scand 109:374-377, 2004

Miller F, Menninger J: Lithium-neuroleptic neurotoxicity is dose dependent. J Clin Psychopharmacol 7:89–91, 1987

Miller LJ: Psychiatric medication during pregnancy: understanding and minimizing risks. Psychiatr Ann 24:69–75, 1994

Milstein V, Small JG, Klapper MH, et al: Uni- versus bilateral ECT in the treatment of mania. Convuls Ther 3:1–9, 1987

Moore CM, Demopulos CM, Henry ME, et al: Brain-to-serum lithium ratio and age: an in vivo magnetic resonance spectroscopy study. Am J Psychiatry 159:1240–1242, 2002

Muly EC, McDonald W, Steffans D, et al: Serotonin syndrome produced by a combination of fluoxetine and lithium (letter). Am J Psychiatry 150:1565, 1993

Nierenberg AA, Papakostas GI, Peterson T, et al: Lithium augmentation of nortriptyline for subjects resistant to multiple antidepressants. J Clin Psychopharmacol 23:92–95, 2003

Obrocea GV, Dunn RM, Frye MA, et al: Clinical predictors of response to lamotrigine and gabapentin monotherapy in refractory affective disorders. Biol Psychiatry 51:253–260, 2002

Oechsner M, Steen C, Sturenburg HJ, et al: Hyperammonaemic encephalopathy after initiation of valproate therapy in unrecognized ornithine transcarbamylase deficiency. J Neurol Neurosurg Psychiatry 64:680–682, 1998

Okuma T: Effects of carbamazepine and lithium on affective disorders. Neuropsychobiology 27:138–145, 1993

O'Reardon J: On antidepressant augmentation. The Carlat Report 2(1):4–5, 2004

Osawa K, Kobayashi K, Noda S, et al: Zonisamide-induced depression and mania in patients with epilepsy. J Clin Psychopharmacol 24:110–111, 2004

Osser D: Hazards of stopping maintenance pharmacotherapy of bipolar disorder. Lecture at Cambridge Hospital, Boston, MA, January 6, 1996

Pariser SF: Women and mood disorders: menarche to menopause. Ann Clin Psychiatry 5:249–254, 1993

Pazzaglia PJ, Post RM, Ketter TA, et al: Preliminary controlled trial of nimodipine in ultra-rapid cycling affective dysregulation. Psychiatry Res 49:257–272, 1993

Perry PJ, Dunner FJ, Hahn RL, et al: Lithium kinetics in single daily dosing. Acta Psychiatr Scand 64:281–294, 1981

Phelan KM, Mosholder AD, Lu S: Lithium interaction with the cycloxygenase-2 inhibitors refecoxib and celecoxib and other nonsteroidal anti-inflammatory drugs. J Clin Psychiatry 64:1328–1334, 2003

Physicians' Desk Reference, 58th Edition. Montvale, NJ, Thomson Healthcare, 2004

Pies R: Psychotropic medication during pregnancy and postpartum. Clinical Advances in the Treatment of Psychiatric Disorders 9:4–7, 1995a

Pies R: Women, mood, and the thyroid. Women's Psychiatric Health 4:4–11, 1995b

Pies R: Combining lithium with mood stabilizers. Ann Clin Psychiatry 14:223–232, 2002a

Pies R: Have we undersold lithium? (editorial). J Clin Psychopharmacol 22:445–449, 2002b

Pies R, Popli AP: Self-injurious behavior: pathophysiology and implications for treatment. J Clin Psychiatry 56:580–588, 1995

Plenge P, Mellerup ET, Bolwig TG, et al: Lithium treatment: does the kidney prefer one daily dose instead of two? Acta Psychiatr Scand 66:121–128, 1982

Pope HG Jr, McElroy SL, Nixon RA: Possible synergism between fluoxetine and lithium in refractory depression. Am J Psychiatry 145:1292–1294, 1988

Popli AP, Tanquary J, Lamparella V, et al: Bupropion and anticonvulsant drug interactions. Ann Clin Psychiatry 7:99–101, 1995

Post RM: Issues in the long-term management of bipolar affective illness. Psychiatr Ann 23:86–93, 1993

Post RM, Frye MA, Denicoff KD, et al: Preliminary algorithms for treatment-resistant bipolar depression, in Treatment-Resistant Mood Disorders. Edited by Amsterdam JD, Hornig M, Nierenberg AA. Cambridge, England, Cambridge University Press, 2001, pp 350–404

Post RM, Leverich GS, Nolen WA, et al: A re-evaluation of the role of antidepressants in the treatment of bipolar depression: data from the Stanley Foundation Bipolar Network. Bipolar Disord 5:296–406, 2003

Potter WZ, Ketter TA: Pharmacological issues in the treatment of bipolar disorder: focus on mood-stabilizing compounds. Can J Psychiatry 38 (suppl 2):51–56, 1993

Price LH, Carpenter LL, Rasmussen SA: Drug combination strategies, in Treatment-Resistant Mood Disorders. Edited by Amsterdam JD, Hornig M, Nierenberg AA. Cambridge, England, Cambridge University Press, 2001, pp 194–222.

Ragheb M: The clinical significance of lithium-nonsteroidal anti-inflammatory drug interactions. J Clin Psychopharmacol 10:350–354, 1990

Reich T, Winokur G: Postpartum psychosis in patients with manic depressive disease. J Nerv Ment Dis 151:60–68, 1970

Reinstein MD, Sonnenberg JG, Mohan SC, et al: Oxcarbazepine: review of 200 subjects treated for mania in a hospital setting. Paper presented at the 155th annual meeting of the American Psychiatric Association, Philadelphia, PA, May 18–23, 2002

Rifkin A, Quitkin F, Curillo C, et al: Lithium carbonate in emotionally unstable character disorders. Arch Gen Psychiatry 27:519–523, 1972

Robillard M, Conn DK: Lamotrigine use in geriatric patients with bipolar depression. Can J Psychiatry 47:767–770, 2002

Rosenblatt JE, Rosenblatt NC: Clinical psychopharmacology: olanzapine-fluoxetine combination for bipolar depression. Currents in Affective Illness 23:1–2, 2004

Sachs GS, Lafer B, Stoll AL, et al: A double-blind trial of bupropion versus desipramine for bipolar depression. J Clin Psychiatry 55:391–393, 1994

Sachs GS, Printz DJ, Kahn DA, et al: The Expert Consensus Guideline Series: medication treatment of bipolar disorders 2000. Postgrad Med Special Report, April 2000, pp 1–104

Sandson NB: Drug Interactions Casebook. Washington, DC, American Psychiatric Publishing, 2003

Sansone MEG, Ziegler DK: Lithium toxicity: a review of neurologic complications. Clin Neuropharmacol 8:242–248, 1985

Sarid-Segal O, Creelman WL, Shader RI: Lithium, in Drug Interactions in Psychiatry, 2nd Edition. Edited by Ciraulo DA, Shader RI, Greenblatt DJ, et al. Baltimore, MD, Williams & Wilkins, 1995, pp 175–213

Schexnayder LW, Hirschowitz J, Sautter FJ, et al: Predictors of response to lithium in patients with psychoses. Am J Psychiatry 152:1511–1513, 1995

Schou M: Hyperlithemia correction: an untraditional view (letter). J Clin Psychiatry 57:42, 1996

Shader RI: Approaches to the treatment of manic-depressive states, in Manual of Psychiatric Therapeutics, 2nd Edition. Edited by Shader RI. Boston, MA, Little, Brown, 1994, pp 247–258

Shelton MD, Calabrese JR: Lamotrigine, in The American Psychiatric Publishing Textbook of Psychopharmacology, 3rd Edition. Edited by Schatzberg AF, Nemeroff CB. Washington, DC, American Psychiatric Publishing, 2004, pp 615–626

Shivakumar G, Suppes T: Bipolar treatment update. Current Psychiatry 3:23–40, 2004

Sillanpaa M: Carbamazepine: pharmacology and clinical uses. Acta Neurol Scand Suppl 88:139–161, 1981

Solomon DA, Ryan CE, Keitner GI, et al: A pilot study of lithium carbonate plus divalproex for the continuation and maintenance treatment of patients with bipolar I disorder. J Clin Psychiatry 58:95–99, 1997

Sovner R: A clinically significant interaction between carbamazepine and valproic acid. J Clin Psychopharmacol 8:448–449, 1988

Sovner R, Davis JM: A potential drug interaction between fluoxetine and valproic acid. (letter). J Clin Psychopharmacol 11:389, 1991

Sporn J, Sachs G: The anticonvulsant lamotrigine in treatment-resistant manic-depressive illness. J Clin Psychopharmacol 17:185–189, 1997

Srisurapanont M, Yatham LN, Zis AP: Treatment of acute bipolar depression: a review of the literature. Can J Psychiatry 40:533–544, 1995

Stahl SM: Psychopharmacology of anticonvulsants: do all anticonvulsants have the same mechanism of action? J Clin Psychiatry 65:149–150, 2004

Sternbach H: The serotonin syndrome. Am J Psychiatry 148:705–713, 1991

Stoll AL, Severus WE: Mood stabilizers: shared mechanisms of action at postsynaptic signal-transduction and kindling processes. Harv Rev Psychiatry 4:77–89, 1996

Stoll AL, Severus WE, Freeman MP, et al: Omega-3 fatty acids in bipolar disorder: a preliminary double-blind, placebo-controlled trial. Arch Gen Psychiatry 56:407–412, 1999

Strakowski SM, McElroy SL, Keck PE Jr: Clinical efficacy of valproate in bipolar illness: comparisons and contrasts with lithium, in Pharmacotherapy for Mood, Anxiety, and Cognitive Disorders. Edited by Halbreich U, Montgomery SA. Washington, DC, American Psychiatric Press, 2000, pp 143–157

Suppes T, Baldessarini RJ, Faedda GL, et al: Risk of recurrence following discontinuation of lithium treatment in bipolar disorder. Arch Gen Psychiatry 48:1082–1088, 1991

Suppes T, Dennehy EB, Swann AC, et al: Report of the Texas Consensus Conference Panel on medication treatment of bipolar disorder 2000. J Clin Psychiatry 63:288–299, 2002

Susman VL, Addonizio G: Reinduction of neuroleptic malignant syndrome by lithium. J Clin Psychopharmacol 7:339–341, 1987

Swann AC, Bowden CL, Calabrese JR, et al: Mania: differential effects of previous depressive and manic episodes on response to treatment. Acta Psychiatr Scand 101:444–451, 2000

Swartz CM, Jones P: Drs Swartz and Jones reply (to letter of M Schou). J Clin Psychiatry 57:42–43, 1996

Taflinski T, Chojnacka J: Sibutramine-associated psychotic episode. Am J Psychiatry 157:2057–2058, 2000

Tiihonen J, Hallikainen T, Tyyananen OP, et al: Lamotrigine in treatment-resistant schizophrenia: a randomized placebo-controlled crossover trial. Biol Psychiatry 54:1241–1248, 2003

Tohen M, Castillo J, Pope HG Jr, et al: Concomitant use of valproate and carbamazepine in bipolar and schizoaffective disorders. J Clin Psychopharmacol 14:67–70, 1994

Tohen M, Vieta E, Calabrese J, et al: Efficacy of olanzapine and olanzapine-fluoxetine combination in the treatment of bipolar I depression. Arch Gen Psychiatry 60:1079–1088, 2003

Tondo L, Baldessarini RJ, Floris G: Long-term clinical effectiveness of lithium maintenance treatment in types I and II bipolar disorders. Br J Psychiatry Suppl 41:S184-S190, 2001

Trannel TJ, Ahmed I, Goebert D: Occurrence of thrombocytopenia in psychiatric patients taking valproate. Am J Psychiatry 158:128–130, 2001

Trimble MR: Anticonvulsants in children and adolescents. J Child Adolesc Psychopharmacol 1:107–124, 1990

Vadnal R, Parthasarathy R: Myo-inositol monophosphatase: diverse effects of lithium, carbamazepine, and valproate. Neuropsychopharmacology 12:277–285, 1995

Venkatakrishnan K, Shader RI, von Moltke LL, et al: Drug interactions in psychopharmacology, in Manual of Psychiatric Therapeutics, 3rd Edition. Edited by Shader RI. Philadelphia, PA, Lippincott Williams & Wilkins, 2003, pp 441–470

Viguera AC, Nonacs R, Cohen LS, et al: Risk of recurrence of bipolar disorder in pregnant and nonpregnant women after discontinuing lithium maintenance. Am J Psychiatry 157:179–184, 2000

Wagner KD: Treatment of childhood and adolescent disorders, in The American Psychiatric Publishing Textbook of Psychopharmacology, 3rd Edition. Edited by Schatzberg AF, Nemeroff CB. Washington, DC, American Psychiatric Publishing, 2004, pp 949–1007

Walton SA, Berk M, Brook S: Superiority of lithium over verapamil in mania: a randomized, controlled single-blind trial. J Clin Psychiatry 57:543–546, 1996

Wang PW, Ketter TA, Becker OV, et al: New anticonvulsant medication uses in bipolar disorder. CNS Spectr 8:941–947, 2003

Weiner RD, Coffey CE: Indications for use of electroconvulsive therapy, in The American Psychiatric Press Review of Psychiatry, Vol 7. Edited by Frances AJ, Hales RE. Washington, DC, American Psychiatric Press, 1988, pp 458–481

Weller E, Weller R, Fristad M: Lithium dosage guide for prepubertal children: a preliminary report. J Am Acad Child Psychiatry 25:92–95, 1986

West SA, Keck PE Jr, McElroy SL: Valproate, in Mania: Clinical and Research Perspectives. Edited by Goodnick P. Washington, DC, American Psychiatric Press, 1998, pp 301–317

Wilder BJ: Pharmacokinetics of valproate and carbamazepine. J Clin Psychopharmacol 12 (suppl):64S-68S, 1992

Yildiz A, Sachs GS: Do antidepressants induce rapid cycling? A gender-specific association. J Clin Psychiatry 64:814–818, 2003

Zerjav-Lacombe S, Tabarsi E: Lamotrigine: a review of clinical studies in bipolar disorders. Can J Psychiatry 46:328–333, 2001

Zornberg GL, Pope HG Jr: Treatment of depression in bipolar disorder: new directions for research. J Clin Psychopharmacol 13:397–408, 1993

CME QUESTIONS AND ANSWERS TO THE *HANDBOOK OF ESSENTIAL PSYCHOPHARMACOLOGY,* SECOND EDITION

Continuing Medical Education Activity
Sponsored by the
American Psychiatric Association

CME Questions and Answers for the *Handbook of Essential Psychopharmacology,* Second Edition

A Continuing Medical Education Activity Sponsored by the American Psychiatric Association

This continuing medical education (CME) activity takes approximately 10 hours to complete. The participant should read the text of the book, consider the objectives below, and answer the questions in the multiple choice test. To receive credit for this activity, complete the evaluation and accompanying attestation form and mail them to

American Psychiatric Association
Department of CME
1000 Wilson Blvd., Suite 1825
Arlington, VA 22209

Accreditation/Designation

The American Psychiatric Association (APA) is accredited by the Accreditation Council for Continuing Medical Education (ACCME) to provide continuing medical education for physicians.

The APA designates this educational activity for a maximum of 10 category 1 credits toward the AMA Physician's Recognition Award and for the CME requirement of the APA. Each physician should claim only those credits that he or she actually spent in the activity.

Target audience: This CME activity is intended for practicing clinical psychiatrists and other physicians who prescribe psychotropic medications.

Objectives: Completion of this activity will improve the participant's knowledge of psychopharmacological treatment of mental health disorders. The participant completes this activity by reading the text of the *Handbook of Es-*

sential Psychopharmacology, Second Edition, noting any new or unfamiliar treatment applications, and testing his or her knowledge by answering the multiple choice questions in this section. Participants should blind the answers to the questions prior to answering.

Estimated time to complete: 10 hours
Date of original release: April 15, 2005
Program review date: April 15, 2008
Program end date: May 1, 2008

APA Disclosure: Neither the American Psychiatric Association (APA) nor American Psychiatric Publishing, Inc. (APPI), received commercial support for the development or production of this CME product.

Faculty Disclosure: Ronald W. Pies, M.D., has indicated that neither he nor an immediate family member has a significant financial interest or affiliation with any commercial organization(s) that may have a direct or indirect interest in this CME product. Dr. Pies also indicated that his text includes discussion of off-label and investigational uses or use of products not yet approved. Specifically, Questions 7, 21, 42, 46, and 49 discuss off-label use of medications.

Evaluation of the *Handbook of Essential Psychopharmacology,* Second Edition, CME Self-Study Activity

Please indicate your reaction to the following statements about this CME self-study activity by circling the appropriate response.

1. Overall, the quality of the CME self-study activity is excellent.
   A. Strongly agree
   B. Agree
   C. Disagree
   D. Strongly disagree

2. The CME self-study activity met its stated objectives.
   A. Strongly agree
   B. Agree
   C. Disagree
   D. Strongly disagree

3. The CME self-study activity provided information that I find useful for my practice.
   A. Strongly agree
   B. Agree
   C. Disagree
   D. Strongly disagree

4. The contents of the CME self-study activity were balanced and free of commercial bias.
   A. Strongly agree
   B. Agree
   C. Disagree
   D. Strongly disagree

I certify that I have read this material and studied the questions for a total of at least ___ hours.

____

Signature

____

Name

____

Address

____

Daytime phone Fax Number

Are you an APA member? ❑ Yes ❑ No

What is your discipline? ❑ Psychiatrist ❑ Other physician
❑ Psychologist ❑ Nurse ❑ Other ________________

To receive your CME credit, return this completed form to

American Psychiatric Association
Department of CME
1000 Wilson Blvd., Suite 1825
Arlington, VA 22209

Program End Date: May 1, 2008 (Self-test will not be accepted for scoring/CME certification after this date.)

CME QUESTIONS AND ANSWERS

1. Which of the following agents, at low doses, work primarily as serotonin *reuptake inhibitors?*

   a. Mirtazapine
   b. Venlafaxine
   c. Sertraline
   d. b and c
   e. None of the above

   ANS: **d**

2. If paroxetine 20 mg qd were added to risperidone 2 mg bid, what would be a possible outcome of this therapy?

   a. Increase in muscle rigidity
   b. Increase in prolactin levels
   c. Akathisia
   d. Tremor
   e. All of the above

   ANS: **e**

3. Expected effects from agents that act as *agonists* at 5-HT_2 and 5-HT_3 receptors include

   a. Anxiety
   b. Sexual dysfunction
   c. Insomnia
   d. Gastrointestinal problems
   e. All of the above

   ANS: **e**

4. Based on postulated effects on serotonin, which of the following agents would cause relatively *little* sexual dysfunction, compared with fluoxetine?

   a. Nefazodone
   b. Mirtazapine
   c. Bupropion
   d. Sertraline
   e. a, b, and c

   ANS: e

5. Which of the following agents has the most potent inhibitory effects on the cytochrome P450 3A4 enzyme?

   a. Nefazodone
   b. Trazodone
   c. Citalopram
   d. Venlafaxine
   e. None of the above

   ANS: a

6. Agents that may decrease the blood levels and/or therapeutic effect of various antidepressants include all of the following *except*

   a. Carbamazepine
   b. Phenytoin
   c. Cimetidine
   d. Rifampin
   e. Phenobarbital

   ANS: c

7. Which of the following agents have been proven useful in the treatment of panic disorder?

   a. Fluoxetine
   b. Paroxetine
   c. Imipramine
   d. Sertraline
   e. All of the above

   ANS: e

8. Therapeutic plasma levels have been established for which of the following agent(s)?

   a. Paroxetine
   b. Mirtazapine
   c. Nortriptyline
   d. None of the above
   e. All of the above

   ANS: c

9. Based on its mechanism of action, which of the following agents has a minimal effect on serotonin?

   a. Citalopram
   b. Mirtazapine
   c. Bupropion
   d. Nefazodone
   e. None of the above

   ANS: c

10. Which of the following antidepressants have FDA-approved labeling for the treatment of borderline personality disorder?

    a. Paroxetine
    b. Fluvoxamine
    c. Sertraline
    d. a and b
    e. None of the above

    ANS: e

11. Which of the following agents have significantly more potent antagonism of dopamine D_2 receptors, compared with olanzapine?

    a. Haloperidol
    b. Risperidone
    c. Clozapine
    d. a and b
    e. None of the above

    ANS: d

12. Aripiprazole is best described as which of the following?

    a. Potent D_2 antagonist
    b. Potent D_1 antagonist
    c. Partial agonist at D_2 receptors
    d. Antagonist at 5-HT_{2A} receptors
    e. c and d

    ANS: **e**

13. With respect to QTc prolongation, which of the following comparisons is correct?

    a. Haloperidol > risperidone > olanzapine > ziprasidone
    b. Pimozide > olanzapine > ziprasidone > quetiapine
    c. Thioridazine > ziprasidone > haloperidol > olanzapine
    d. Ziprasidone > thioridazine > olanzapine > quetiapine
    e. None of the above

    ANS: **c**

14. Which of the following agents or actions are most likely to *increase* plasma clozapine levels?

    a. Cigarette smoking
    b. Carbamazepine
    c. Phenytoin
    d. None of the above
    e. All of the above

    ANS: **d**

15. An increased risk of cerebrovascular adverse events has been associated with which of the following scenarios?

    a. Use of atypical antipsychotic agent in delirious patients
    b. Use of atypical antipsychotic agent in dementia patients
    c. Use of typical neuroleptic agent in bipolar patients
    d. Use of atypical antipsychotic agent in schizophrenia patients
    e. None of the above

    ANS: **b**

16. Which of the following agents have the best-established correlation between plasma blood levels and therapeutic response?

    a. Haloperidol
    b. Risperidone
    c. Quetiapine
    d. Aripiprazole
    e. All of the above

   ANS: a

17. With respect to clinically significant anticholinergic effects, which of the following statements is most accurate?

    a. Ziprasidone has greater anticholinergic effects than clozapine
    b. Haloperidol has greater anticholinergic effects than risperidone
    c. Risperidone has greater anticholinergic effects than quetiapine
    d. Clozapine has greater anticholinergic effects than risperidone
    e. None of the above

   ANS: d

18. Which of the following represents an FDA-approved indication for use of some atypical antipsychotic agents?

    a. Acute treatment of schizophrenia
    b. Acute treatment of mania
    c. Maintenance treatment of bipolar disorder
    d. Treatment of bipolar depression, combined with fluoxetine
    e. All of the above

   ANS: e

19. Agranulocytosis with clozapine most often has its onset

    a. Within 2 days of starting clozapine
    b. Within 6 months of starting clozapine
    c. After 2 years of clozapine treatment
    d. After 4 years of clozapine treatment
    e. None of the above

   ANS: b

20. A patient receiving clozapine has an absolute neutrophil count (ANC) of $800/mm^3$. Which of the following is correct?

    a. Continue clozapine if the patient remains psychotic
    b. Hold clozapine for 1 week; rechallenge; monitor ANC weekly
    c. Hold clozapine for 1 week; restart clozapine if next ANC is normal ($>2,000/mm^3$)
    d. Hold clozapine; consider infection precautions; do not rechallenge
    e. None of the above

    ANS: **d**

21. A patient with schizophrenia taking an atypical antipsychotic is started on carbamazepine for possible manic symptoms. Which of the following is *most* likely?

    a. The patient will show immediate psychotic decompensation
    b. The patient's carbamazepine blood level will rise much higher than expected, owing to the presence of the antipsychotic
    c. The patient's antipsychotic blood level will decrease significantly, owing to the effect of carbamazepine
    d. The patient's antipsychotic blood level will triple, owing to the effect of carbamazepine
    e. None of the above

    ANS: **c**

22. The incidence of serious (nonbenign) rash is increased significantly when lamotrigine is used concomitantly with which of the following agents?

    a. Olanzapine
    b. Lithium
    c. Risperidone
    d. All of the above
    e. None of the above

    ANS: **e**

23. Which of the following agents have FDA-approved labeling for the short-term and maintenance treatment of bipolar I disorder?

    a. Carbamazepine
    b. Topiramate
    c. Olanzapine
    d. a and c
    e. All of the above

    ANS: c

24. Pharmacokinetic interactions with valproic acid would most likely be seen with which of the following medications?

    a. Lithium
    b. Gabapentin
    c. Lamotrigine
    d. a and c
    e. None of the above

    ANS: c

25. Once-daily (qd) dosing of lithium results in which of the following, in comparison to twice daily (bid) dosing, assuming the same total daily dose and clearance?

    a. Higher average steady-state lithium levels
    b. Lower average steady-state lithium levels
    c. Marked increase in polyuria and polydipsia
    d. No change in average steady-state lithium levels
    e. None of the above

    ANS: d

26. Which of the following are "black box warnings" for patients taking divalproex (valproic acid)?

    a. Pancreatitis
    b. Hepatotoxicity
    c. Teratogenicity
    d. None of the above
    e. All of the above

    ANS: e

27. When added to lithium, which of the following medications can significantly increase plasma lithium levels?

    a. Lisinopril (Prinivil)
    b. Celecoxib (Celebrex)
    c. Haloperidol
    d. a and b
    e. All of the above

    ANS: **d**

28. Carbamazepine has which of the following interactions with clozapine?

    a. Increased hepatic clearance of clozapine
    b. Decreased hepatic clearance of clozapine
    c. Possible increased risk of agranulocytosis
    d. a and c
    e. None of the above

    ANS: **d**

29. After how many days following drug initiation, or dosage increase, should a lithium blood level ordinarily be obtained?

    a. After about 4–5 lithium half-lives, or roughly 1 day
    b. After about 4–5 lithium half-lives, or roughly 5 days
    c. After about 2–3 lithium half-lives, or roughly 2 days
    d. After about 6–7 lithium half-lives, or roughly 12 days
    e. None of the above

    ANS: **b**

30. Which of the following statements regarding lamotrigine are correct?

    a. Lamotrigine has FDA-approved labeling for maintenance treatment in bipolar disorder
    b. Lamotrigine probably has greater efficacy in delaying relapse of bipolar depression than in treating or preventing manic episodes
    c. Lamotrigine causes serious rash in approximately 8% of treated patients
    d. a and b
    e. None of the above

    ANS: **d**

31. The neurotransmitter affected most by lorazepam and diazepam is
    a. Chloride
    b. Serotonin
    c. GABA
    d. Dopamine
    e. None of the above

ANS: c

32. Which of the following benzodiazepines has the shortest elimination half-life?
    a. Lorazepam
    b. Alprazolam
    c. Temazepam
    d. Triazolam
    e. Estazolam

ANS: **d**

33. In a patient with severe cirrhosis, which benzodiazepine(s) would be the preferred agent(s), all other factors being equal?
    a. Lorazepam
    b. Oxazepam
    c. Temazepam
    d. All of the above
    e. None of the above

ANS: **d**

34. In converting a patient from diazepam 10 mg/day, which choice would be the most appropriate?
    a. Clonazepam 0.5 mg/day
    b. Lorazepam 4 mg/day
    c. Alprazolam 3 mg/day
    d. Oxazepam 5 mg/day
    e. None of the above

ANS: a

35. The proposed mechanism of action for buspirone is

    a. Potentiation of GABA
    b. Inhibition of serotonin reuptake
    c. 5-HT_{1A} receptor partial agonism
    d. 5-HT_2 receptor antagonism
    e. None of the above

ANS: c

36. Which statement is most accurate with respect to documented risks of benzodiazepine (BZD) administration?

    a. BZDs are absolutely contraindicated for use beyond 3 weeks
    b. BZDs have been proven ineffective for insomnia, after 2 weeks of use
    c. BZDs are usually contraindicated in patients with a strong history of alcohol/substance abuse
    d. BZDs do not pose a risk of withdrawal symptoms if suddenly discontinued
    e. None of the above

ANS: c

37. Which statement regarding zolpidem is *incorrect*?

    a. Zolpidem interacts with the same major binding site as diazepam
    b. Its actions can be reversed by flumazenil
    c. Zolpidem acts as a GABA antagonist
    d. Zolpidem acts with high affinity at $GABA_A$ receptors with α_1 subunits
    e. None of the above

ANS: c

38. Which of the following statements regarding benzodiazepine (BZD) use in the elderly are correct?

    a. BZD use is associated with increased risk of hip fracture in the elderly
    b. BZD use is associated with increased risk of cognitive impairment in dementia patients
    c. BZD use is associated with increased risk of disinhibition in dementia patients
    d. a, b, and c
    e. None of the above

    ANS: d

39. Pharmacokinetic interactions with benzodiazepines can be seen with which of the following medications?

    a. Fluoxetine
    b. Erythromycin
    c. Cimetidine
    d. Phenytoin
    e. All of the above

    ANS: e

40. Clonidine's mechanism of action most resembles that of which of the following agents?

    a. Guanfacine
    b. Mirtazapine
    c. Terazosin
    d. Doxepin
    e. None of the above

    ANS: a

41. Which laboratory abnormalities are required for the diagnosis of serotonin syndrome?

    a. Elevation of creatine phosphokinase (CPK)
    b. Elevation of white blood cell count (WBC)
    c. Elevation of liver function tests (LFTs)
    d. Reduction in 5-hydroxyindoleacetic acid (5-HIAA)
    e. None of the above

    ANS: e

42. Extrapyramidal side effects of antipsychotics may respond to which of the following medications?
    a. Biperiden
    b. Trihexyphenidyl
    c. Amantadine
    d. All of the above
    e. None of the above

    ANS: **d**

43. Which of the following statements regarding monthly haloperidol decanoate is correct?
    a. Peak plasma level after injection is reached around day 6; steady state is reached after about 3 months
    b. Peak plasma level after injection is reached around day 2; steady state is reached after about 2 weeks
    c. Peak plasma level after injection is reached around day 30; steady state is reached after about 6 months
    d. Peak plasma level after injection is reached around day 6; steady state is reached after about 1 month
    e. None of the above

    ANS: **a**

44. Which of the following statements are true regarding risperidone microspheres (long-acting risperidone)?
    a. It is given every 4 weeks
    b. All oral antipsychotics should be discontinued prior to the first injection
    c. A 3-week overlap between oral antipsychotic and injection is recommended
    d. Routine plasma level monitoring is required
    e. All of the above

    ANS: **c**

45. Which of the following are likely to result in an increase in serum lithium levels?

    a. Increase in sodium intake
    b. Increase in fluid intake
    c. Levothyroxine
    d. Ibuprofen
    e. All of the above

ANS: d

46. Which of the following agents has been proven useful as monotherapy for panic attacks (panic disorder)?

    a. Buspirone
    b. Lithium
    c. Fluoxetine
    d. Aripiprazole
    e. None of the above

ANS: c

47. Which of the following statements is *incorrect* with respect to medication use during the first trimester of pregnancy?

    a. Benzodiazepines are associated with increased incidence of cleft lip or palate
    b. SSRI use is associated with a markedly increased incidence of major fetal malformations
    c. Valproic acid and carbamazepine are associated with increased risk of spinal cord or craniofacial abnormalities
    d. There are very few controlled, prospective studies of psychotropic use during pregnancy
    e. Most antipsychotics do not appear to be major teratogens, but controlled data are lacking

ANS: b

48. Which of the following statements regarding treatment of bipolar disorder is correct?
    a. Divalproex appears to be superior to lithium for mixed/dysphoric mania
    b. Divalproex appears to be superior to lithium for classic, euphoric mania
    c. Lamotrigine is superior to lithium for prophylaxis of mania
    d. Oxcarbazepine has been proven effective for bipolar depression
    e. None of the above

    ANS: a

49. Which of the following statements regarding augmentation of antidepressants are correct?
    a. Lithium may potentiate the effects of some antidepressants in unipolar depression
    b. Some data indicate that thyroid hormone may potentiate the effects of tricyclic antidepressants in unipolar depression
    c. Olanzapine may augment the effects of fluoxetine in unipolar, nonpsychotic major depression
    d. Combining bupropion with an SSRI may be a useful augmentation strategy, though controlled data are lacking
    e. All of the above

    ANS: e

50. Which of the following agents have been shown effective in bipolar depression (acute or maintenance treatment) on the basis of controlled studies?
    a. Lamotrigine
    b. Lithium
    c. Combination of olanzapine and fluoxetine
    d. a, b, and c
    e. None of the above.

    ANS: d

INDEX

Page numbers printed in ***boldface*** type refer to tables or figures.

AA (Alcoholics Anonymous), **356**
Abilify. *See* Aripiprazole
Absorption of drugs, 6–7
ACE (angiotensin-converting enzyme) inhibitor interactions
  with antipsychotics, **176**
  with lithium, **370**, 419
Acetaminophen interactions
  with antidepressants, **60**, 102
  with lithium, 418
Acetazolamide interactions
  with lithium, **370**
  with topiramate, 402, 420
Acetophenazine, **148**
Acetylcholine
  lithium actions on, 340
  receptors for, 5
Acne, lithium-induced, **367**
Adapin. *See* Doxepin
Adderall, Adderall XR, 74
ADHD. *See* Attention-deficit/hyperactivity disorder
Adolescents. *See* Children and adolescents
α_1-Adrenergic receptors
  antidepressant actions at, **37**
  antipsychotic actions at, 143, **159**, 197
α_2-Adrenergic receptors
  antidepressant actions at, **37**, 88
  antipsychotic actions at, 141
ADs. *See* Antidepressants
Aggressive behavior
  antidepressants for
    selective serotonin reuptake inhibitors, **33**
    tricyclics, **35**
  antipsychotics for, 140, **155**
    alternatives to, **155**, 194
    beta-blocker augmentation of, **178**
  buspirone for, **262**
  in dementia patients, 194

Aggressive behavior *(continued)*
mood stabilizers for, 339, 400
lithium, **349**, 399–400
Aging. *See* Elderly patients
Agitation
drug-induced
antidepressants, **49–50**
aripiprazole, 390
management of, **58**
antipsychotics in, 140, 193
barbiturates in, 298
benzodiazepines in, **58**, 293
beta-blockers in, **58**, 254, **271**
buspirone in, 225, **262**
clonidine in, 254
gabapentin in, **58**
guanfacine in, 254
trazodone in, 194
Agonists, 2
inverse, 3
partial, 3
Agoraphobia. *See also* Panic disorder
tiagabine for, 299
Agranulocytosis, drug-induced
clozapine, 143, 206–207
management of, **173–174**
mirtazapine, 96–97
AISD. *See* Sexual dysfunction, antidepressant-induced
Akathisia, antipsychotic-induced, 143, **164**, 203–204
atypical antipsychotics and, 202, 208
definition of, 203
management of, **171**
benzodiazepines in, 204, 234, **268**
beta-blockers in, **171**, 202, 204, 233–234
pathophysiology of, 203–204
prevalence of, 203
prophylaxis for, 202
treatment response and, 203
Akineton (biperiden), **165**
Alcohol
actions on $GABA_A$ receptors, **272**
interaction with benzodiazepines, 257, **283**, 310
metabolism of, 10
withdrawal from
benzodiazepines for, 254, **269**
kindling and, 405
Alcoholics Anonymous (AA), **356**
Alcoholism
lithium for, **350**, 400
support groups for, **356**
Alogia, in schizophrenia, 195, 197
Alopecia, drug-induced
carbamazepine, 342
lithium, **368**
valproate, **181**, 342, **364**, 415–416
Alprazolam
abuse liability of, 307–308
in relatives of substance abusers, 308
cost of, **265**
discontinuation of, 309
dosage of, **260**
drug interactions with, **282, 283**
antidepressants, 312
fluvoxamine, 120
antipsychotics, **176**
carbamazepine, 429
formulations of, **260**
indications for
antipsychotic augmentation, **178**
avoidant personality disorder, **266**
depression, **268**, 291, 297–298
panic disorder, **266**, 429
posttraumatic stress disorder, **267**

Alprazolam *(continued)*
indications for *(continued)*
social phobia, **266**
suicidality, 298
pharmacokinetics of, 256, **274**
metabolic pathway, **277**, 305, 311
side effects of, 306
mania, 297
sublingual, 290
switching to clonazepam from, 321
use in special populations
elderly and/or dementia patients, **288**
pregnancy, 315
withdrawal from, 289, 308
Alzheimer's disease.
See also Dementia
antipsychotics in, 193
vs. buspirone for agitation, 225
Amantadine
for antidepressant-induced sexual dysfunction, 99
for extrapyramidal side effects, **165, 171**
Ambien. *See* Zolpidem
Amino acid neurotransmitters, 3, 4
receptors for, 4
γ-Aminobutyric acid (GABA), 2, 4
anticonvulsant actions on, 340, **357**
carbamazepine, 405
valproate, 404
antipsychotic actions on, 145
γ-Aminobutyric acid (GABA) receptors
$GABA_A$ receptor, 255
anxiolytic and sedative-hypnotic actions at, 255, **272–273**, 303–304
fluoxetine actions at, 256
subunits of, 255, 304
$GABA_B$ receptor, baclofen actions at, 302
Amiodarone, interaction with antipsychotics, 144
Amitriptyline
age effects on metabolism of, 90
dosage of, **28**
drug interactions with
benzodiazepines, **283**, 312
lithium, **372**
formulations of, **28**
indications for, **33–35**
depressed cancer patients, 111
panic disorder, 82
intramuscular, 79, 113
mechanism of action of, **27**, **36**
plasma levels of, **48**
in pregnancy, 114
rectal, 113
side effects of, **49**
seizures, 95
use in borderline personality disorder, 81
use in hepatic disease, 92
Amnesia. *See* Memory, drug-induced impairment of
Amobarbital, 298
Amoxapine, **28**
for psychotic depression, **157**
Amphetamine, **73–74**
Amphetamine mixed salts, **74**
Amytal interview, 298
Anafranil. *See* Clomipramine
Androgens, interaction with antidepressants, 102
Angiotensin-converting enzyme (ACE) inhibitor interactions
with antipsychotics, **176**
with lithium, **370**, 419

Anhedonia, in schizophrenia, 195, 197
Anorexia nervosa, fluoxetine for, **32**
Anorgasmia. *See* Sexual dysfunction
Antacids
  during carbamazepine therapy, **373**
  drug interactions with
    antipsychotics, 145, **175**
    benzodiazepines, **283**, 304, 311
    valproate, **378**
Antagonists, 2
  neutral, 2
Antiarrhythmic drug interactions, 10
  with antidepressants, 114
    selective serotonin reuptake inhibitors, **61**, 103, 112, 114
    tricyclics, 101
Anticholinergic agents. *See also specific drugs*
  drug interactions with
    antipsychotics, 144, **175**, 203
    benzodiazepines, 257, **283**
    tricyclic antidepressants, **60**
  for extrapyramidal side effects, 144, **165, 171**
    akathisia, 204
    benzodiazepine augmentation of, **286**
    dosage of, **165**
    prophylactic, 201–202
  for hypersalivation, 144, 205–206
Anticholinergic effects
  of antidepressants, **49–50, 53, 56**
    in cancer patients, 111–112
    tricyclics, 22, 111–112
  of antihistamines, **262**
  of antipsychotics, 143, 144, 145, **162–163, 171**, 208
  central anticholinergic syndrome, **67–69**, 112, 234–235
  management of, **56, 171**
Anticoagulant interactions, 10
  with antidepressants, 103
    selective serotonin reuptake inhibitors, **61**
    tricyclics, **60**
  with benzodiazepines, 311
  with carbamazepine, 343, **373**
Anticonvulsants. *See also* Mood stabilizers; *specific drugs*
  combination of, **385–386**
  combined with lithium, **381–384**
  drug interactions with, **373–380**
    antidepressants, 24, 102
    antipsychotics, **175**
    benzodiazepines, 257
  indications for
    antipsychotic augmentation, 216–217
    anxiety disorders, 254, 299–300
    behavioral disturbances in dementia, **155**
    bipolar disorder, 338–433
  in kindling, 405–406
  mechanisms of action of, 340, **357**, 404–405
  side effects of, 342–343, **362–365**
  tolerance to, 406
  use in special populations, 345, **387–388**
Antidepressants (ADs), 19–122. *See also specific drugs and classes*
  adequate duration of trial for, 103
  choice of, 79–80
  class of, 19
  classification of, 19, 21, **27**
  comparative efficacy of, 104
  cost of, **31**, 80

Antidepressants (ADs) *(continued)*
discontinuation of, 91–92
cholinergic rebound syndrome after, 91
elimination half-life and, 91–92
relapse after, 80
tapering schedule for, 91
dosage of, **28–30**
for children and adolescents, **78**
drug interactions with, 23–24, **60–65**, 80, 101–103, 118–120
anticonvulsants, 102
antipsychotics, 102, **175**, 212–213
benzodiazepines, **283**, 311–312, 314
carbamazepine, **375**
nonpsychotropic medications, 113–114
serotonin syndrome due to, 24
food interactions with, **63**, 103
formulations of, **28–30**
generic names of, **28–30**
heterocyclic, 19
heterogeneity of, 19
indications for, 20, **32–35**, 79–85
antipsychotic augmentation, **178**
anxiety disorders, 253, 254, 302
bipolar disorder, 20, 97–98, 338, 339, **353**, 391–393
borderline personality disorder, 81
depression with atypical features, 83–84
dysthymic disorder, 84–85
maintenance therapy, 80–81
mixed anxiety-depressive states, 83
obsessive-compulsive disorder, 82
postpartum depression, 26
intramuscular, 79, 113
intravenous, 79
mechanisms of action of, 4, 20–21, **27**, **36**, 85–90
drugs in development, 88, 89
effects of reuptake blockade and receptor antagonism, **37**
effects of serotonin receptor stimulation, **38**
predicting response based on, 89
speeding up, 89–90
neurotropic effects of, 21
onset of action of, 89–90
pharmacodynamics of, **42–47**
pharmacokinetics of, 21–22, **39–47**, 90–94
age effects on, 90–91
food effects on, 93
metabolism, 10, 21–22
protein binding, 21, 93
in renal and hepatic disease, 92–93
plasma levels of, 22, **48**, 94
potentiation of, 24–25, **71–72**, 103–110
vs. switching to another class of agent, 104–106
questions and answers about, 79–116
rectal, 113
side effects of, 22–23, **37**, **38**, **49–55**, 94–101
management of, **56–58**
mania or rapid cycling in bipolar disorder, 97–98, 391, 393, 394–395
risk factors for, **369**
seizures, 94–96
sexual dysfunction, **51**, **53**, 99–100
suicidality in children and adolescents, 121–122

Antidepressants (ADs) *(continued)*
trade names of, **28–30**
use in special populations, 75–77, 111–116
breastfeeding, 26, 116
cancer/medically ill patients, 111–114
children and adolescents, 26, **78**
elderly patients, 25
pregnancy, 26, 114–116
vignettes/puzzlers about, 117–122
withdrawal symptoms with, 91–92
Antidepressants, tricyclic (TCAs)
cost of, **31**, 80
dosage of, **28–29**
drug interactions with, **60**, 101–102
antipsychotics, 102, 144, **175**, 212
benzodiazepines, **283**, 312
carbamazepine, **60**, 343, **375**, 428–429
lithium, **372**
monoamine oxidase inhibitors, 24, **65**, 101, 109–110
selective serotonin reuptake inhibitors, 23, 24, **62**, 101
valproate, 343
efficacy of, 104
elimination half-lives of, 21, 92
drug discontinuation and, 91–92
formulations of, **28–29**
indications for, 20, **33–35**
aggression, **35**
antipsychotic augmentation, **178**
anxiety disorders, 302
borderline personality disorder, **34**
dementia-related syndromes, **35**
eating disorders, **34**
generalized anxiety disorder, **34**
hypochondriasis, **34**
insomnia, **34**
monoamine oxidase inhibitor potentiation, 109–110
obsessive-compulsive disorder, 20, **33**, 82
pain syndromes, **34**
panic disorder, **33**, 82
postpartum depression, 26
posttraumatic stress disorder, **34**, 302
social phobia, **34**
somatization disorder, **34**
mechanism of action of, **27**, **36**
overdose of, 80, 100–101
pharmacokinetics of, 10, 22, **40**
in renal and hepatic disease, 92–93
plasma levels of, 22, **48**, 94, 100–101, 117
potentiation of, 24, 25, **71–72**
selective serotonin reuptake inhibitors, 107
side effects of, 22–23, **49**
in elderly persons, 25
in medically ill patents, 111–112
seizures, 94–95
switching from selective serotonin reuptake inhibitors to, 104–106
therapeutic windows for, 22, **48**
use in special populations, **76**
cancer/medically ill patients, 111–113
children and adolescents, 26
elderly persons, 25
pregnancy, 114–115
withdrawal symptoms with, 91–92
Antidiarrheal agents, interaction with antipsychotics, **175**

Antihistamines, 254, **262**
side effects of, 257
memory impairment, 307
tolerance to, 257
Antihypertensive interactions
with antipsychotics, **176**
with monoamine oxidase inhibitors, 24, **65**
Antimicrobial interactions, 10
with antidepressants, 102–103, 114
selective serotonin reuptake inhibitors, **61**
with antipsychotics, 144, **177**, 214
with benzodiazepines, 257, **282**
with carbamazepine, 343, **374**
Antiparkinsonian agents
benzodiazepine augmentation of, **286**
for extrapyramidal side effects, 144, **165**, **171**
akathisia, 204
dosage of, **165**
prophylactic, 201–202
interaction with antipsychotics, 144
Antipsychotics (APs), 139–235. *See also specific drugs*
active metabolites of, 142
atypical, 25, 140
combination of, 145, 215–216
efficacy of, 197–198
side effects of, 207–208
class of, 139
combination of, 145, **180**, 214–216
cost of, **152**
depot, conversion from oral drug to, 186–188, 230–231
dosage of, **148–151**
drug interactions with, 144–145, **175–177**, 212–214
anticholinergic agents, 144, **175**, 203
benzodiazepines, **284**
carbamazepine, 145, **175**, **177**, **179**, 213, 343, **374**
lithium, 144, **176**, **179**, **371**, 418
other antipsychotics, **176**
phenytoin, 145, **175**, **177**, 232
selective serotonin reuptake inhibitors, 23–24, **62**, 102, 212–213, 232–233
tricyclic antidepressants, **60**, 102, 212
valproate, 343, **377**
elimination half-lives of, 142, **160–161**
dosing schedules and, 200–201
formulations of, **150**, **151**, 186–188
generic names of, **148–149**
indications for, 140, **153–158**, 188–195
antidepressant augmentation, 25, **71**, 140
anxiety disorders, 301
bipolar disorder, **156**, 190–192, 337, 338
maintenance therapy, **356**
mania, 140, **156**, 188–189, 337, 344, **351**, **352**, 389–390
brief psychotic disorder, **153**
delusional disorder, **153**, 195
dementia, 140, 146, **155**, 193–194
mental retardation with behavioral dyscontrol, **157**, **184**
obsessive-compulsive disorder, 140, **157**, 194–195, 301

Antipsychotics (APs) *(continued)*
indications for *(continued)*
personality disorders, **154**, 192–193
posttraumatic stress disorder, 301
psychotic depression, 140, **157**
rapid neuroleptization, 195
schizoaffective disorder, 140, **154**, 190–191
schizophrenia, **153**
schizophreniform disorder, **153**
substance-induced psychosis, **154**
Tourette's syndrome, 140, **158**
intramuscular, 142, 188
intravenous, 186
mechanisms of action of, 140–142, **159**, 195–199, 340
onset of action of, 195–196
pharmacokinetics of, 10, 142–143, **160–161**, 200–201
plasma levels of, 142–143, **148–149**, 200
potentiation of, 145, **178–181**, 214–219
questions and answers about, 186–227
receptor affinities of, **159**, 196–197
side effects of, 143–144, **162–164**, 201–212, 301
atypical agents, 207–208
cardiotoxicity, 132–144, **180**, 211–212, 235
electroencephalogram abnormalities, 220
extrapyramidal symptoms, **162–164**
akathisia, 203–204
prophylaxis for, 201–202
glucose and lipid abnormalities, 144, **172**, 208–209
management of, 144, **165**, **171–172**
neuroleptic malignant syndrome, **67–69**, **166–170**, 209–211
quetiapine-induced cataract, 212
related to dosing schedule, 200
sexual dysfunction, 143, **172**, 204–205
terminology for, 139
trade names of, **148–149**
use in special populations, 145–147, **182–185**, 219–227
breastfeeding, **185**, 220
children and adolescents, 146, **182**, 225–227
dementia patients, 146, **155**, **183**, 193, 223–225
developmentally disabled persons, **184**
elderly patients, 145–146, **183**, 221–223
Lewy body dementia, **155**, 194, 225
Parkinson's disease, 224–225
pregnancy, 146–147, **184–185**, 220–221
seizure disorders, 219–220
vignettes/puzzlers about, 227–235
withdrawal syndromes from, 207
Antiretroviral agents, 229
drug interactions with
antidepressants, 114
selective serotonin reuptake inhibitors, **64**, 120
antipsychotics, **176**, 214, 229
benzodiazepines, 257
zolpidem, **285**
zopiclone, **285**

Anxiety
drug-induced
antidepressants, **38**
benzodiazepines, **178**, **278**
buspirone, **278**
yohimbine, **59**
rebound, after benzodiazepine discontinuation, 309
Anxiety disorders. *See also specific anxiety disorders*
anticonvulsants for, 254, 299–300
antidepressants for, 20, 77, 82–83, 253, 254, 255, 302
monoamine oxidase inhibitors, 302
selective serotonin reuptake inhibitors, **32**, 82, 83, 253, 255, **270**, 291–292
combined with benzodiazepines, 292
trazodone, 302
tricyclics, 302
anti-noradrenergic agents for, 254
antipsychotics for, 301
barbiturates for, 298
beta-blockers for, 254, **271**
buspirone for, 254
clonidine for, 254, **271**
cognitive-behavioral therapy for, 292–293, 316
guanfacine for, 299
mood stabilizers for, 299, 300, 400
treatment in pregnancy, 258, **287**, 315–316
World Council of Anxiety treatment guidelines for, 291–292
Anxiolytics and sedative-hypnotics, 253–323. *See also* Benzodiazepines; *specific drugs*
abuse liability of, 307–308, 310
antidepressant effects of, 254
antihistamines, 254, **262**
barbiturates, **262**
benzodiazepines, 253–259
buspirone, **262**
class of, 253–254
discontinuation of, 308–310
dosage of, **260–261**
drug interactions with, 257–258, **282–285**, 310–313
tricyclic antidepressants, **60**
formulations of, **260–261**
generic names of, **260–261**
indications for, 254–255, **266–269**, 290–299
mechanisms of action of, 255–256, **272–273**, 302–304
meprobamate, **262**
pharmacokinetics of, 256, **274–277**, 304–306
potentiation of, 258, **286**, 313–315
questions and answers about, 289–319
receptor affinities of, 255, **272–273**
side effects of, 256–257, **278**
management of, **279–281**
trade names of, **260–261**
use in special populations, 258–259, **287–288**, 315–319
breastfeeding, **287**, 317
children and adolescents, 259
elderly and/or dementia patients, 258–259, **288**
medically ill patients, 258
pregnancy, 258, **287**, 315–316
vignettes/puzzlers about, 320–323
withdrawal from, 308–310
zaleplon, **263**
zolpidem, **263**

Apathy
in schizophrenia, 195, 197
selective serotonin reuptake inhibitor–induced, 100
APD. *See* Avoidant personality disorder
Aplastic anemia, carbamazepine-induced, 343, 431
Appetite changes, drug-induced
antidepressants, **37**, 112
lithium, **366**
valproate, **364**, **365**
APs. *See* Antipsychotics
Aripiprazole, 139
cost of, **152**
dosage of, **148**, **151**, 199
drug interactions with, **175**, 177, 214
carbamazepine, **373**
elimination half-life of, 142, **161**
dosing schedule and, 200
formulations of, **151**
indications for
bipolar disorder, **156**, 338, **356**
mania, 140, 190, 389
dementia-related syndromes, 193
schizophrenia, 198
mechanism of action of, 142, 198–199
pharmacokinetics of, **161**
receptor affinities of, **159**
side effects of, **163**, 208
agitation, 390
extrapyramidal symptoms, 202
sexual dysfunction, 205
use in special populations
elderly patients, 222, 223
pregnancy, **185**
Arrhythmias, drug-induced
antidepressants, **37**, **49–50**
management of, **56**
tricyclics, 22, 100, 112
lithium, **367**
pimozide, **158**
Artane. *See* Trihexyphenidyl
Asendin (amoxapine), **28**, **157**
Aspartate, 4
Aspirin interactions
with lithium, 418
with valproate, **377**
Asthenia, carbamazepine-induced, **362**
Ataxia, drug-induced
benzodiazepines, 257, **278**, 306
management of, **279**
buspirone, **278**
carbamazepine, **179**, 342, **363**
lamotrigine, **364**
lithium, **361**
Atenolol, for akathisia, **171**, 204
Ativan. *See* Lorazepam
Atomoxetine, **74**
for attention-deficit/hyperactivity disorder, 21
for depression, 21
mechanism of action of, 21
Atropine
for hypersalivation, 205
interaction with monoamine oxidase inhibitors, **65**
Attention-deficit/hyperactivity disorder (ADHD)
antidepressants for, **76**
atomoxetine for, 21
guanfacine for, 299
Autism, antipsychotics in, **184**
Autoinduction
of carbamazepine, 341, 407–408
of lamotrigine, 341
of valproate, 410

Autonomic effects
of antidepressants, 22, **52**
of bethanechol, **59**
Autoreceptors, 3
Aventyl. *See* Nortriptyline
Avoidant personality disorder (APD), benzodiazepines for, 254, **266**
Azapirone anxiolytic. *See* Buspirone

Baclofen, for posttraumatic stress disorder, 302
Barbiturates, 254, **262**. *See also specific drugs*
drug interactions with
antidepressants, 103
selective serotonin reuptake inhibitors, 24
tricyclics, **60**
antipsychotics, **176**
indications for, 298
mechanism of action of, 255, **272**
metabolism of, 10
BDD (body dysmorphic disorder), fluoxetine for, **33**
BDNF (brain-derived neurotrophic factor), 4, 21, 90
Befloxatone, 88
Behavioral disinhibition
antidepressants for, 20
drug-induced
benzodiazepines, **178**, 257, 258, **280, 288**, 293
selective serotonin reuptake inhibitors, 100
Benadryl. *See* Diphenhydramine
Benign prostatic hypertrophy, antihistamines in, **262**
Bentyl. *See* Dicyclomine
Benzisoxazoles, 139, **148**. *See also* Antipsychotics
Benzodiazepine receptor, 2, 255
Benzodiazepines (BZDs), 2, 253–259. *See also specific drugs*
abuse liability of, 307–308
in relatives of substance abusers, 308
choice of, 289
combined with buspirone, 313
cost of, **265**
dependence on, 257
discontinuation of, 257, **281**, 292, 308, 309
dosage of, **260–261**
drug interactions with, 257, **282–284, 288**, 289, 310–313, 320–322
antacids, 304, 311
antidepressants, 311–312, 314
nefazodone, 24, 257, **283**, 289, 311, 320–321
selective serotonin reuptake inhibitors, 24, **62**
tricyclic antidepressants, **60**
antipsychotics, **176, 178**
clozapine, 222, 310
carbamazepine, 257, **282**, 322, 429
disulfiram, **282**, 322
L-dopa, **284**, 321
elimination half-lives of, 256, **274–275**, 305
formulations of, **260–261**
generic names of, **260–261**
"hangover" effects from, 258, **288**
indications for, 254, **266–269**, 290–298
agitation, **58**, 293
alcohol withdrawal, 254, **269**
antidepressant augmentation, 313–314

Benzodiazepines (BZDs) *(continued)*
indications for *(continued)*
antipsychotic augmentation, **178**, 196, 217, 258, **286**, 314
augmentation of mood stabilizers, **286**, 313–314
avoidant personality disorder, 254, **266**
bipolar disorder, 296–297, 338, 344
depressed phase, 297
mania, **156**, 254, **267**, **286**, 296–297, 313
depression, 110, 254, **268**, **286**, 291, 297–298, 313
extrapyramidal side effects, **171**, 254
akathisia/dyskinesia, 204, 234, **268**
generalized anxiety disorder, 254, **266**, 290–291, 292
insomnia, **57**, 254, **267**, 294–295
neuroleptic malignant syndrome, **169**, 210
night terrors, 254, **268**
nocturnal myoclonus, 254, **268**
obsessive-compulsive disorder, 254, **266**, 291, 293
panic disorder, 254, **266**, 321–322, 429
periodic leg movements of sleep, 296, 322
posttraumatic stress disorder, 254, **267**
psychosis, **153**, **154**, **268**, **286**, 314
in emergency setting, 293
schizophrenia, 145, **178**, 196, 217, 294
social phobia, 254, **266**
intermediate-acting, 256
intramuscular, 293, 304
intravenous, 290, 305
long-acting, 256
mechanism of action of, 255, **272–273**, 302–303
onset of action of, **274**, 305, 320
overdose of, flumazenil for, 2–3
pharmacokinetics of, 256, **274–277**, 304–306, 320
absorption, 304
food effects on, 304, 311
in hepatic disease, 256, 289, 305
lipophilicity and onset of action, 305, 320
metabolic pathways, 10, **277**, 305
single-dose kinetics, 305–306, 320
potentiation of, 258
receptor affinity of, 255, **272–273**
short-acting, 256
side effects of, **178**, 256–257, **278**, 306–307
management of, **279–281**
sublingual, 290
switching to buspirone from, 312–313
tolerance to, **178**, 292, 296
trade names of, **260–261**
use in special populations, 258–259, **287–288**
breastfeeding, **287**, 317
children and adolescents, 259, 318–319
elderly and/or dementia patients, 258–259, **288**, 317

Benzodiazepines (BZDs) *(continued)*
use in special populations *(continued)*
medically ill patients, 258
respiratory disease, 318
pregnancy, 258, **287**, 315–316
substance-abusing patients, 292, 307–308
withdrawal from, 257, **281**, 308–309
antidepressants for, 20
management of, 309
symptoms of, 309
Benztropine
benzodiazepine augmentation of, **286**
for extrapyramidal side effects, **165**, **171**
prophylaxis, 201
for hypersalivation, **171**, 205
interaction with antipsychotics, 144
Beta-blockers, 10
combined with benzodiazepines, 258
contraindications to, 234
drug interactions with
antidepressants, 102
selective serotonin reuptake inhibitors, 112, 114
antipsychotics, **176**, **178**
indications for
agitation and anxiety, **58**, 254, **271**
akathisia, **171**, 202, 204, 233–234
antipsychotic augmentation, **178**
behavioral disturbances in dementia, 194
bipolar disorder, 344
hypersalivation, 205
mental retardation with behavioral dyscontrol, **157**
schizophrenia, 145
tremor, **364**
side effects of, **178**
withdrawal from, 307
Beta-carbolines, 3
Bethanechol
for anticholinergic drug effects, **56**, 144, **171**
for drug-induced sexual dysfunction, **59**, 99, **172**
side effects of, **59**
Biogenic amine neurotransmitters, 3
receptors for, 1, 2
Biperiden, for extrapyramidal side effects, **165**
Bipolar disorder. *See also* Mania
antidepressants in, 20, 97–98, 338, 391–395
mania or rapid cycling induced by, 97–98, 391, 393
recommendations for use of, 98, 394–395
antipsychotics in, 140, **156**, 188–192, 337, 338, 344, 389–390
atypical agents, 190–191, **356**
maintenance therapy, 192
mania, 188–189
augmenting strategies in, 344, **381–386**
benzodiazepines in, 296–297, 344
calcium channel blockers in, 338, 344, **355**, 400–401, 421–422
in children and adolescents, 345, **387**, 425–426
combining mood stabilizers in, 344, **381–386**
diabetes mellitus and, 208
kindling in, 405–406
maintenance therapy for, 140, 192, 339, **356**

Bipolar disorder *(continued)*
- mood stabilizers in, 337–343 (*See also* Mood stabilizers)
- omega-3 fatty acids in, 403
- postpartum, 424–425
- preferred treatments for, **351–356**
  - depressive episodes, **353–354**, 391–393, 422
  - maintenance therapy, **356**
  - mania or mixed episodes, **351–352**, 389
  - in pregnancy, **351**, **353**
  - rapid cycling, **355**, 390–391, 421
  - Texas Medication Algorithm, **156**, 339, 389, 401

Bleeding, selective serotonin reuptake inhibitor–induced, 23, 96

Body dysmorphic disorder (BDD), fluoxetine for, **33**

Borderline personality disorder (BPD)
- antidepressants in, **81**
  - monoamine oxidase inhibitors, 81
  - selective serotonin reuptake inhibitors, **33**, 81
  - tricyclics, **34**
- antipsychotics in, 140, **154**, 192
- mood stabilizers in, 339, 400
  - lithium, **350**, 400

Bowel obstruction, antipsychotic-induced, 145

BPD. *See* Borderline personality disorder

BPRS (Brief Psychiatric Rating Scale), 192

Bradycardia, drug-induced
- anxiolytics, **278**
- beta-blockers, **178**
- lithium, **367**, 411

Brain-derived neurotrophic factor (BDNF), 4, 21, 90

Breastfeeding
- antidepressants during, 26, 116
- antipsychotics during, **185**, 220
- benzodiazepines during, **287**, 317
- buspirone during, 317

Brief Psychiatric Rating Scale (BPRS), 192

Brief psychotic disorder, antipsychotics for, 140, **153**

Bromocriptine, for neuroleptic malignant syndrome, **69**, **169**, 210

Bulimia nervosa
- fluoxetine for, **32**
- tricyclic antidepressants for, **34**

Bupropion, 21, **46**
- combined with a selective serotonin reuptake inhibitor, 24, 107–108
- cost of, **31**
- dosage of, **28**
  - for children and adolescents, **78**
- drug interactions with, **46**
  - antipsychotics, **175**, 214
  - carbamazepine, **373**
  - valproate, **377**
- extended-release, **28**, **31**
- formulations of, **28**
- indications for
  - antidepressant-induced sexual dysfunction, **59**, **76**, 99
  - bipolar disorder, 338, **353**, 394
  - smoking cessation, **46**, **76**
- mechanism of action of, **27**, **36**
- pharmacodynamics of, **46**
- pharmacokinetics of, **39**, **46**, 91
- side effects of, **46**, **49**, **51–54**, **59**
  - mania, 98
  - seizures, **46**, **59**, 95
- sustained-release, **28**, **31**

Bupropion *(continued)*
use in obsessive-compulsive disorder, 82
use in panic disorder, 83
use in special populations, 75–77
cancer patients, 112
elderly patients, 25
BuSpar. *See* Buspirone
Buspirone, 254, **262**
antidepressant activity of, 291
combined with benzodiazepines, 313
drug interactions with, 258, 312
monoamine oxidase inhibitors, **65**, 258
selective serotonin reuptake inhibitors, 24, 322–323
serotonin syndrome due to, 312, 322–323
indications for, **262**, 291
antidepressant augmentation, **71**, 256, **262**
antidepressant-induced sexual dysfunction, 100
anxiety in children and adolescents, 318
behavioral disturbances in dementia, **155**, 194
vs. antipsychotics, 225
benzodiazepine augmentation, 258, **286**
generalized anxiety disorder, 254, 291, 292
mental retardation with behavioral dyscontrol, **157**
mechanism of action of, 3, 255–256, **272**, 303, 322
onset of action of, **262**
overdose of, **262**
pharmacodynamics of, 291
pharmacokinetics of, 256
side effects of, 257, **278**
switching from benzodiazepine to, 312–313
use in special populations
breastfeeding, 317
elderly and medically ill patients, 259
pregnancy, 258, 316
respiratory disease, 318
Butyrophenones, 139, **148**. *See also* Antipsychotics
BZDs. *See* Benzodiazepines

CAEs (cerebrovascular adverse events), antipsychotic-associated, 146, **155**, **183**, 193
Caffeine, 10
for drug-induced sedation, **57**
interaction with lithium, 343, 431
for orthostatic hypotension, **56**
Calcium channel blockers (CCBs). *See also specific drugs*
for bipolar disorder, 338, 344, **355**, 400–401, 421–422
drug interactions with, 10
antidepressants, **63**, 102, 114
antipsychotics, 235
carbamazepine, 343, **373**, 401
lithium, 343, **370**, 401, 422
Calcium ion flux, 4
cAMP (cyclic AMP), 4
cAMP response binding protein (CREB), 90
Cancer-related depression, 111–114
antidepressants for, 111–113
drug interactions with, 113–114
psychostimulants for, 113
Captopril interactions
with antipsychotics, **176**
with lithium, **370**, 419

Carbamazepine (CBZ)
autoinduction of, 341, 407–408
combined with other mood stabilizers, 344
lithium, **381**
valproate, **385**, 406, 416–417, 430
dosage of, **346**, 407
drug interactions with, 341, 343, **373–376**, 428–429
antidepressants, 102, 114
monoamine oxidase inhibitors, 417
nefazodone, 119, 341
selective serotonin reuptake inhibitors, **61**
tricyclics, **60**, 343, **375**, 428–429
antipsychotics, 145, **175**, **177**, **179**, 213, 343
benzodiazepines, 257, **282**, 322, 429
calcium channel blockers, 343, **373**, 401
ketoconazole, 341
mood stabilizers
lamotrigine, **379**
lithium, **370**
topiramate, 419
valproate, 343, **376**, **377**, 416–417, 430
elimination half-life of, 341, **358**, 407
extended-release, 338, **346**, 414
formulations of, **346**
indications for, 339, 400
antipsychotic augmentation, **179**, 216
benzodiazepine withdrawal, 309
bipolar disorder, 338
maintenance therapy, **356**
mania, **351**
predicting response to, 396, 406
rapid cycling, **355**
mechanism of action of, **357**, 405
pharmacokinetics of, 341, **358**, 407–408
plasma levels of, **346**, 407
rectal, 113
side effects of, **179**, 342–343, **362**
in children, 426
hepatotoxicity, 343, **363**, 415
hyponatremia, 343, **363**, 413–414
leukopenia, 343, **363**, 426, 431
management of, **363**
tolerance to, 406
use in special populations
children and adolescents, **387**, 425, 426
elderly or medically ill patients, 345, **388**, 427
pregnancy, 345, **387**, 423
Carbidopa, interaction with antipsychotics, **176**
Carbonic anhydrase inhibitor interactions
with lithium, 343, **370**
with topiramate, 402, 420
Cardiac disease
antidepressants in, **75**, 112
tricyclics, 25, 112
antipsychotics in, 146
Cardiovascular effects
of antidepressants, **49–50**, **52**
management of, **56**
tricyclics, 22, 100

Cardiovascular effects *(continued)*
of antipsychotics, 143–144, **180**, 211–212, 235
when used with selective serotonin reuptake inhibitors, **178**
of benzodiazepines, **278**
of methylphenidate, **59**
of mood stabilizers
carbamazepine, 343
combined with nortriptyline, 428–429
lithium, 344–345, **367**
of sildenafil, **59**
of verapamil, 401
Cataract, quetiapine-induced, 212
Catatonia
benzodiazepines for, 217, 314
lethal
causes/mechanisms of, **68, 168**
differential diagnosis of, **67–68, 166–168**
management of, **69, 169**
CBT (cognitive-behavioral therapy)
for anxiety disorders, 292–293
for bipolar depression, **353**
CBZ. *See* Carbamazepine
CCBs. *See* Calcium channel blockers
Celecoxib, interaction with lithium, **370**, 418
Celexa. *See* Citalopram
Central anticholinergic syndrome, 112, 234–235
causes/mechanisms of, **68, 168**
differential diagnosis of, **67–68, 166–168**
management of, **69, 169**
Central nervous system depressants, benzodiazepine interactions with, 257, **283**
Central nervous system depression, antidepressant-induced, **37**
Central pontine myelinolysis, 414
Centrax. *See* Prazepam
Cerebrovascular adverse events (CAEs), antipsychotic-associated, 146, **155, 183**, 193, 223–224
Chest pain, anxiolytic-induced, **278**
Children and adolescents
antidepressants for, 25
dosage of, **78**
pharmacokinetics of, 90
precautions for use of, 121–122
antipsychotics for, 146, **182**, 225–227
benzodiazepines for, 259, 318–319
mood stabilizers for, 345, **387**, 425–426
treatment of anxiety disorders in, 318–319
Chloral hydrate, 254
for insomnia, 298–299
therapeutic index for, 298–299
tolerance to, 299
Chloramphenicol, interaction with tricyclic antidepressants, **60**
Chlordiazepoxide
abuse liability of, 307
cost of, **265**
dosage of, **260**
drug interactions with, **282**
disulfiram, 322
formulations of, **260**
indications for
generalized anxiety disorder, 290
periodic leg movements of sleep, 322
pharmacokinetics of, **274**
metabolic pathway, **277**, 305
Chloride ion flux, 2, 4

m-Chlorophenylpiperazine (m-CPP), 322
Chlorpromazine, 139
  active metabolites of, 142
  in Alzheimer's disease, 193
  combined with verapamil in mania, 422
  dosage of, **148, 150**
  drug interactions with, **175–176**
    antidepressants, 102
    valproate, 343, **377**
  formulations of, **150**
  pharmacokinetics of, **160**
  plasma levels of, **148**
  side effects of, 143, **162**
    sexual dysfunction, 204
  withdrawal syndromes with, 207
Chlorprothixene, **149**
Cholinergic rebound syndrome, after antidepressant discontinuation, 91
Choreoathetosis, lithium-induced, **361**
Chronic obstructive pulmonary disease (COPD)
  antidepressants in, **76**
  benzodiazepines in, 318
  beta-blockers in, **178**
  buspirone in, 318
Cimetidine interactions
  with antipsychotics, **175, 177**, 214
  with benzodiazepines, 257, **282**
  with carbamazepine, **373**
  with tricyclic antidepressants, **60**
  with valproate, 343, 377
  with zaleplon, **285**
Ciprofloxacin interactions
  with antipsychotics, **177**, 214
  with selective serotonin reuptake inhibitors, **61**
Circadian rhythms, in depression, 21
Cirrhosis. *See also* Hepatic dysfunction
  antidepressant metabolism in, 92–93
Citalopram, **44**
  cost of, **31**
  dosage of, **28**
    for children and adolescents, **78**
  drug interactions with, **44**
    benzodiazepines, **283**
    protease inhibitors, 120
  formulations of, **28**
  indications for
    anxiety in children and adolescents, 318
    tricyclic antidepressant potentiation, 107
  intravenous, 79
  mechanism of action of, **27, 36,** 86
  pharmacodynamics of, **44**
  pharmacokinetics of, 10, **39, 44**
  in pregnancy, 115
  side effects of, 23, **49, 55**
    sexual dysfunction, 99
Clarithromycin interactions
  with antipsychotics, **177**, 214
  with carbamazepine, **374**
  with selective serotonin reuptake inhibitors, **61**
Clearance of drugs, 8
Cleft lip/palate, benzodiazepine-induced, 258, **287**, 315
Clinical Global Impression scale, 226
Clomipramine
  combined with antipsychotics, 218
  dosage of, **28**
  formulations of, **28**
  indications for
    anxiety disorders, 302
    obsessive-compulsive disorder, 20, **33**, 82
      in psychotic patients, 218

Clomipramine *(continued)*
- indications for *(continued)*
  - panic disorder, 82
- interaction with monoamine oxidase inhibitors, 24
- intravenous, 79
- in pregnancy, 114
- side effects of, **49**
  - seizures, 23

Clonazepam
- cost of, **265**
- depression induced by, 321
- dosage of, **260**
- drug interactions with
  - carbamazepine, 322, 429
  - clozapine, 310
  - lithium, 297
- formulations of, **260**
- indications for
  - antipsychotic augmentation, **178**
  - bipolar disorder, 296–297, 338, 344
    - depressed phase, 297
    - mania, **267**, 296–297
  - catatonic schizophrenia, 217, 314
  - depression, 291
  - extrapyramidal side effects, **165**
  - obsessive-compulsive disorder, **266**, 293
  - panic disorder, **266**
  - periodic leg movements of sleep, 296
  - REM sleep behavioral disorder, **268**
  - social phobia, **266**, 300
- pharmacokinetics of, 256, **274**
  - metabolic pathway, **277**, 305
- in pregnancy, 315–316
- switching from alprazolam to, 321
- tolerance to, 296

Clonidine
- drug interactions with
  - monoamine oxidase inhibitors, **65**
  - tricyclic antidepressants, **60**
- indications for
  - anxiety or agitation, 254, **271**
  - bipolar disorder, 344
  - hypersalivation, 205
  - Tourette's syndrome, **158**

Clorazepate
- cost of, **265**
- dosage of, **260**
- drug interactions with, **283**
  - antacids, 304
- formulations of, **260**
- for generalized anxiety disorder, 292
- metabolism of, **277**, 304
- pharmacokinetics of, **274**

Clozapine, 139
- combining with other antipsychotics, **180**, 214–216
- cost of, **152**
- dosage of, **148, 151**
- drug interactions with, 144, **175–177**
  - antidepressants, 102, 212–213
  - benzodiazepines, 222, 257, **284**, 310
  - carbamazepine, **374**
  - fluvoxamine, 232–233
  - lamotrigine, 432
  - valproate, 432
- formulations of, **151**
- indications for, 189–190
  - borderline personality disorder, **154**, 192
  - dementia-related syndromes, 194
  - mania, 189–190, **351**

Clozapine *(continued)*
indications for *(continued)*
mental retardation with behavioral dyscontrol, **157**
obsessive-compulsive disorder, 194
posttraumatic stress disorder, 301
psychotic depression, **157**
schizoaffective disorder, **154**
schizophrenia, **153,** 190, 198
mechanism of action of, 141
onset of action of, 196
pharmacokinetics of, 10, 142, **161**
in elderly patients, 221
plasma levels of, 142–143, **148**
effect of smoking on, 230
therapeutic response and, 201
potentiation of, 214–216
lithium, **179**
receptor affinities of, **159,** 197
side effects of, 143–144, **163,** 205–208
agranulocytosis, 143, **173–174,** 206–207
in children and adolescents, 226
in elderly persons, 222
glucose and lipid abnormalities, 209
neuroleptic malignant syndrome, 210
"restart" effects after surgery, 231–232
seizures, 205, 219–220
sexual dysfunction, 205
use in special populations
children and adolescents, **182,** 226–227
developmentally disabled persons, **184**
elderly patients, 145–146, **183,** 222
medically ill patients, 145–146
Parkinson's disease, 145, **155,** 194, 224–225
pregnancy, **185**
withdrawal syndromes from, 207
Clozaril. *See* Clozapine
Clumsiness, anxiolytic-induced, **278**
Cocaine abuse, lamotrigine for, 400
Codeine, 10
interaction with antidepressants, 102
selective serotonin reuptake inhibitors, **63**
Cogentin. *See* Benztropine
Cognitive effects
of antidepressants, 22, **37, 51, 54**
of antipsychotics, 144, 145
of anxiolytics and sedative-hypnotics
benzodiazepines, **178,** 257, 258, **278–279, 288,** 306–307
buspirone, **279**
nonbenzodiazepine hypnotics, 257
zaleplon, **263**
zolpidem, **263**
in central anticholinergic syndrome, **67, 166**
in lethal catatonia, **67, 166**
of mood stabilizers
carbamazepine, 342
lithium, 342, 345, **361, 367,** 411
in children, 425–426
combined with antipsychotics, 418
in elderly patients, 427
tiagabine, 299
topiramate, 402
valproate, 345

Cognitive effects *(continued)*
in neuroleptic malignant syndrome, **67**, **166**
in serotonin syndrome, **67**, **70**, **166**
Cognitive-behavioral therapy (CBT)
for anxiety disorders, 292–293, 316
for bipolar depression, **353**
Coma, lithium-induced, **361**, 411
Combivir (lamivudine/zidovudine), 229
Concerta. *See* Methylphenidate
Confusion. *See also* Cognitive effects
drug-induced
antipsychotics, 144, 145
benzodiazepines, 257, 258, **278**, **279**
buspirone, **279**
lithium, **361**, 411
topiramate, 402
tricyclic antidepressants, 22
zolpidem, **263**
in serotonin syndrome, **70**
Conjugation, 9
Constipation, drug-induced
antidepressants, **37**, **51**, **53**, **56**
reboxetine, 97
selective serotonin reuptake inhibitors, **55**
tricyclics, 22, 111
antipsychotics, 144, **171**
clozapine, 205, 231
anxiolytics, **278**
management of, **56**, **171**
topiramate, 402
verapamil, 401
Continuing Medical Education questions and answers, 449–468
COPD. *See* Chronic obstructive pulmonary disease
Corticosteroids
for carbamazepine-induced rash, **363**
interaction with antidepressants, 102, 114
Corticotropin-releasing hormone, in depression, 21
Cost
of antidepressants, **31**, 80
of antipsychotics, **152**
of benzodiazepines, **265**
Coumadin. *See* Warfarin
COX-2 (cyclooxygenase-2) inhibitor interactions, with lithium, **370**, 418
m-CPP (*m*-chlorophenylpiperazine), 322
CREB (cAMP response binding protein), 90
Cyclic AMP (cAMP), 4
Cyclooxygenase-2 (COX-2) inhibitor interactions, with lithium, **370**, 418
Cyclosporine, 10
Cymbalta. *See* Duloxetine
CYP. *See* Cytochrome enzymes
Cyproheptadine
for drug-induced sexual dysfunction, **59**, 99, 100, **172**
for serotonin syndrome, **69**, **169**
side effects of, **59**
Cytochrome (CYP) enzymes, 1, 9–15
age-related changes in activity of, 90
in antidepressant metabolism, 22, **39–41**
in antipsychotic metabolism, 142
in anxiolytic and sedative-hypnotic metabolism, 256
in benzodiazepine metabolism, 305, 311–312

Cytochrome (CYP) enzymes *(continued)*
in carbamazepine metabolism, 341
in drug–drug interactions, 16
families of, 10
CYP 1A2, 10
CYP 2B, 10
CYP 2C, 10
CYP 2D6, 10
CYP 2E1, 10
CYP 3A4/5, 10
functions of, 9
inducers of, **14**, 15
inhibitors of, **13**, 15
sites of, 9
steroidogenic, 9, 22
substrates of, **11–12**, 15
zenobiotic, 9–10, 22

DA. *See* Dopamine
Dalmane. *See* Flurazepam
Dantrolene
for malignant hyperthermia, **69**, **169**
for neuroleptic malignant syndrome, **69**, **169**, 210
Delavirdine, interaction with selective serotonin reuptake inhibitors, **64**
Delirium
antipsychotics for, 140
intravenous, 186
lithium-induced, 427
Delirium tremens, benzodiazepines for, 7, **269**, 304
Delusional disorder
antipsychotics for, **153**, 195
selective serotonin reuptake inhibitors for, 195
subtypes of, **153**
Demeclocycline, for carbamazepine-induced hyponatremia, 414
Dementia patients
antidepressants in, 20
selective serotonin reuptake inhibitors, **33**
tricyclics, 25, **35**
antipsychotics in, 140, 146, **155**, 193–194
vs. buspirone for agitation, 225
cerebrovascular adverse events and, 146, **155**, **183**, 193, 223–224
Lewy body dementia, **155**, 194, 225
Parkinson's disease, 145, **155**, 194, 224–225
anxiolytics and sedative-hypnotics in
benzodiazepines, **288**
buspirone, **262**
zolpidem, **263**
mood stabilizers in, 345, 426–428
Demerol. *See* Meperidine
Demethylation reactions, 9
Depakene. *See* Valproate
Depakote, Depakote-ER, Depakote Sprinkle. *See* Divalproex
Depersonalization disorder, lamotrigine for, 400
Depolarization, 4
L-Deprenyl, **30**
transdermal, 88
Depression
antidepressants for, 19–122 (*See also* Antidepressants)
with atypical features, **75**, 83–84
benzodiazepines in, 110, 254, **268**, **286**, 291, 297–298
bipolar, treatment of, **43**, **353–354**, 391–395, 422
circadian rhythms in, 21

Depression *(continued)*
- "double," 105
- drug-induced
  - benzodiazepines, **178,** 257, **268, 278, 280,** 297, 321
  - beta-blockers, **178**
  - buspirone, **278**
- glucocorticoids in, 5
- maintenance therapy for, 80–81
- neuroendocrine abnormalities in, 20–21
- norepinephrine in, 20
- postpartum, 26
- with psychotic features, 25
  - antidepressants for, 25
  - antipsychotics for, 140, **157**
- recurrent, 80–81
- refractory, 24–25
  - adding a psychostimulant to a selective serotonin reuptake inhibitor in, 108
  - adding a tricyclic antidepressant to a selective serotonin reuptake inhibitor in, 107
  - adding bupropion to a selective serotonin reuptake inhibitor in, 107–108
  - antidepressant potentiation in, 24–25, **71–72,** 103–110
  - antipsychotics in, **157**
  - augmentation of monoamine oxidase inhibitors in, 109–110
  - benzodiazepines in, 110
  - changing from one selective serotonin reuptake inhibitor to another in, 106–107
  - crossover monotherapy in, 104–106
  - efficacy of tricyclics vs. other antidepressants in, 104
  - lithium as augmenting agent in, 109, 398–399
  - modafinil as augmenting agent in, 108–109
- serotonin in, 20

Dermatological effects
- of antipsychotics, 143
- of carbamazepine, 342, **362, 363,** 414
- of lamotrigine, 342, 345, **364, 387,** 412–413, 426, 431–432
- of lithium, **368**

Desipramine
- age effects on metabolism of, 90–91
- dosage of, **28**
- formulations of, **28**
- indications for, **33–34**
  - panic disorder, 82
  - selective serotonin reuptake inhibitor potentiation, 107
- interaction with benzodiazepines, **283,** 312
- mechanism of action of, **27, 36**
- overdose of, 80
- plasma levels of, **48**
- in pregnancy, 114, 115
- side effects of, 23, **49**
  - mania, 394, 395
- sudden death in children linked to, 26
- use in obsessive-compulsive disorder, 82
- use in seizure disorders, **76**

Desmethyldiazepam, 256, 277, **283,** 304, 320

Desmethylimipramine, **40,** 92

Desmethylsertraline, **41,** 92, 312

Desmethylvenlafaxine, **41,** 91, 93

Desyrel. *See* Trazodone
Developmentally disabled patients
antipsychotics for, **157**, **184**
buspirone for, **262**
Dexedrine, Dexedrine Spansules. *See* Dextroamphetamine
Dexmethylphenidate, **73**
Dextroamphetamine, **73–74**
for antidepressant-induced sexual dysfunction, 100
Dextromethorphan, interaction with monoamine oxidase inhibitors, **65**, 101
Diabetes mellitus
antidepressants in, **76**
for neuropathy, 20
selective serotonin reuptake inhibitors, **32**
tricyclics, **34**
antipsychotic-induced, 144, **172**, 209, 235
beta-blockers in, **178**
mental illness and, 208
Diabetic insipidus, lithium-induced, 342, **366**
Diarrhea
drug-induced
antidepressants, **49–51**, **53**
selective serotonin reuptake inhibitors, 23, **55**, 112
anxiolytics, **278**
bethanechol, **59**
lithium, **179**, **360**, **361**, **366**, 411
valproate, **364**
in serotonin syndrome, **70**
Diazepam
abuse liability of, 307
in relatives of substance abusers, 308
cost of, **265**
dosage of, **260**
drug interactions with, **282**, **283**
antidepressants, 312
duration of action of, 7
elimination half-life of, 7, 320
formulations of, **260**
indications for
antipsychotic augmentation, **178**
catatonic schizophrenia, 217, 314
delirium tremens, 7, **269**
generalized anxiety disorder, 290–291
panic disorder, **266**
intravenous, 290
pharmacokinetics of, **274**, 320
lipophilicity and onset of action, 7, 305, 320
metabolic pathway, 10, **277**, 305, 311
use in special populations
breastfeeding, 317
children and adolescents, 318
pregnancy, 315
withdrawal from, 309
Dibenzodiazepines, 139, **148**. *See also* Antipsychotics
Dibenzothiazepines, 139, **148**. *See also* Antipsychotics
Dibenzoxapines, 139, **148**. *See also* Antipsychotics
Diclofenac, interaction with lithium, 417–418
Dicyclomine, 234
Digoxin, interaction with benzodiazepines, **283**
Dihydroindolones, 139, **148**. *See also* Antipsychotics
Dilantin. *See* Phenytoin

Diltiazem interactions
with carbamazepine, 343, **373**
with lithium, **370**
with selective serotonin reuptake inhibitors, **63**
Diphenhydramine, **262**
for extrapyramidal side effects, **165**
interaction with antipsychotics, 214
side effects of, 257
Diphenylbutylpiperidines, 139, **148**. *See also* Antipsychotics
Diplopia. *See* Visual disturbances
Discontinuation of drugs, 9. *See also* Withdrawal syndromes
antidepressants, 91–92
antipsychotics, 207, **281**, 292
benzodiazepines, 257, **282**, 292, 308, 309
beta-blockers, 307
lithium, 397–398, 412
zaleplon, **263**, 309
zolpidem, 309–310
Disorientation, anxiolytic-induced, **278**
Distribution of drugs, 7–8
after initial dose, 7
lipophilicity and, 7
Disulfiram interactions
with benzodiazepines, **282**, 322
with tricyclic antidepressants, **60**
Ditropan (oxybutynin), 206
Diuretic interactions
with lithium, 343, **366**, **372**
with monoamine oxidase inhibitors, **65**
Divalproex sodium. *See also* Valproate
dosage of, **346**, 409
extended-release, 409
formulations of, **346**, 409
pharmacokinetics of, **358**, 409
therapeutic blood level of, **346**
Dizziness, drug-induced
antidepressants, 22, **37**, **52**
antipsychotics, **171**, 188
clozapine, 205, 231
quetiapine, 223
benzodiazepines, **278**, 306
mood stabilizers
carbamazepine, **362**, **363**, 414
gabapentin, 300
lamotrigine, **364**
oxcarbazepine, **364**
pregabalin, 300
tiagabine, 299
verapamil, 401
DNA, 4
Donepezil, interaction with selective serotonin reuptake inhibitors, 114
L-Dopa
drug interactions with
antipsychotics, **176**
benzodiazepines, **284**, 321
monoamine oxidase inhibitors, **65**
tricyclic antidepressants, **60**
psychosis induced by, 224
Dopamine (DA), 2
antidepressant actions on, **27**, **36**, 86, 87
effects of, **37**
benzodiazepine actions on, 302
in schizophrenia, 141
Dopamine receptors
antipsychotic actions at, 140–141, **159**, 196–197, 340
akathisia and, 203
aripiprazole, 198–199
onset of action related to, 196
buspirone actions at, 303
families of, 141
lithium actions at, 340, 403
pramipexole actions at, 422

Doral. *See* Quazepam
Doxepin
  dosage of, **28**
  formulations of, **28**
  indications for, **33–34**
    cancer patients, 111
    insomnia, 295
  intramuscular, 79, 113
  in pregnancy, 114
  rectal, 113
  side effects of, **49**
Doxycycline
  for carbamazepine-induced hyponatremia, 414
  interaction with tricyclic antidepressants, **60**
Dreams, anxiolytic-induced, **278**
Droperidol, 186
Drowsiness, drug-induced. *See also* Sedation
  antidepressants, **51, 54, 55**
  benzodiazepines, 256, **279**, 306
  carbamazepine, **362**, 426
  lithium, **360**
Drug–drug interactions, 15–16. *See also specific drugs*
  with antidepressants, 23–24, **60–65**, 80, 101–103, 118–120
    monoamine oxidase inhibitors, 24, **65**, 101
    selective serotonin reuptake inhibitors, 23–24, **61–64**
    tricyclics, 23, 24, **60**
  with antipsychotics, 144–145, **175–177**, 212–214
  with anxiolytics and sedative-hypnotics, 257–258, **282–285**
    benzodiazepines, 257, **282–284**, **288**, 289, 310–312, 320–322
    buspirone, 258, 312
  with mood stabilizers, 341, 343–344, **370–380**, 416–420
    carbamazepine, **373–376**
    lamotrigine, **379–380**
    lithium, **370–372**
    valproate, **377–378**
Dry mouth, drug-induced, 2
  antidepressants, **37, 51, 53, 56**
    selective serotonin reuptake inhibitors, **55**
    tricyclics, 22, 111
  antipsychotics, 144, **171**
  anxiolytics, **278**
  cyproheptadine, **59**
  gabapentin, 300
  management of, **56, 171**
Duloxetine
  cost of, **31**
  dosage of, **28**
  efficacy of, 104
  formulation of, **28**
  mechanism of action of, 21, **27**, **36**, 88
  pharmacokinetics of, **39**
  side effects of, 97
Dysarthria, lithium-induced, **361**
Dyskinesia
  benzodiazepines for, **268**
  tardive, 140, 143, **164**, 189, 192, 228
    in elderly patients, 143, **183**
    incidence of, 143
Dyslipidemia, antipsychotic-induced, 144, 208–209
  management of, **172**
Dysmorphic birth defects, benzodiazepine-induced, 258, **287**, 315
Dyspnea, anxiolytic-induced, **278**

Dysthymic disorder
antidepressants for, 84–85
character spectrum subtype of, 84–85
depression comorbid with, 105
interpersonal therapy for, 85
subaffective, 84
Dystonia, antipsychotic-induced, 143, **164**
prophylaxis for, 202

Eating disorders, antidepressants for, 20
selective serotonin reuptake inhibitors, **32**
tricyclics, **34**
Ebstein's anomaly, lithium-induced, 344, **387**, 423
ECG. *See* Electrocardiography
ECT. *See* Electroconvulsive therapy
Edema, lithium-induced, **366**
EEG (electroencephalography), antipsychotic-induced abnormalities on, 220
Efavirenz, 229
interaction with selective serotonin reuptake inhibitors, **64**
Effexor, Effexor XR. *See* Venlafaxine
Ejaculatory dysfunction. *See* Sexual dysfunction
Elavil. *See* Amitriptyline
Eldepryl (L-deprenyl), **30**, 88
Elderly patients
antidepressants for, 25
dosage of, **28–29**
pharmacokinetics of, 21, 90–91
antipsychotics for, 145–146, **183**, 221–223
atypical agents, 222–223
pharmacodynamics of, 221–222
pharmacokinetics of, 221
tardive dyskinesia from, 143
anxiolytics and sedative-hypnotics for, 258–259
benzodiazepines, 258, **288**, 317
buspirone, 259
zaleplon, **263**
zolpidem, **263**
elimination half-life of drug in, 8
glucuronidation in, 15
mood stabilizers for, 345, **388**, 426–428
Electrocardiography (ECG)
during carbamazepine therapy, 428–429
during intramuscular ziprasidone therapy, 188
during lithium therapy, **367**, 411
in tricyclic antidepressant overdose, 100
Electroconvulsive therapy (ECT)
actions on 5-HT_2 receptors, 20, 87
indications for
bipolar disorder
depressive episodes, **353**, **354**
maintenance therapy, **356**
mania, **351**, **352**
in postpartum period, 425
in pregnancy, 424
lethal catatonia, **69**, **169**
neuroleptic malignant syndrome, **69**, **169**, 210
psychotic depression, 25, **157**
schizoaffective disorder, **154**
schizophreniform disorder, **153**
in pregnancy, 26, 147, 424
Electroencephalography (EEG), antipsychotic-induced abnormalities on, 220
Elimination of drugs, 8–9
presystemic, 6–7

Elimination half-life of drugs, 8–9
calculation of, 8
vs. duration of action, 7
in elderly patients, 8
Enalapril, interaction with lithium, **370**, 419
Encainide, interaction with selective serotonin reuptake inhibitors, 103, 112, 114
Endep. *See* Amitriptyline
Enuresis, drug-induced
clozapine, 205, 206
lithium, 425
Epinephrine, interaction with tricyclic antidepressants, **60**
EPS. *See* Extrapyramidal side effects
Equetro (carbamazepine, extended-release), 338, **346**, 414
Erectile dysfunction. *See* Sexual dysfunction
Erythromycin interactions, 10
with antidepressants, 114
selective serotonin reuptake inhibitors, **61**
with antipsychotics, 144, **177**
with benzodiazepines, 257, **282**
with carbamazepine, 343, **374**
Escitalopram, **44**
cost of, **31**
dosage of, **28**
for children and adolescents, **78**
drug interactions with, **44**
formulations of, **28**
indications for, **32**
generalized anxiety disorder, **266**, 292
tricyclic antidepressant potentiation, 107
mechanism of action of, **27**
pharmacodynamics of, **44**
pharmacokinetics of, **39**, **44**
side effects of, 23, **55**
Eskalith, Eskalith-CR. *See* Lithium
Estazolam
cost of, **265**
dosage of, **261**
formulations of, **261**
pharmacodynamics of, **273**
pharmacokinetics of, 256, **275**
Estorra. *See* Eszopiclone
Estrogen
for antidepressant augmentation, **71**
interaction with antidepressants, 102
Eszopiclone, 253, **264**
discontinuation of, 257
dosage of, **261**
drug interactions with, **285**
formulations of, **261**
for insomnia, **264**, 296
mechanism of action of, 255, **272**, 303–304
pharmacodynamics of, **273**
pharmacokinetics of, 256, **276**
use in elderly and/or dementia patients, **288**
Ethanol. *See* Alcohol
Ethosuximide, interaction with valproate, 417
Extended-release drug formulations, 6
Extrapyramidal side effects (EPS)
antidepressant-induced
selective serotonin reuptake inhibitors, 23, 112
tricyclics, 23
antipsychotic-induced, 139, 143, **162–163**, **180**
akathisia, 203–204, 233–234
atypical agents, 197, 202, 208, 223

Extrapyramidal side effects (EPS) *(continued)*
antipsychotic-induced *(continued)*
in children and adolescents, **182**, 226
differential diagnosis of, **164**
in elderly patients, **183**
lithium exacerbation of, **367**, 418
mental and motor symptoms of, **164**
prophylaxis for, 201–202
risk factors for, 202
when used with selective serotonin reuptake inhibitors, **178**
management of, 144, **165**, **171**
benzodiazepines for, **171**, 254
hydroxyzine for, **262**
types of, 143

Fainting, anxiolytic-induced, **278**
Falls, drug-associated
benzodiazepines, 257, 258, **279**, **288**, 317
zolpidem, **263**
Famotidine
during carbamazepine therapy, **373**
during valproate therapy, **364**
Fatigue, drug-induced
benzodiazepines, 256, **278**, **279**, 306
buspirone, **278**
carbamazepine, 342
lithium, **360**
oxcarbazepine, **364**
selective serotonin reuptake inhibitors, **55**
Felbamate, interaction with valproate, 417
Fenfluramine, interaction with monoamine oxidase inhibitors, **65**
Fentanyl, interaction with monoamine oxidase inhibitors, **65**
Fibromyalgia, antidepressants for, 20
First-pass extraction of drugs, 7
Flecainide, interaction with selective serotonin reuptake inhibitors, **61**
"Floppy baby syndrome," benzodiazepine-induced, 258, **287**
Florinef. *See* Fludrocortisone
Fluconazole, interaction with antipsychotics, **177**
Fludrocortisone, for orthostatic hypotension, **56**, **171**
Flumazenil
for benzodiazepine overdose, 2–3
mechanism of action of, 2
Fluoxetine, **42**
anticonvulsant effect of, 95
combined with bupropion, 108
combined with olanzapine (*See* Olanzapine/fluoxetine combination)
combined with psychostimulants, 108
cost of, **31**
dosage of, **28**
for children and adolescents, **78**
drug interactions with, **42**, 114
antipsychotics, 102, 144, **175**, **177**, 212, 214
benzodiazepines, 257, **283**, 312
carbamazepine, **375**
encainide, 112
lithium, **371**, 430
tricyclic antidepressants, 23
valproate, 343, **377**
elimination half-life and discontinuation of, 92

Fluoxetine *(continued)*
- formulations of, **28**
- indications for, **32–33**
  - anxiety in children and adolescents, 318
  - dysthymic disorder, 84
  - obsessive-compulsive disorder, 194
    - in psychotic patients, 218
  - panic disorder, 82, 83
  - postpartum depression, 26
  - posttraumatic stress disorder, 291
  - tricyclic antidepressant potentiation, 107
  - venlafaxine withdrawal symptoms, 92
- mechanism of action of, **27**, **36**, 256
- pharmacodynamics of, **42**
- pharmacokinetics of, **39**, **42**
  - age effects on, 91
- side effects of, 23, **42**, **49**, **51–55**
  - frontal lobe syndrome, 100
  - sexual dysfunction, 99
- switching to paroxetine from, 106
- use in special populations, **75–76**
  - breastfeeding, 116
  - cancer patients, 112
  - children and adolescents, 26, **78**
  - pregnancy, 26, **42**, 114–116
- withdrawal symptoms with, 92

Fluphenazine
- dosage of, **148**, **150**
- formulations of, **150**
- onset of action of, 195
- pharmacokinetics of, **160**
- plasma levels of, **148**
- side effects of, 143, **162**
  - sexual dysfunction, 204

Fluphenazine decanoate
- conversion from oral drug to, 186–187
- dosage of, **150**

Flurazepam
- cost of, **265**
- dosage of, **261**
- formulations of, **261**
- pharmacodynamics of, **273**
- pharmacokinetics of, **275**
  - metabolic pathway, **277**, 305
- use in elderly and/or dementia patients, **288**

Fluvoxamine, **44**
- cost of, **31**
- dosage of, **28**
- drug interactions with, **44**, 114
  - alprazolam, 120
  - antipsychotics, 102, 144, **177**, **178**, 195, 212–213, 218
    - clozapine, 232–233
    - olanzapine, 24, 232–233
  - benzodiazepines, 257, **283**, 289, 311–312
  - carbamazepine, **375**
  - lithium, **371**
  - methadone, 122
  - theophylline, 120
  - tricyclic antidepressants, 23
- formulations of, **28**
- indications for, **32**
  - borderline personality disorder, 81
  - dysthymic disorder, 85
  - obsessive-compulsive disorder, 194
  - social phobia, 292
- mechanism of action of, **27**
- metabolism of, 22
- pharmacodynamics of, **44**
- pharmacokinetics of, **39**, **44**

Fluvoxamine *(continued)*
side effects of, 23, **44, 55**
frontal lobe syndrome, 100
use in special populations
breastfeeding, 116
pregnancy, 115
Focalin. *See* Methylphenidate
Folic acid supplementation in pregnancy, 423
Food
antidepressant interactions with, 103
monoamine oxidase inhibitors, **66**
effects on drug absorption, 6
of antidepressants, 93
of benzodiazepines, 304, 311
Fracture, benzodiazepine-associated, 258, **288,** 317
Free drug, steady-state concentration of, 8
Free fraction of drug, 8
Frontal lobe syndrome, selective serotonin reuptake inhibitor–induced, 100

GABA. *See* γ-Aminobutyric acid
Gabapentin
combined with other mood stabilizers, **386**
indications for
agitation, **58**
anxiety disorders, 254
bipolar disorder, 338
insomnia, **57**
mixed anxiety-depressive states, 314
social phobia, 300
mechanism of action of, 340, **357**
side effects of, 300
Gabitril. *See* Tiagabine
GAD. *See* Generalized anxiety disorder
GAF (Global Assessment of Functioning) Scale, 108
Galactorrhea, antipsychotic-induced, 204
GAS (Global Assessment Scale), 192
Gastrointestinal effects
of antidepressants, **37, 49–51, 53, 56**
reboxetine, 97
selective serotonin reuptake inhibitors, 23, **37, 38, 55,** 112
tricyclics, 22, 111
venlafaxine, **45**
of antipsychotics, 144, **171**
clozapine, 205, 231
ziprasidone, 188
of anxiolytics
benzodiazepines, **278, 280**
chloral hydrate, 299
of bethanechol, **59**
of mood stabilizers
carbamazepine, **179,** 342, **362, 363**
lamotrigine, **364**
lithium, **179, 360, 361, 366,** 411
oxcarbazepine, **364**
topiramate, 402
valproate, **181,** 342, **364**
Generalized anxiety disorder (GAD)
anticonvulsants for
pregabalin, 300
tiagabine, 315
antidepressants for, 20
in children and adolescents, 318
selective serotonin reuptake inhibitors, **32,** 255, **270,** 292
trazodone, 302

Generalized anxiety disorder (GAD) *(continued)*
antidepressants for *(continued)*
tricyclics, **34,** 302
venlafaxine, **32,** 255
benzodiazepines for, 254, **266,** 290–291, 292
combined with buspirone, 313
buspirone for, 254, **262,** 291, 292
Geodon. *See* Ziprasidone
Gepirone, 88
Glaucoma
antidepressants in, 77, 117–118
antihistamines in, **262**
Global Assessment of Functioning (GAF) Scale, 108
Global Assessment Scale (GAS), 192
Glomerular dysfunction, lithium-induced, 342, **366,** 410
Glomerular filtration rate, 8
Glucocorticoids. *See also* Corticosteroids
in depression, 5
receptors for, 5
Glucose dysregulation, antipsychotic-induced, 144, 208–209, 235
management of, **172**
Glucuronidation, 1, 9, 15
Glutamate, 4
anticonvulsant actions on, 340, **357**
carbamazepine, 405
lamotrigine, 405
valproate, 404
antipsychotic actions on, 340
in schizophrenia, 142
Glycine, 4
for antipsychotic augmentation, 217
Glycogen synthase kinase–3 (GSK-3), lithium inhibition of, 340, **357,** 403
Glycopyrrolate, for hypersalivation, 144, 205
G-protein–linked receptors, 3–4, 5
Grapefruit juice interactions, 10
with antidepressants, 103
selective serotonin reuptake inhibitors, **63**
with antipsychotics, 214
with buspirone, 312
GSK-3 (glycogen synthase kinase–3), lithium inhibition of, 340, **357,** 403
Guanethidine interactions
with antipsychotics, **176**
with monoamine oxidase inhibitors, **65**
with tricyclic antidepressants, **60**
Guanfacine, 299
for anxiety or agitation, 254
for attention-deficit/hyperactivity disorder, 299
for posttraumatic stress disorder, 299
for Tourette's syndrome, **158,** 299
Gynecomastia, antipsychotic-induced, 143, 204

Hair loss, drug-induced
carbamazepine, 342
lithium, **368**
valproate, **181,** 342, **364,** 415–416
Halazepam
abuse liability of, 307
dosage of, **260**
formulations of, **260**
metabolism of, **277**
pharmacokinetics of, **274**
Halcion. *See* Triazolam
Haldol. *See* Haloperidol

Hallucinations, 228, 230
  drug-induced
    anxiolytics, **278**
    zolpidem, 323
Haloperidol, 139
  active metabolites of, 142
  combined with lorazepam, **268**, 293
  combined with other antipsychotics, **180**
    clozapine, 215
  dosage of, **148**, 195–196
  drug interactions with, **175–176**
    antidepressants, 102
    carbamazepine, 213, 343, **374**
    lithium, **371**, 418
  indications for
    borderline personality disorder, 192
    dementia syndromes, **155**, 225
    drug-induced psychosis, **154**
    obsessive-compulsive disorder, 194
    rapid neuroleptization, 195
    schizophrenia, **153**
    Tourette's syndrome, **158**
  intravenous, 186
  pharmacokinetics of, **160**
  plasma levels of, 142, **148, 153**
  receptor affinities of, **159**, 196
  side effects of, 143, **162**
    anticholinergic prophylaxis for, 201–202
    related to dosing schedule, 200
    sexual dysfunction, 204
  therapeutic window for, 142
  use in special populations
    children and adolescents, **182**, 226
    developmentally disabled persons, **184**
    elderly patients, **183**
    pregnancy, 220
Haloperidol decanoate
  conversion from oral drug to, 186–187, 230–231
  dosage of, **150**
Haloperidol pyridinium, 142
Hamilton Rating Scale for Depression, 85, 108, 428
Headache, drug-induced
  antidepressants, **51, 54**
    selective serotonin reuptake inhibitors, 23, **32, 55**
  benzodiazepines, **278**, 306
  mood stabilizers
    carbamazepine, 342, 414
    lamotrigine, 342
    oxcarbazepine, **364**
  verapamil, 401
Heart block, tricyclic antidepressant–induced, 22, 100
  management of, **56**
  when combined with carbamazepine, 429
Hemodialysis, for lithium toxicity, 412
Heparin, interaction with diazepam, 311
Hepatic drug metabolism, 9
Hepatic dysfunction
  antidepressants in, 92–93
  antipsychotics in, 142
  benzodiazepines in, 256, 289, 305
  drug-induced
    antipsychotics, 143
    carbamazepine, 343, **363**, 415
    isocarboxazid, 93
    nefazodone, 23, 93, 314
    tranylcypromine, 93
    tricyclic antidepressants, 23
    valproate, 341, 342, **358, 365**, 415

Herbal preparations, interaction with selective serotonin reuptake inhibitors, **63**
Heteroreceptors, 3
5-HIAA (5-hydroxyindoleacetic acid), 89
Hip fracture, benzodiazepine-associated, 258, **288,** 317
Histamine H_2 antagonists, for antipsychotic-induced weight gain, **172**
Histaminic receptors
  antidepressant actions at, **37**
  antipsychotic actions at, 143, **159,** 197
Hostility, anxiolytic-induced, **278**
5-HT. *See* Serotonin
Hydralazine interactions
  with antipsychotics, 214
  with zaleplon, **285**
Hydrochlorothiazide, interaction with lithium, **372**
Hydroxybupropion, **39**
5-Hydroxyindoleacetic acid (5-HIAA), 89
Hydroxylation reactions, 9, 10
Hydroxynefazodone, **40**
11-Hydroxynortriptyline, 93
Hydroxyzine, **262**
Hyperammonemic encephalopathy, valproate-induced, 342, 433
Hypercortisolemia, in depression, 21
Hyperpolarization, 4, 255
Hyperprolactinemia, antipsychotic-induced, 143, **163,** 204, 208
Hyperreflexia
  lithium-induced, 411
  in serotonin syndrome, **70**
Hypersalivation, drug-induced
  anxiolytics, **278**
  clozapine, 143, **171,** 205–206
  management of, 144, **171,** 205
Hypertension, drug-induced
  antidepressants
    bupropion, **59**
    duloxetine, 97
    management of, **56**
    tricyclics, 22
    venlafaxine, **56**
  anxiolytics, **278**
  clozapine, 205
  yohimbine, **59**
Hypertensive crisis, monoamine oxidase inhibitor–induced, **56**
Hyperthermia
  in central anticholinergic syndrome, **67, 166**
  drug-induced
    lithium, 411
    topiramate, 402
  in lethal catatonia, **67, 166**
  malignant, **67–68, 166–168,** 209–211
  in neuroleptic malignant syndrome, **67, 166**
Hypnotic agents. *See* Anxiolytics and sedative-hypnotics
Hypochondriasis
  selective serotonin reuptake inhibitors for, **33**
  tricyclic antidepressants for, **34**
Hypomania. *See also* Mania
  drug-induced
    antidepressants, 97–98
    ziprasidone, 390
  in serotonin syndrome, **70**

Hyponatremia
central pontine myelinolysis from rapid overcorrection of, 414
drug-induced
carbamazepine, 343, **363**, 413–414
oxcarbazepine, 343, **364**, 414
selective serotonin reuptake inhibitors, 112
from excessive water drinking, clozapine for, 190
Hypotension, drug-induced, 2
antidepressants, **37**, **49–50**
management of, **56**
tricyclics, 22
antipsychotics, 144, 145, 146, **162–163**, **171**, 208
clozapine, 205, 231
droperidol, 186
quetiapine, 223
benzodiazepines, **278**, 306
intramuscular lorazepam, 293
beta-blockers, **178**
buspirone, **278**
management of, **56**, **171**
sildenafil, **59**
verapamil, 401
Hypothyroidism, lithium-induced, 342, **367**, 427

Ibuprofen interactions
with antidepressants, 102
with lithium, 343, 417–418
Idazoxan, 88
Imipramine
dosage of, **28**
drug interactions with
benzodiazepines, **283**, 312
chlorpromazine, 102
lithium, **372**
monoamine oxidase inhibitors, 24
formulations of, **28**
indications for, **34–35**
anxiety disorders, 302
dysthymic disorder, 84
panic disorder, 82, 83
intramuscular, 79, 113
mechanism of action of, **27**
pharmacokinetics of, **40**
in hepatic disease, 92
plasma levels of, **48**
in pregnancy, 114
side effects of, **49**, **51–54**
Imipramine pamoate, 79
IMPase (inositol monophosphatase)
carbamazepine stimulation of, 405
lithium inhibition of, 403
Incoordination
drug-induced
anxiolytics, **278**
lithium, **361**
in serotonin syndrome, **70**
Indapamide, interaction with lithium, 343
Indomethacin, interaction with lithium, 417–418
Inositol monophosphatase (IMPase)
carbamazepine stimulation of, 405
lithium inhibition of, 403
Inositol triphosphate, 4
Insomnia
antidepressants for, 20, **76**, 295
selective serotonin reuptake inhibitors, **33**
tricyclics, **34**
antihistamines for, 257
benzodiazepines for, **57**, 254, **267**
long-term use of, 294–295

Insomnia *(continued)*
  chloral hydrate for, 298–299
  drug-induced
    antidepressants, **49–51**, **54**
      management of, **57**
      reboxetine, 97
      selective serotonin reuptake inhibitors, 23, **33**, **38**, **55**
    anxiolytics, **278**
  nonbenzodiazepine hypnotics for, 295–296
    eszopiclone, **264**, 296
    zaleplon, **263**, 296
    zolpidem, **57**, **263**, 295–296
    zopiclone, **264**
  rebound, after drug discontinuation
    benzodiazepines, 257, 309
    zolpidem, 310
Insulin, interaction with monoamine oxidase inhibitors, **65**
Insulin resistance, antipsychotic-induced, 208–209
Interpersonal therapy
  for bipolar depression, **353**
  for dysthymic disorder, 85
Intramuscular drug administration
  antidepressants, 79, 113
  antipsychotics, 142, 188
  benzodiazepines, 293, 304
Intrauterine growth impairment, benzodiazepine-induced, 258, **287**, 315
Intravenous drug administration
  antidepressants, 79
  antipsychotics, 186
  benzodiazepines, 290, 305
Inverse agonists, 3
Ion channels, 4
  chloride, 2, 255
Ionotropic receptors, 3–4
Ipratropium spray, for hypersalivation, **171**, 206
Irritability, anxiolytic-induced, **278**
Isocarboxazid
  mechanism of action of, 27
  tablet strength and dosage of, **30**
Isoniazid interactions
  with benzodiazepines, **282**
  with carbamazepine, **374**
  with tricyclic antidepressants, **60**
Itraconazole interactions
  with antipsychotics, **177**
  with selective serotonin reuptake inhibitors, **62**

Janimine. *See* Imipramine
Jitteriness, antidepressant-induced, **37**
  management of, **58**

Kemadrin. *See* Procyclidine
Ketoconazole interactions
  with antidepressants, 103
    selective serotonin reuptake inhibitors, **62**
  with antipsychotics, **177**, 214
  with anxiolytics and sedative-hypnotics
    benzodiazepines, 257, **282**
    buspirone, 312
    zolpidem, **285**
    zopiclone, **285**
  with carbamazepine, 341
Ketorolac, interaction with lithium, 418
Kindling, 405–406
Klonopin. *See* Clonazepam

Lamictal. *See* Lamotrigine
Lamivudine/zidovudine, 229

Lamotrigine
autoinduction of, 341
combined with other mood stabilizers, 344
lithium, **383**
dosage of, **346**
drug interactions with, **379–380**
antidepressants, 102
antipsychotics, **175**
clozapine, 432
carbamazepine, **374**
oxcarbazepine, **374**
topiramate, 419–420
valproate, 341, 342, 343, **378, 380,** 417
elimination half-life of, **359**
formulations of, **346**
indications for, 400
antipsychotic augmentation, 145, **179,** 216–217
anxiety disorders, 254, 300, 400
bipolar disorder, 98, 338, 339
depressive episodes, **353,** 392
maintenance therapy, **356**
rapid cycling, **355,** 391
posttraumatic stress disorder, 300, 400
psychosis, 400
mechanism of action of, 340, **357,** 405
pharmacokinetics of, 15, 341, **359**
side effects of, 342
management of, 364
rash, 342, 345, **364, 387,** 412–413, 426, 431–432
use in special populations
children and adolescents, 345, **387,** 426
elderly patients, **388,** 427–428
pregnancy, **387**
Laryngospasm, barbiturate-induced, 298
LBD (Lewy body dementia), antipsychotics in, **155,** 194, 225
Leukocytosis, clozapine-induced, 205
Leukopenia, carbamazepine-induced, 343, **363,** 426, 431
Levetiracetam, for bipolar disorder, 338, 402–403
Lewy body dementia (LBD), antipsychotics in, **155,** 194, 225
Lexapro. *See* Escitalopram
Librium. *See* Chlordiazepoxide
Lidocaine, interaction with antidepressants, 114
Ligand-gated channels, 3–4
Ligands, 2–3
Lightheadedness, drug-induced
benzodiazepines, 257, 306
management of, **279**
carbamazepine, 342
Lipid irregularities, antipsychotic-induced, 144, 208–209
Lipophilicity of drugs, 7
antidepressants, 21
benzodiazepines, 305, 320
Lisinopril, interaction with lithium, **370,** 419
Lithium
brain-to-serum concentration ratio of, 426
combined with other drugs
carbamazepine, **381**
gabapentin, **386**
lamotrigine, **383**
thyroxine, **385,** 420, 421
topiramate, **384**
valproate, 344, 345, **382,** 419
in children, 426

Lithium *(continued)*
discontinuation of, 397–398, 412, 423
dosage of, **346**
drug interactions with, 343, **370–372**, 417–419
angiotensin-converting enzyme inhibitors, **370**, 419
antipsychotics, 144, **176**, **179**, **371**, 418
caffeine, 343, 431
calcium channel blockers, 343, **370**, 401, 422
clonazepam, 297
nonsteroidal anti-inflammatory drugs, 343, **372**, 417–418
selective serotonin reuptake inhibitors, 24, 430
elimination half-life of, 340, **358**
formulations of, **346**
indications for, 339, **349–350**, 398–400
alcoholism, **350**, 400
antidepressant augmentation, 24, **71**, 109, 110, **349**, 398–399
antipsychotic augmentation, 145, **179**
bipolar disorder, 337–339
depressive episodes, **349**, **353**, 392
maintenance therapy, **356**
mania, **156**, **349**, **351**, 389
mixed episodes, 389
predicting response to, 396, 406
prophylaxis, **349**
rapid cycling, **355**, 390
relapse after discontinuation of, 397–398, 423
borderline personality disorder, **350**, 400
impulsive aggression, **349**, 399–400
mental retardation with behavioral dyscontrol, **157**
obsessive-compulsive disorder, **350**
schizoaffective disorder, **349**, 399
schizophrenia, **350**, 399
schizophreniform disorder, **153**, 398, 399
mechanism of action of, 340, **357**, 403–404
pharmacokinetics of, 340–341, **358**, 408–409
potentiation of, 420
benzodiazepines, 313
side effects of, **179**, 342, **360**, 410–412
in children, 425
dosing schedule and, 410–411
management of, **366–368**
noncompliance due to, 411
slow-release, 6, **347**
therapeutic blood level of, **346**
dosing schedule and, 408–409
toxicity of
management of, 411–412
stages of, **361**
use in special populations, 344–345
children and adolescents, 345, **387**, 425
elderly or medically ill patients, 345, **388**, 426–427
pregnancy, 344–345, **387**, 423–424
withdrawal from, 397–398, 412

Lithium citrate syrup, **347**
Lithobid. *See* Lithium
Liver function test abnormalities. *See* Hepatic dysfunction
Loratadine, 429
  interaction with antidepressants, 114
Lorazepam
  abuse liability of, 307–308
  combined with haloperidol, **268,** 293
  cost of, **265**
  dosage of, **260**
  drug interactions with, **282**
    sertraline, 289
  elimination half-life of, 320
  formulations of, **260**
  indications for
    akathisia, 204, 234
    antipsychotic augmentation, **178**
    bipolar disorder, 338, 344
    catatonic patients, **69, 169,** 217, 314
    mania, **267,** 296
    panic disorder, **266**
    psychosis, **154,** 293
  intramuscular, 293, 304
  intravenous, 290
  metabolism of, 15, 256, **277,** 305
    in hepatic disease, 289
  pharmacokinetics of, **274,** 320
    absorption, 289
    lipophilicity and onset of action, 305, 320
  side effects of, 306
  sublingual, 290
  use in special populations
    breastfeeding, 317
    children and adolescents, 318
    elderly and/or dementia patients, 258–259, **288**
    pregnancy, 315
  withdrawal from, 308
Loxapine, 139
  for children and adolescents, **182,** 226
  dosage of, **148**
  pharmacokinetics of, **160**
  side effects of, **162**
Loxitane. *See* Loxapine
Ludiomil (maprotiline), **28,** 95
Lunesta. *See* Eszopiclone
Luvox. *See* Fluvoxamine

MADRS (Montgomery-Åsberg Depression Rating Scale), 393
Major tranquilizers. *See* Antipsychotics
Malignant hyperthermia
  causes/mechanisms of, **68, 168**
  differential diagnosis of, **67–68, 166–168**
  management of, **69, 169**
Manerix. *See* Moclobemide
Mania. *See also* Bipolar disorder
  antipsychotics for, 140, **156,** 188–189, 337, 344, 389–390
    aripiprazole, 140, 190, 389
    chlorpromazine-verapamil combination, 422
    clozapine, 189–190
    intramuscular olanzapine, 188
    olanzapine, 140, 190, 339, **351,** 389
    quetiapine, 140, 190, **351**
    risperidone, 140, 190, **351,** 389
    ziprasidone, 140, 190–191, 389
  benzodiazepines for, **156,** 254, **267, 286,** 296–297, 313

Mania *(continued)*
- calcium channel blockers for, 400–401
- drug-induced
  - alprazolam, 297
  - antidepressants, 22, **37**, 97–98, 391, 393, 394–395
    - prevention of, 395
    - risk factors for, **369**
  - atypical antipsychotics, 189, 390
- mood stabilizers for, 337–433
  - lithium, **156**, 188, 339, **349**, 389
  - valproate, 339, **351**, 389
  - valproate-lithium combination, 344
- preferred treatments of, **351–352**

MAOIs. *See* Monoamine oxidase inhibitors

Maprotiline, **28**
- seizures induced by, 95

Marplan. *See* Isocarboxazid

MEC (minimal effective concentration), 6

Mechanism of action (MOA), 1, 2–6, **5**
- of antidepressants, 4, 20–21, **27**, **36**, 85–90
- of antipsychotics, 140–142, **159**, 195–199, 340
- of anxiolytics and sedative-hypnotics, 255–256, **272–273**, 302–304
- of mood stabilizers, 4, 340, **357**, 403–406

Medically ill patients
- antihistamines for, **262**
- antipsychotics for, 145–146
- benzodiazepines for, 258, 318
- buspirone for, 259
- depression treatment in, 111–114
- mood stabilizers for, **388**
- psychostimulants for, 113

Mellaril. *See* Thioridazine

Memory
- components of, 306
- drug-induced impairment of (*See also* Cognitive effects)
  - antihistamines, 307
  - benzodiazepines, **178**, 257, **279**, 306–307
  - carbamazepine, 342
  - lithium, 342, **360**, **367**
  - tricyclic antidepressants, 22, 23
- long-term, 4

Menstrual dysfunction, drug-induced
- antipsychotics, 143, 204, 208
- valproate, 342

Mental retardation with behavioral dyscontrol
- antipsychotics for, **157**, **184**
- buspirone for, **262**

Meperidine, interaction with monoamine oxidase inhibitors, **65**, 101

Meprobamate, 254, **262**

Meridia (sibutramine), **368**

Mesoridazine
- dosage of, **149**
- side effects of, **162**

Messenger RNA (mRNA), 4, **5**

Metabolic acidosis, topiramate-induced, 402

Metabolic syndrome, antipsychotic-induced, 208–209

Metabolism of drugs, 1, 9–15
- antidepressants, 21–22
  - age effects on, 90–91
- antipsychotics, 142
- benzodiazepines, 10, **277**, 305

Metabolism of drugs *(continued)*
cytochrome enzymes in, 9–15, **11–14**
glucuronidation, 15
phase I reactions, 9
phase II reactions, 9
Metadate ER, Metadate CD. *See* Methylphenidate
Methadone interactions
with antipsychotics, 214
with monoamine oxidase inhibitors, **65**
with nefazodone, 122
with selective serotonin reuptake inhibitors, **63**, 122
with tricyclic antidepressants, **60**
with zaleplon, **285**
3-Methoxy-4-hydroxyphenylglycol (MHPG), 89
N-Methyl-D-aspartate (NMDA) receptors, 4, 90
antipsychotic actions at, 197
Methyldopa interactions
with antipsychotics, **176**
with lithium, **371**
with monoamine oxidase inhibitors, **65**
Methylin, Methylin ER. *See* Methylphenidate
Methylphenidate, 73
indications for
antidepressant augmentation, 24, 71, 108
monoamine oxidase inhibitors, 110
antidepressant-induced sexual dysfunction, **59**
selective serotonin reuptake inhibitor–induced apathy, 100
interaction with tricyclic antidepressants, **60**
side effects of, **59**
Methysergide, for serotonin syndrome, **69, 169**
Metoprolol, interaction with benzodiazepines, **282**
Metronidazole, interaction with lithium, **371**
Mexiletine interactions
with antipsychotics, 144
with selective serotonin reuptake inhibitors, **61**, 103
MHPG (3-methoxy-4-hydroxyphenylglycol), 89
Mianserin, 88
Midazolam
drug interactions with, **282**
elimination half-life of, 256
intramuscular, 304
intravenous, 290
metabolism of, 305, 311
Migraine
selective serotonin reuptake inhibitors for, **32**
valproate prophylaxis for, 400
Milnacipran, **27**, 88
Minimal effective concentration (MEC), 6
Mirtazapine, 19, **47**
combined with venlafaxine, 24
cost of, **31**
dosage of, **28**
for children and adolescents, **78**
drug interactions with, **47**
efficacy of, 104
formulations of, **28**
mechanism of action of, 3, 21, **27**, **36**, 87–88

Mirtazapine *(continued)*
for mixed anxiety-depression states, 314
pharmacodynamics of, 47
pharmacokinetics of, 10, **40**, **47**
side effects of, 23, **47**, **49**, **51**, 96
agranulocytosis, 96–97
seizures, 95
sexual dysfunction, 99
use in special populations, **75–76**
children and adolescents, **78**
elderly patients, 25
MOA. *See* Mechanism of action
Moban. *See* Molindone
Moclobemide, **30**
Modafinil
for antidepressant augmentation, **71**, 108–109
for drug-induced sedation, **57**, **171**
Molindone, 139
dosage of, **148**
side effects of, **162**
sexual dysfunction, 204
Monoamine oxidase inhibitors (MAOIs), 19
combined with tricyclic antidepressants, 24–25
drug interactions with, 24, **65**, 101
buspirone, 258, 312
carbamazepine, 417
selective serotonin reuptake inhibitors, 24, 101
serotonin syndrome due to, 24
tricyclic antidepressants, **60**, 101, 109–110
food restrictions for use of, **66**
indications for
anxiety disorders, 20
atypical depression, 83–84
bipolar depression, **353**
borderline personality disorder, 81
dysthymic disorder, 85
mixed anxiety-depressive states, 83
panic disorder, 20, 82
posttraumatic stress disorder, 302
mechanism of action of, 21, **27**
potentiation of, 109–110
reversible, 88
side effects of
hepatotoxicity, 93
hypertensive crisis, **56**
hypotension, **56**
tablet strengths and dosage of, **30**
transdermal, 88
use in seizure disorders, **76**
Montgomery-Åsberg Depression Rating Scale (MADRS), 393
Mood stabilizers, 337–433. *See also specific drugs*
class of, 337–338
combination of, 344
definition of, 344–345
dosage of, **346–348**
drug interactions with, 343–344, **370–380**, 416–420
formulations of, **346–348**
generic names of, **346–348**
indications for, 338–339, 389–403
bipolar disorder, 337–339
depressive episodes, **353–354**, 392
maintenance therapy, **356**
mania or mixed episodes, **351–352**, 389
predicting response to, 396, 406
rapid cycling, **355**
psychotic states, 339

Mood stabilizers *(continued)*
indications for *(continued)*
schizoaffective disorder, 145, **154**, 339
schizophrenia, 145
mechanisms of action of, 4, 340, **357**, 403–406
pharmacokinetics of, 340–341, **358–359**, 407–410
potentiation of, 344, **381–386**, 420–422
benzodiazepines, **286**, 313–314
questions and answers about, 389–428
side effects of, 342–343, **360–369**, 410–416
management of, **363–368**
risk factors for antidepressant-induced mania or cycling, **369**
therapeutic blood level of, **346–348**
trade names of, **346–348**
use in special populations, 344–345, **387–388**, 423–428
children and adolescents, 345, **387**, 425–426
elderly or medically ill patients, 345, **388**, 426–428
pregnancy and postpartum period, 344–345, **387**, 423–425
vignettes/puzzlers about, 428–433
Morphine, 15
interaction with monoamine oxidase inhibitors, **65**
mRNA (messenger RNA), 4, 5
Muscarinic receptors, 5
antidepressant actions at, **37**
antipsychotic actions at, 143, **159**, 197
Muscle fasciculations, lithium-induced, 411
Myoclonus
drug-induced
fluoxetine, **33**
tricyclic antidepressants, 23
nocturnal, benzodiazepines for, 254, **268**
in serotonin syndrome, **70**

Nadolol, for akathisia, 204
Naproxen interactions
with antidepressants, 102
with valproate, **377**
Nardil. *See* Phenelzine
Nausea/vomiting, drug-induced
antidepressants, **51, 53**
selective serotonin reuptake inhibitors, 23, **38, 55**, 112
management of, 112
antipsychotics
clozapine, 205
ziprasidone, 188
anxiolytics, **278**
mood stabilizers
carbamazepine, **362**, 426
lamotrigine, **364**
lithium, **361, 366**, 411
oxcarbazepine, **364**
topiramate, 402
Navane. *See* Thiothixene
NE. *See* Norepinephrine
Nefazodone, **47**
dosage of, **28**, 119
for children and adolescents, **78**
drug interactions with, 24, **47**
antipsychotics, **175, 177**, 214
benzodiazepines, 24, 257, **283**, 289, 311, 320–321
buspirone, 312

Nefazodone *(continued)*
drug interactions with *(continued)*
carbamazepine, 119, 341, **375**
methadone, 122
zolpidem, **285**
zopiclone, **285**
formulations of, **28**
indications for
mixed anxiety-depressive states, 83, 314
obsessive-compulsive disorder, 82
panic disorder, 83
mechanism of action of, 27, **36**, 87
metabolism of, 10
pharmacodynamics of, **47**
pharmacokinetics of, **40, 47**
plasma levels of, 119
side effects of, 23, **47, 49, 51–54**
hepatic dysfunction, 23, 93, 314
seizures, 95
sexual dysfunction, 99
use in special populations, **75–77**
Neonatal effects. *See also* Pregnancy
of antidepressants, 114, 116
of antipsychotics, **184–185**, 220
of benzodiazepines, 258, **287**, 315–316
Nervousness, drug-induced
antidepressants, **51, 54**
selective serotonin reuptake inhibitors, **55**
anxiolytics, **278**
tiagabine, 299
topiramate, 402
Neurobehavioral effects. *See* Cognitive effects
Neuroendocrine abnormalities, in depression, 20–21
Neuroleptic malignant syndrome (NMS), 143, 209–211
antipsychotic rechallenge after, 210–211
causes/mechanisms of, **68, 168**
clozapine-induced, 205
differential diagnosis of, **67–68, 166–168**
electroconvulsive therapy for, **69, 169**, 210
lithium reactivation of, **367**, 418
management of, **69, 169–170**, 210
symptoms of, **67, 166–167**, 209–210
Neuroleptics, 139. *See also* Antipsychotics
Neuropathic pain, antidepressants for, 20
monoamine oxidase inhibitors, 20
selective serotonin reuptake inhibitors, **32**
tricyclics, **34**
Neurosteroids, mechanism of action of, 255
Neurotransmitters, 3–6. *See also specific neurotransmitters*
amino acids, 3, 4
antidepressant actions on, 20, 21, 27, **36–38**, 85–90
antipsychotic actions on, 140–142
benzodiazepine actions on, 255, **272–273**, 302–303
biogenic amines, 3, 5
classes of, 3
mood stabilizer actions on, 340, **357**, 403–405
neuronal adaptation to actions of, 6
peptides, 3, 5
receptors for, 3–5
autoreceptors and heteroreceptors, 3
G-protein–linked, 3–4
ligand-gated channels, 3–4

Neurotrophic factors, 4, **5**
antidepressant effects on, 21
Neutral antagonists, 2
Nicardipine, 235
Nicotine dependence, bupropion for, **46, 76**
Nicotinic receptors, 5
Nifedipine, interaction with selective serotonin reuptake inhibitors, **63**
Night terrors, benzodiazepines for, 254, **268**
Nimodipine, for bipolar disorder, 338, **355,** 401, 422
Nitric oxide, 3
NMDA (*N*-methyl-D-aspartate) receptors, 4, 90
antipsychotic actions at, 197
NMS. *See* Neuroleptic malignant syndrome
Non-nucleoside reverse transcriptase inhibitors, and selective serotonin reuptake inhibitors, **64**
Nonsteroidal anti-inflammatory drug (NSAID) interactions
with antidepressants, 102
with lithium, 343, **372,** 417–418
with valproate, **377**
Norepinephrine (NE), 3
antidepressant actions on, 20, 21, **27, 36,** 86, 87, 88
effects of, **37**
antipsychotic actions on, 141–142
benzodiazepine actions on, 303
in depression, 20
lithium actions on, 340
receptors for, 6
valproate actions on, 404
Norepinephrine reuptake inhibitors (NRIs), 21
Norfluoxetine, **39,** 91, 92, 214, **283,** 312
Norpramin. *See* Desipramine
Nortriptyline
cost of, **31**
dosage of, **28**
drug interactions with
carbamazepine, 428–429
chlorpromazine, 102
formulations of, **28**
indications for, **33–34**
depressed cancer patients, 112
panic disorder, 82
selective serotonin reuptake inhibitor potentiation, 107
mechanism of action of, **27, 36**
pharmacokinetics of, **40**
age effects on, 91
dosing and, 118
plasma levels of, **48,** 117
in pregnancy, 114, 115
side effects of, **49**
narrow-angle glaucoma, 117–118
therapeutic window for, 22
NRIs (norepinephrine reuptake inhibitors), 21
NSAIDs. *See* Nonsteroidal anti-inflammatory drug interactions
Nystagmus, carbamazepine-induced, 426

Obese patients, antidepressants for, **75**
Obsessional disorder, 227–228
Obsessive-compulsive disorder (OCD)
antidepressants for, 20, 82
intravenous formulations, 79
monoamine oxidase inhibitors, 20

Obsessive-compulsive disorder (OCD) *(continued)*
- antidepressants for *(continued)*
  - selective serotonin reuptake inhibitors, **32**, 82, 228, 255, **270**, 291
    - in children and adolescents, 318
  - trazodone, 302
  - tricyclics, 20, **33**, 302
- antipsychotic exacerbation of, 218
- antipsychotics for, 140, **157**, 194–195, 218, 301
- benzodiazepines for, 254, **266**, 291, 293
- lithium for, **350**
- schizophrenia and, 218

OCD. *See* Obsessive-compulsive disorder

OFAs (omega-3 fatty acids), for bipolar disorder, 403

OFC. *See* Olanzapine/fluoxetine combination

Olanzapine, 139
- combining with other antipsychotics, **180**
- cost of, **152**
- dosage of, **149**, **151**, **347**
- drug interactions with, 144, **175**, **177**
  - antipsychotics, **178**
  - fluvoxamine, 24, 102, 212–213, 232–233
- elimination half-life of, **358**
- formulations of, **151**, **347**
- indications for, 339
  - bipolar disorder, **156**, 190–191, 338
    - maintenance therapy, 140, 191
    - mania, 140, 190, 339, **351**, 389
    - mixed episodes, 389
  - borderline personality disorder, **154**, 192
  - dementia-related syndromes, **155**, 193
  - obsessive-compulsive disorder, 194
  - posttraumatic stress disorder, 301
  - psychotic depression, **157**
  - refractory schizophrenia, 190
  - schizophrenia, 198
  - Tourette's syndrome, **158**
- intramuscular, 188
- mechanism of action of, 340
- metabolism of, 10, 15
- onset of action of, 196
- pharmacokinetics of, 142, **161**, **358**
- plasma levels of, 143, **149**, **347**
  - effect of smoking on, 230
- receptor affinities of, **159**, 197
- side effects of, 144, **163**, 188, 207–208
  - cerebrovascular adverse events, 223
  - electroencephalogram abnormalities, 220
  - glucose and lipid abnormalities, 209
  - sexual dysfunction, 205
- use in special populations
  - children and adolescents, **182**, 226, 345
  - developmentally disabled persons, **184**
  - elderly patients, 146, **183**, 222, 223, 345, **388**
  - Parkinson's disease, 225
  - pregnancy, **185**, 221

Olanzapine/fluoxetine combination
for bipolar depression, **156**, 191, 338, **353**, 393–394
for lithium augmentation, 420
for refractory depression, **157**
Oligohydrosis, topiramate-induced, 402
Omega-3 fatty acids (OFAs), for bipolar disorder, 403
Omeprazole interactions
with antidepressants, 103
with antipsychotics, **175**, **177**
with benzodiazepines, **282**
Ondansetron, for nausea, 112
Opioid interactions
with antipsychotics, **176**
with benzodiazepines, 257, **283**, 310
with monoamine oxidase inhibitors, 24, **65**
with selective serotonin reuptake inhibitors, **63**, 114
Oral contraceptive interactions
with benzodiazepines, **282**
with carbamazepine, 343, **375**
with lamotrigine, **378**
with oxcarbazepine, 343, 429
with tricyclic antidepressants, **60**
Orap. *See* Pimozide
Orlistat, for drug-induced weight gain, **172**, **368**
Orthostatic hypotension. *See* Hypotension
Osteoporosis
lithium and, **367**
thyroxine and, 421
Overdose of drug
barbiturates, **262**
benzodiazepines, 2–3
selective serotonin reuptake inhibitors, 112
tricyclic antidepressants, 80, 100–101
Oxazepam
abuse liability of, 307
cost of, **265**
dosage of, **260**
drug interactions with, **282**
sertraline, 289
formulations of, **260**
metabolism of, 15, 256, **277**, 305
in hepatic disease, 289
pharmacokinetics of, **274**
absorption, 289
use in special populations
breastfeeding, 317
elderly and/or dementia patients, 258–259, **288**
Oxcarbazepine
for bipolar disorder, 338
efficacy of, 397
maintenance therapy, **356**
mania, **351**
predictors of response to, 396
rapid cycling, **355**
dosage of, **347**
drug interactions with, 341, 343–344
antipsychotics, 213
benzodiazepines, 257
lamotrigine, **374**, **379**
oral contraceptives, 343, 429
selective serotonin reuptake inhibitors, **61**
elimination half-life of, **358**
formulations of, **347**
mechanism of action of, **357**
pharmacokinetics of, 341, **358**
side effects of, 343
management of, **364**

Oxcarbazepine *(continued)*
therapeutic blood level of, **347**
use in special populations, **387–388**
pregnancy, 423
Oxidative metabolism of drugs, 9, 10
Oxybutynin, for clozapine-induced enuresis, 206
Oxygen therapy, for malignant hyperthermia, **69, 169**

Pain syndromes, antidepressants for, 20
selective serotonin reuptake inhibitors, **32,** 111
tricyclics, **34**
Palpitations, drug-induced
antidepressants, **52**
anxiolytics, **278**
methylphenidate, **59**
Pamelor. *See* Nortriptyline
Pancreatitis, drug-induced
antipsychotics, 143
valproate, 342, 426
Panic disorder
antidepressants for, 20, 82–83
monoamine oxidase inhibitors, 20, 82
selective serotonin reuptake inhibitors, **32,** 82, 83, 255, **270,** 291
in children and adolescents, 319
tricyclics, **33,** 82, 302
benzodiazepines for, 254, **266,** 321–322, 429
combined with buspirone, 313
switching from alprazolam to clonazepam, 321
mood stabilizers for
tiagabine, 299, 315
valproate, 299, 400
PANSS (Positive and Negative Syndrome Scale), 199, 400
Paranoid personality disorder, antipsychotics for, **154,** 193
Paresthesias, topiramate-induced, 402
Parkinsonism, antipsychotic-induced, 143, **164**
prophylaxis for, 202
Parkinson's disease
antidepressants in, **76**
antipsychotics in, **155,** 224–225
clozapine, 145, 194, 224–225
Parnate. *See* Tranylcypromine
Paroxetine, **43**
combined with bupropion, 107
combined with psychostimulants, 108
controlled-release, **29, 31**
cost of, **31**
dosage of, **28–29**
for children and adolescents, **78**
drug interactions with, **43,** 114
antipsychotics, 144, **175, 177,** 212, 214
tamoxifen, 103
tricyclic antidepressants, 23
elimination half-life and discontinuation of, 92
formulations of, **28–29**
indications for, **32–33**
anxiety in children and adolescents, 318, 319
bipolar depression, **43, 353,** 394
generalized anxiety disorder, **266,** 292
panic disorder, 82
posttraumatic stress disorder, 291
social phobia, 292, 319
mechanism of action of, **27, 36,** 86
pharmacodynamics of, **43**

Paroxetine *(continued)*
pharmacokinetics of, **40, 43**
age effects on, 91
in pregnancy, 115
side effects of, 23, **43, 49, 51–55**
sexual dysfunction, 99
switching to fluoxetine from, 106
use in hepatic disease, 93
use in special populations
breastfeeding, 116
children and adolescents, **78,** 121
withdrawal symptoms from, 92
Partial agonists, 3
Paxil, Paxil CR. *See* Paroxetine
Paxipam. *See* Halazepam
Pediatric patients. *See* Children and adolescents
Pemoline
combined with fluoxetine, 108
combined with monoamine oxidase inhibitors, 110
Pentazocine, interaction with selective serotonin reuptake inhibitors, **63**
Peptic ulcer disease, antidepressants in, **76**
Peptide neurotransmitters, 3
Pergolide, for antidepressant augmentation, **71**
Periodic leg movements of sleep (PLMS)
benzodiazepines for, 296, 322
pergolide for, 296
Permitil. *See* Fluphenazine
Perphenazine
dosage of, **148, 150**
formulations of, **150**
interaction with antidepressants, 102
pharmacokinetics of, 142, **160**
plasma levels of, **148**
side effects of, **162**
Personality disorders. *See also specific personality disorders*
antidepressants for, 20
selective serotonin reuptake inhibitors, **32**
tricyclics, **34**
antipsychotics for, **154,** 192–193
Pertofrane. *See* Desipramine
P-glycoprotein (P-gp), 1, 7
Pharmacodynamics, 2–6
of antidepressants, **42–47**
definition of, 1
drug side effects and, 2
of hypnotic agents, **273**
ligands and receptors, 2–3
neurotransmitters and signal transduction, 3–6
Pharmacokinetics, 6–9
absorption, 6–7
of antidepressants, 21–22, **39–47,** 90–94
of antipsychotics, 142–143
of benzodiazepines, 256, **274–277,** 304–306, 320
definition of, 1, 6
distribution, 7–8
elimination, 8–9
of mood stabilizers, 340–341, **358–359,** 407–410
single-dose kinetics
of benzodiazepines, 305–306
definition of, 305
Phase I reactions, 9
Phase II reactions, 9
Phenacetin, 10
Phenelzine
drug interactions with
carbamazepine, 417
succinylcholine, **65**

Phenelzine *(continued)*
- indications for
  - depression with atypical features, 84
  - panic disorder, 82
  - social phobia, 300
- mechanism of action of, **27**
- tablet strength and dosage of, **30**

Phenobarbital
- for benzodiazepine withdrawal, 309
- drug interactions with
  - antipsychotics, 145, **176**
  - benzodiazepines, 257
  - carbamazepine, **375**
  - lamotrigine, **379**
  - valproate, 343, **378**, 417

Phenothiazines, 139, **148–149**. *See also* Antipsychotics

Phentermine, interaction with monoamine oxidase inhibitors, **65**

Phenylbutazone, interaction with tricyclic antidepressants, **60**

Phenytoin interactions, 10
- with antipsychotics, 145, **175**, **177**, 232
- with benzodiazepines, 257, **282**
- with carbamazepine, **375**
- with lamotrigine, **378**
- with oxcarbazepine, 343
- with topiramate, 419
- with tricyclic antidepressants, **60**
- with valproate, 343, 417

Phosphatidylinositol (PI) signaling, lithium effects on, 404

Photosensitivity, antipsychotic-induced, 143

Physostigmine, for central anticholinergic syndrome, **69**, **169**

PI (phosphatidylinositol) signaling, lithium effects on, 404

Pilocarpine, for anticholinergic drug effects, **56**

Pimozide, 139
- dosage of, **148**
- indications for
  - delusional disorder, 195
  - obsessive-compulsive disorder, 194
  - Tourette's syndrome, **158**
- pharmacokinetics of, **160**
- side effects of, **162**

Pindolol, for selective serotonin reuptake inhibitor potentiation, 89–90

Plasma levels
- of antidepressants, 94
  - nefazodone, 119
  - tricyclics, 22, **48**, 94, 100–101, 117
- of antipsychotics, 142–143, **148–149**
  - elimination half-life and, 200
  - therapeutic response to clozapine and, 201
- of mood stabilizers, **346–348**
  - carbamazepine, **346**, 407
  - lithium, **346**, 408–409
  - valproate, **348**, 409–410

Platelet abnormalities, valproate-induced, 342, 345, **365**

PLMS (periodic leg movements of sleep)
- benzodiazepines for, 296, 322
- pergolide for, 296

PMDD (premenstrual dysphoric disorder), selective serotonin reuptake inhibitors for, **33**

Polycystic ovarian disease, valproate-induced, 342

Polydipsia
- clozapine for, 190
- lithium-induced, 342, **360**, 425

Polyphagia, lithium-induced, 425
Polyuria, lithium-induced, **179**, 342, **360**, 410, 425
Positive and Negative Syndrome Scale (PANSS), 199, 400
Postpartum period
  depression in, 26
  mood stabilizers for bipolar disorder in, 424–425
Posttraumatic stress disorder (PTSD)
  antidepressants for, 20, 302
    selective serotonin reuptake inhibitors, **32**, 255, **267**, **270**, 291–292
    tricyclics, **34**, 302
  antipsychotics for, 301
  baclofen for, 302
  benzodiazepines for, 254, **267**
  buspirone for, **262**
  guanfacine for, 299
  mood stabilizers for, 300, 339
    lamotrigine, 400
    tiagabine, 258, 315
    valproate, 400
  treatment in children and adolescents, 319
Postural hypotension. *See* Hypotension
Pramipexole
  for antidepressant augmentation, **71**
  for bipolar depression, 422
Prazepam
  dosage of, **260**
  formulations of, **260**
  metabolism of, **277**
  pharmacokinetics of, **274**
Prednisone, interaction with carbamazepine, 343
Pregabalin, 300
  for anxiety disorders, 300
  mechanism of action of, 300, 340, **357**
  side effects of, 300
Pregnancy
  antidepressants in, 26, 114–116
  antipsychotics in, 146–147, **184–185**, 220–221
  anxiolytics and sedative-hypnotics in
    benzodiazepines, 258, **287**, 315–316
    buspirone, 258, 316
    zaleplon, 258, 316
    zolpidem, 258, 316, 323
  electroconvulsive therapy in, 26, 147
  mood stabilizers in, 344–345, **387**, 423–424
Premenstrual dysphoric disorder (PMDD), selective serotonin reuptake inhibitors for, **33**
Priapism, drug-induced, 99. *See also* Sexual dysfunction
  antipsychotics, 204, 205
  trazodone, **37**, 99
Primidone interactions
  with carbamazepine, **375**
  with lamotrigine, **379**
Procainamide, interaction with tricyclic antidepressants, **60**
Procyclidine, for extrapyramidal side effects, **165**
Prolixin. *See* Fluphenazine
Promazine, **148**
Propafenone interactions
  with antipsychotics, 144
  with selective serotonin reuptake inhibitors, **61**, 114
Propantheline bromide, for tricyclic antidepressant withdrawal symptoms, 91–92

Propoxyphene, interaction with benzodiazepines, **282**

Propranolol
- for akathisia, **171**, 204, 233–234
- drug interactions with
  - antipsychotics, **176**
  - benzodiazepines, **282**
- for serotonin syndrome, **69**, **169**

2-Propyl-4-pentanoic acid, **358**

ProSom. *See* Estazolam

Protease inhibitor interactions, 10
- with antidepressants, 114
  - selective serotonin reuptake inhibitors, **64**, 120
- with antipsychotics, **176**
- with benzodiazepines, 257

Protein binding of drug, 7–8

Protein kinase A, 90

Protein kinase C, lithium actions on, 411

Protein kinases, 4, **5**

Protein phosphorylation, 4, **5**

Protriptyline
- dosage of, **29**
- elimination half-life of, 21
- formulations of, **29**
- side effects of, 23

Prozac. *See* Fluoxetine

Pruritus, lithium-induced, **368**

Pseudotumor cerebri, and lithium, **367**

Psoriasis, lithium exacerbation of, **368**

Psychodynamic psychotherapy, for bipolar depression, **353**

Psychomotor effects
- of antidepressants, 23, **37**
- of antipsychotics, 143, **164** (*See also* Extrapyramidal side effects)
- of benzodiazepines, 257, **279**

Psychosis
- antidepressant-induced, 22, **37**
- antipsychotics for, 139–235 (*See also* Antipsychotics)
- benzodiazepines for, **153**, **154**, 254, **268**, **286**, 314
- mood stabilizers for, 339
  - lithium, **153**, **349**, **350**, 398, 399
- in pregnancy, **184**

Psychostimulants, **73–74**
- for antidepressant augmentation, 24, **71**, 108, 110
- for depression in medically ill patients, 113

Psychotherapy
- for anxiety disorders, 292–293, 316
- for bipolar disorder, **353**, **356**
- for dysthymic disorder, 85
- for schizophrenia, 218–219

Psychotic depression
- antidepressants for, 25
- antipsychotics for, 140, **157**
  - clozapine, 189–190
- electroconvulsive therapy for, 25, **157**

Psychotropic medications
- antidepressants, 19–122
- antipsychotics, 139–235
- anxiolytics and sedative-hypnotics, 253–323
- discontinuation of, 9
- drug interactions with, 15–16
- mechanisms of action of, 1, 2–6, **5**
- metabolism of, 9–15
- mood stabilizers, 337–433
- pharmacodynamics of, 2–6
- pharmacokinetics of, 6–9

PTSD. *See* Posttraumatic stress disorder

QT interval prolongation, drug-induced, 144
  antipsychotics, 143–144, 188, 211–212, 235
    management of, **172**
  calcium channel blockers, 235
  tricyclic antidepressants, 22
Quazepam
  dosage of, **261**
  formulations of, **261**
  metabolism of, **277**
  pharmacodynamics of, **273**
  side effects of, 306
Quetiapine, 139
  cost of, **152**
  dosage of, **148, 151**
  drug interactions with, **177**, 214
    nefazodone, 24
  formulations of, **151**
  indications for
    bipolar disorder, **156**, 338
      mania, 140, 190, **351**
    dementia with psychotic features, **155**
    posttraumatic stress disorder, 301
    schizophrenia, 198
    Tourette's syndrome, **158**
  metabolism of, 10
  pharmacokinetics of, 142, **161**, 200
  receptor affinities of, **159**, 197
  side effects of, 142–143, **163**, 207–208
    cataracts, 212
    related to dosing schedule, 200
    sexual dysfunction, 205
  use in special populations
    children and adolescents, **182**, 226
    elderly patients, **183**, 222, 223
    Parkinson's disease, 224–225
    pregnancy, **185**
Quinidine interactions
  with antidepressants, 103, 114
    tricyclics, **60**
  with antipsychotics, 144, **177**, 214
Quinolinones, 139.
  See also Antipsychotics

Ranitidine
  during carbamazepine therapy, **373**
  interaction with benzodiazepines, **282**
Rapid neuroleptization, 195
Rash, drug-induced
  antipsychotics, 143
  carbamazepine, 342, **363**, 414, 426
  lamotrigine, 342, 345, **364**, **387**, 412–413, 426, 431–432
Reboxetine
  dosage of, **29**
  mechanism of action of, 21, **27**, **36**
  side effects of, 97
Receptors, 3
  amino acid, 4
  autoreceptors, 3
  benzodiazepine, 2, 255
  for biogenic amines, 1, 2
  glucocorticoid, 5
  G-protein–linked, 3–4, 5
  heteroreceptors, 3
  ionotropic (ligand-gated channels), 3–4
  metabotropic, 4
  muscarinic, 5
  nicotinic, 5
  NMDA, 4
  norepinephrine, 6
Rectal administration, of antidepressants, 113

REM sleep behavioral disorder, clonazepam for, **268**
Remeron. *See* Mirtazapine
Renal dysfunction
  antidepressants in, 91, 93
  lithium in, 345
  lithium-induced, 342, **366,** 410
Reserpine, interaction with monoamine oxidase inhibitors, **65**
Respiratory disease
  antidepressants in, **76**
  benzodiazepines in, 318
  beta-blockers in, **178**
  buspirone in, 318
Respiratory suppression, drug-induced
  baclofen, 302
  barbiturates, 298
  benzodiazepines, 257, **280,** 290, 318
Restless leg syndrome, 296
Restlessness, in serotonin syndrome, **70**
Restoril. *See* Temazepam
Rifampin interactions
  with benzodiazepines, 257, **282**
  with tricyclic antidepressants, **60**
  with zaleplon, **285**
  with zolpidem, **285**
Rigidity, lithium-induced, 411
Risperdal. *See* Risperidone
Risperdal Consta, 187–188, 228
Risperidone, 139
  combined with other antipsychotics, **180**
    clozapine, 215–216
  cost of, **152**
  dosage of, **148, 151**
  drug interactions with, **175–177,** 214, 222
    antidepressants, 102, 222
  formulations of, **151**
  indications for
    bipolar disorder, **156,** 191, 338
      mania, 140, 190, **351,** 389
    dementia-related syndromes, 193
    obsessive-compulsive disorder, 194, 228, 301
    posttraumatic stress disorder, 301
    schizophrenia, 198
    Tourette's syndrome, **158**
  long-acting, 187–188, 228
  mechanism of action of, 141
  metabolism of, 10
  onset of action of, 196
  pharmacokinetics of, 142, **161**
  plasma levels of, **148**
  receptor affinities of, **159**
  side effects of, 143, **163,** 208
    cerebrovascular adverse events, 146, **155, 183,** 193, 223–224
    electroencephalogram abnormalities, 220
    extrapyramidal symptoms, 202
    neuroleptic malignant syndrome, 210
    related to dosing schedule, 200
    sexual dysfunction, 205
  use in special populations
    children and adolescents, **182,** 226
    developmentally disabled persons, **184**
    elderly patients, 146, **183,** 193, 222–223, 345
    Parkinson's disease, 225
Ritalin, Ritalin SR, Ritalin LA. *See* Methylphenidate

Ritonavir interactions
with antidepressants, **64**, 114, 120
with antipsychotics, **176**, 214
with zolpidem, **285**
with zopiclone, **285**
RNA, messenger (mRNA), 4, **5**
Rofecoxib, interaction with lithium, **370**, 418

St. John's wort, interaction with selective serotonin reuptake inhibitors, **63**
Salicylates, interaction with valproate, 343
Saline diuresis, for lithium toxicity, 412
Saquinavir, interaction with antidepressants, **64**, 114
Schizoaffective disorder
antidepressants for, 20
antipsychotics for, 140, **154**, 190–191
electroconvulsive therapy for, **154**
mood stabilizers for, 145, **154**, 339
lamotrigine, 400
lithium, **349**, 399
Schizoid personality disorder, antipsychotics for, **154**
Schizophrenia
anticonvulsants for, 145, **179**, **181**, 216–217
antipsychotics for, 140, **153**
clozapine
combined with neuroleptic, 214–215
vs. olanzapine, 190
combining atypical antipsychotics, 215–216
potentiation of, 145, **178–181**, 214–219
psychotherapy and, 218–219
benzodiazepines for, 145, **178**, 196, 217, 294, 314
beta-blockers for, 145
childhood, 225–226
in children and adolescents, 146
diabetes mellitus and, 208
dopamine hypothesis of, 141, 142
glutamate dysfunction in, 142
glycine for, 217
mood stabilizers for, 145
lamotrigine, 400
lithium, **350**, 399
valproate, 400
negative symptoms of, 195, 197–198
efficacy of atypical antipsychotics for, 197–198
obsessive-compulsive symptoms in, 218
Schizophrenia Outpatient Health Outcomes (SOHO) study, 198
Schizophreniform disorder
antipsychotics for, 140, **153**
lithium for, **179**, 398, 399
Schizotypal personality disorder, antipsychotics for, **154**, 193
Scopolamine, transdermal, for hypersalivation, 205
Secondary messengers, 4, **5**
Sedation, drug-induced
antidepressants, **37**, **49–50**, **57**
mirtazapine, 23
nefazodone, 23
tricyclics, 23
antipsychotics, **162–163**, **171**
clozapine, 205
quetiapine, 223
ziprasidone, 188

Sedation, drug-induced *(continued)*
benzodiazepines, **178**, 256, 306
cyproheptadine, **59**
management of, **57**, **171**
mood stabilizers
carbamazepine, **363**
valproate, **181**
Sedative-hypnotics. *See* Anxiolytics and sedative-hypnotics
Seizure disorders
antidepressants in, **76**, 95
antipsychotics in, 219–220
tiagabine in, 299–300
Seizures
benzodiazepine-withdrawal, 257, 308
drug-induced
antidepressants, **76**, 94–96
bupropion, **46**, **59**, 95
maprotiline, 95
mirtazapine, 95
nefazodone, 95
predisposing factors for, 95–96
selective serotonin reuptake inhibitors, 95
tricyclics, 23, 94–95
venlafaxine, 95
antipsychotics, 143, **175**, 219–220
clozapine, 205, 219–220
lithium, **361**
tiagabine, 299
kindling and, 405
Selective serotonin reuptake inhibitors (SSRIs). *See also specific drugs*
cost of, **31**
dosage of, **28–29**
for children and adolescents, 78
drug interactions with, 23–24, **61–64**, 114
antipsychotics, 23–24, 102, 144, **175**, **177**, **178**, 212–214
benzodiazepines, **283**, 311–312
beta-blockers, 112
buspirone, 24, 322–323
carbamazepine, **375**
lamotrigine, **379**
lithium, **371**, 430
monoamine oxidase inhibitors, 24, **65**, 101
tricyclic antidepressants, 23, 24, **60**, 101
efficacy of, 104
elimination half-lives of, 22
drug discontinuation and, 92
formulations of, **28–28**
heterogeneity of, 19
indications for, 20, **32–33**
aggression, **33**
antipsychotic augmentation, **178**
anxiety disorders, 253, 255, **270**, 291–292
in children and adolescents, 318–319
behavioral disturbances in dementia, **33**, **155**, 194
bipolar disorder, 98, 338, **353**, 394
body dysmorphic disorder, **33**, 81
borderline personality disorder, **32**, 81
delusional disorder, 195
dysthymic disorder, 84–85
eating disorders, **32**
generalized anxiety disorder, **32**, 255, **270**
hypochondriasis, **33**
insomnia, **33**

Selective serotonin reuptake inhibitors (SSRIs) *(continued)*
indications for *(continued)*
mental retardation with behavioral dyscontrol, **157**
mixed anxiety-depressive states, 83
combined with benzodiazepines, 314
obsessive-compulsive disorder, **32,** 82, 228, 255, **270,** 291
pain syndromes, **32,** 111
panic disorder, **32,** 82, 83, 255, **270,** 291
posttraumatic stress disorder, 255, **270,** 291–292
premenstrual dysphoric disorder, **33**
social phobia, **32,** 255, **270,** 292
mechanism of action of, 27, **36,** 85–86
metabolism of, 10
overdose of, 112
pharmacokinetics of, **39–40**
in hepatic disease, 92–93
for postpartum depression, 26
potentiation of, 24, 71–72
benzodiazepines, **286**
bupropion, 24, 107–108
lithium, 109
psychostimulants, 108
tricyclic antidepressants, 107
side effects of, 23, **49–55,** 112
apathy, 100
bleeding, 23, 96
in children and adolescents, 319
in elderly patients, 25
seizures, 95
sexual dysfunction, 23, 37, **38,** 99–100
slow-release, 6
switching between, 106–107
switching from tricyclic antidepressant to, 104–106
use in special populations, 75–77
breastfeeding, 116
cancer/medically ill patients, 111, 112
children and adolescents, 26, **78,** 318–319
elderly patients, 25
pregnancy, 26, 114–116
withdrawal symptoms with, 92
Selegiline, **30**
transdermal, 88
Selenium supplementation, for valproate-induced hair loss, 415
Self-injurious behavior. *See also* Suicidality
antidepressant-induced, in children and adolescents, 121
in mental retardation
antipsychotics for, **184**
buspirone for, **262**
mood stabilizers for, 339
Serax. *See* Oxazepam
Serentil (mesoridazine), **149, 162**
Seroquel. *See* Quetiapine
Serotonin (5-HT), 2, 3
antidepressant actions on, 20, 21, **27, 36,** 85–88
effects of, **37**
benzodiazepine actions on, 303
in depression and suicidality, 20
lithium actions on, 340
Serotonin receptors
antidepressant actions at, 20, 85–87
antagonism, **37**
mirtazapine, 88–89
stimulation, **38**

Serotonin receptors *(continued)*
autoreceptors, 3
desensitization of, 4, 85–86
5-HT_{1A}, buspirone actions at, 255–256, **262**, 303
5-HT_2
antidepressant down-regulation of, 20, 87
antipsychotic actions at, 141, 142, **159**, 197, 340
aripiprazole, 199
electroconvulsive therapy actions at, 20, 87
in etiology of depression, 86–87
heteroreceptors, 3
Serotonin syndrome, 24, **37**, **65**, 120
with buspirone, 312, 322–323
causes/mechanisms of, **68**, **168**
from combining lithium and fluoxetine, 430
differential diagnosis of, **67–68**, **166–168**
management of, **69**, **169**
symptom frequency in, **70**
Serotonin-norepinephrine reuptake inhibitors (SNRIs), 21
indications for, **32–33**
mechanism of action of, 27, 86, 88
Seroxat. *See* Paroxetine
Sertraline, **42**
in breastfeeding, **42**
combined with bupropion, 107–108
cost of, **31**
dosage of, **29**
for children and adolescents, **78**
drug interactions with, **42**
benzodiazepines, **283**, 289, 312
lamotrigine, 102, **379**
zolpidem, **285**
zopiclone, **285**
elimination half-life and discontinuation of, 92
formulations of, **29**
indications for, **32–33**
anxiety in children and adolescents, 318
dysthymic disorder, 84, 85
panic disorder, 82
posttraumatic stress disorder, 291
social phobia, 292
tricyclic antidepressant potentiation, 107
mechanism of action of, **27**, **36**, 86
metabolism of, 10
pharmacodynamics of, **42**
in hepatic disease, 92–93
pharmacokinetics of, **40**, **42**
in pregnancy, 115
side effects of, 23, **50**, **51–55**
withdrawal symptoms with, 92
Serzone. *See* Nefazodone
Sexual dysfunction
antidepressant-induced (AISD), **51**, **53**, 99–100
duloxetine, 97
management of, **59**, 99–100
selective serotonin reuptake inhibitors, 23, **37**, **38**, 99–100
tricyclics, 23
antidepressants for patients with, **76**
antipsychotic-induced, 143, 204–205
management of, **172**
anxiolytic-induced, **278**
Shivering, in serotonin syndrome, **70**

SIADH (syndrome of inappropriate antidiuretic hormone), drug-induced
  carbamazepine, **179**, 343
  selective serotonin reuptake inhibitors, 25
Sibutramine, **368**
Signal transduction, 3–6, **5**
Sildenafil
  for sexual dysfunction, **59**, 100, **172**
  side effects of, **59**
Sinequan. *See* Doxepin
Single-dose kinetics
  of benzodiazepines, 305–306
  definition of, 305
Sleep disorders. *See also* Insomnia
  benzodiazepines for, 254, **268**, **296**
Sleep-related breathing disorders, benzodiazepines in, **268**, 294
Slow-release drug formulations, 6
Smoking
  antipsychotic interaction with, 145, **177**, 230
  bupropion for cessation of, **46**, **76**
SNRIs. *See* Serotonin-norepinephrine reuptake inhibitors
Social phobia
  anticonvulsants for
    gabapentin, 300
    pregabalin, 300
  antidepressants for
    phenelzine, 300
    selective serotonin reuptake inhibitors, **32**, 255, **266**, **270**, 292
      in children and adolescents, 319
    venlafaxine, **32**
  anxiolytics for
    benzodiazepines, 254, **266**, 300
    buspirone, **262**
Social withdrawal, in schizophrenia, 195, 197
Sodium bicarbonate, for malignant hyperthermia, **69**, **169**
Sodium chloride, for orthostatic hypotension, **56**, 144, **171**
Sodium ion flux, 4
SOHO (Schizophrenia Outpatient Health Outcomes) study, 198
Somatoform disorders, antidepressants for, 20, **33**, **34**
Sonata. *See* Zaleplon
Sotalol, interaction with antipsychotics, 144
Sparine (promazine), **148**
Speech slurring, benzodiazepine-induced, **279**
Spina bifida, valproate-induced, 342, 345, 423
SS (steady-state) concentration of drug, 8–9
SSRIs. *See* Selective serotonin reuptake inhibitors
Status epilepticus, tiagabine-induced, 299
Steady-state (SS) concentration of drug, 8–9
Stelazine. *See* Trifluoperazine
Steroid hormones, 10
Stevens-Johnson syndrome, drug-induced
  carbamazepine, **363**
  lamotrigine, 342, 413, 431–432
Stokes-Adams attack, 429
Stomatitis in cancer patients, 111, 113
Strattera. *See* Atomoxetine

Stroke, antipsychotic-associated, 146, **155**, **183**, 193, 223–224
Sublingual administration, of benzodiazepines, 290
Substance-abusing patients, use of benzodiazepines in, 292, 307–308
Substance-induced psychosis, antipsychotics for, **154**
Succinylcholine, interaction with phenelzine, **65**
Suicidality.
See also Self-injurious behavior
antidepressant-induced, in children and adolescents, 121–122, 319
benzodiazepines and, 297–298
serotonin in, 20
Sulindac, interaction with lithium, 418
Sumatriptan, interaction with monoamine oxidase inhibitors, **65**
Surmontil (trimipramine), **29**, **49**
Sweating
antidepressant-induced, **37**, **52**, 97
in serotonin syndrome, **70**
Symbyax. *See* Olanzapine/fluoxetine combination
Symmetrel. *See* Amantadine
Sympathomimetic agent interactions
with monoamine oxidase inhibitors, 24, **65**, 101
with tricyclic antidepressants, **60**
Syndrome of inappropriate antidiuretic hormone (SIADH), drug-induced
carbamazepine, **179**, 343, 413–414
selective serotonin reuptake inhibitors, 25
T_4. *See* Thyroxine
Tachycardia, drug-induced
antidepressants, **37**
management of, **56**
reboxetine, 97
tricyclics, 22
anxiolytics, **278**
clozapine, 205
methylphenidate, **59**
Tacrine, 10
Tamoxifen, interaction with antidepressants, 103
Taractan (chlorprothixene), **149**
Tardive dyskinesia (TD), antipsychotic-induced, 140, 143, **164**, 189, 192, 228
in elderly patients, 143, **183**
incidence of, 143
TCAs. *See* Antidepressants, tricyclic
TD. *See* Tardive dyskinesia
TED (thromboembolic disease) stockings, for orthostatic hypotension, 144, **171**
Tegretol. *See* Carbamazepine
Temazepam
cost of, **265**
dosage of, **261**
for elderly patients, 258–259
formulations of, **261**
metabolism of, 256, **277**, 305
pharmacodynamics of, **273**
pharmacokinetics of, **275**
sertraline interaction with, 289
use in elderly and/or dementia patients, **288**
Teratogenicity. *See* Pregnancy
Terazosin, for hypersalivation, **171**, 205
Tertiary messengers, 4

Texas Medication Algorithm, **156**, 339, 389, 401
Theophylline (Theo-dur) interactions, 10
with antidepressants, 103, 120
with carbamazepine, 343
with lithium, 343, **372**
Therapeutic window
for haloperidol, 142
for tricyclic antidepressants, 22, **48**
Thiazide diuretic interactions
with lithium, 343, **366, 372**
with monoamine oxidase inhibitors, **65**
Thienobenzodiazepines, 139, **149**
Thioridazine
in Alzheimer's disease, 193
dosage of, **149, 150**, 234
formulations of, **150**
pharmacokinetics of, 142, **160**
side effects of, 143, **162**
cardiotoxicity, 235
sexual dysfunction, 204
Thiothixene, 139
for borderline personality disorder, 192
combined with clozapine, 215
dosage of, **149, 150**
formulations of, **150**
interaction with antidepressants, 102
plasma levels of, **149**
side effects of, **162**
Thioxanthenes, 139, **149**. *See also* Antipsychotics
Thorazine. *See* Chlorpromazine
Thrombocytopenia, valproate-induced, 342, 345, **365, 388**
Thromboembolic disease (TED) stockings, for orthostatic hypotension, 144, **171**
Thyroid dysfunction, drug-induced
carbamazepine, **363**
lithium, 342, **367**
Thyroxine (T_4)
for antidepressant augmentation, 24, **72**
for bipolar disorder, 338, 344, **355, 385**, 420, 421
for lithium-induced hypothyroidism, **367**
Tiagabine
for anxiety disorders, 254, 258, 299, 315
mechanism of action of, 255, **357**
side effects of, 299
Tic douloureux, 429
Tindal. *See* Acetophenazine
Tofranil. *See* Imipramine
Tolerance to drug effects
anticonvulsants, 406
antihistamines, 257
baclofen, 302
benzodiazepines, **178**, 292, 296
chloral hydrate, 299
Topamax. *See* Topiramate
Topiramate
combined with lithium, **384**
drug interactions with, 419–420
lamotrigine, **379**
valproate, **378**, 419, 433
indications for
bipolar disorder, 338, 402–403
drug-induced weight gain, **172**, 402
posttraumatic stress disorder, 300
mechanism of action of, **357**
side effects of, 402

Tourette's syndrome
antipsychotics for, 140, **158**
clonidine for, **158**
guanfacine for, **158**, 299
Toxic epidermal necrolysis, lamotrigine-induced, 342
Tramadol, interaction with selective serotonin reuptake inhibitors, **63**
Transcription, genetic, 4, **5**
Tranxene. *See* Clorazepate
Tranylcypromine
interaction with carbamazepine, 417
mechanism of action of, **27**
tablet strength and dosage of, **30**
Trazodone
dosage of, **29**
formulations of, **29**
indications for
antidepressant-induced sexual dysfunction, 99
anxiety disorders, 302
behavioral disturbances in dementia, **155**, 194
depressed cancer patients, 111
insomnia, **57**, 295
mechanism of action of, **27**
priapism induced by, **37**, 99
Tremin (trihexyphenidyl), 144, **165**, **171**
Tremor
drug-induced
antidepressants, **37**
selective serotonin reuptake inhibitors, 112
tricyclics, 23
carbamazepine, 342
lithium, **179**, 342, **360**, **361**, **367**, 411, 425, 427
tiagabine, 299
topiramate, 402
valproate, 342, **364**
in serotonin syndrome, **70**
Triazolam
cost of, **265**
dosage of, **261**
drug interactions with, **282**
nefazodone, 320–321
elimination half-life of, 256
formulations of, **261**
memory impairment induced by, **279**, 307
pharmacodynamics of, **273**
pharmacokinetics of, **275**
metabolic pathway, **277**, 305, 311
sublingual, 290
use in elderly and/or dementia patients, **288**
withdrawal from, 308
Trifluoperazine
dosage of, **148**, **150**
formulations of, **150**
plasma levels of, **148**
side effects of, **162**
Triflupromazine, **148**
Trigeminal neuralgia, 429
Trihexyphenidyl
for extrapyramidal side effects, **165**, **171**
interaction with antipsychotics, 144
Trilafon. *See* Perphenazine
Trileptal. *See* Oxcarbazepine
Trimipramine, **29**
side effects of, **49**

Troleandomycin, interaction with carbamazepine, **374**
12-Step programs, **356**
Twitching, lithium-induced, 411
Tyramine, interaction with monoamine oxidase inhibitors, **65**

Urecholine. *See* Bethanechol
Urinary hesitancy/retention, drug-induced
  antidepressants, **37**
    duloxetine, 97
    reboxetine, 97
    tricyclics, 22, 111
  antipsychotics, 144, 145

Valdecoxib, interaction with lithium, **370**
Valium. *See* Diazepam
Valproate
  autoinduction of, 410
  combined with other mood stabilizers
    carbamazepine, **385**, 406, 416–417, 430
    gabapentin, **386**
    lithium, 344, 345, **382**, 419
      in children, 426
  dosage of, **348**, 409
  drug interactions with, 343, 377–**378**
    antidepressants, 102
    antipsychotics, 144–145, **175**, **181**
      clozapine, 432
    benzodiazepines, **282**
    carbamazepine, 343, **376**, **377**, 416–417, 430
    ethosuximide, 417
    felbamate, 417
    lamotrigine, 341, 342, 343, **378**, **380**, 417
    phenobarbital, 343, **378**, 417
    phenytoin, 343, 417
    selective serotonin reuptake inhibitors, **61**
    topiramate, **378**, 419, 433
  elimination half-life of, 341, 409, 410
  formulations of, **348**, 409–410
  indications for, 339, 400
    antipsychotic augmentation, 145, **181**, 216
    anxiety disorders, 254, 299–300, 400
    behavioral disturbances in dementia, 194
    bipolar disorder, 338, 339
      depressive episodes, 392
      maintenance therapy, **356**
      mania, 339, **351**, 389
      mixed episodes, 389
      predictors of response to, 396
      rapid cycling, **355**, 390
    borderline personality disorder, 400
    mental retardation with behavioral dyscontrol, **157**
    migraine prophylaxis, 400
    schizophrenia, 400
  mechanism of action of, 340, **357**, 404
  pharmacokinetics of, 15, 341, 409–410
  side effects of, **181**, 342
    in children, 426
    hair loss, **181**, 342, **364**, 415–416

Valproate *(continued)*
side effects of *(continued)*
hepatotoxicity, 341, 342, **358**, **365**, 415
hyperammonemic encephalopathy, 342, 433
management of, **364–365**
therapeutic blood level of, **348**, 409–410
tolerance to, 406
use in special populations
children and adolescents, 345, **387**, 425, 426
elderly or medically ill patients, 342, 345, **388**, 427
pregnancy, 342, 345, **387**, 423
Vasopressin, 3
nasal, for clozapine-induced enuresis, 206
Venlafaxine, **45**
combined with mirtazapine, 24
cost of, **31**
dosage of, **29**
for children and adolescents, **78**
drug interactions with, 118
antipsychotics, **175**
efficacy of, 104
extended-release, **29**
formulations of, **29**
indications for
anxiety in children and adolescents, 318
bipolar depression, **353**
generalized anxiety disorder, **32**, 255, **266**, 292
obsessive-compulsive disorder, 82
panic disorder, 83
social phobia, 292
mechanism of action of, **27**, **36**, 86, 87
speeding up, 89
pharmacodynamics of, **45**
pharmacokinetics of, **41**, **45**
side effects of, 23, **45**, **50**, **51–54**, 82
hypertension, **56**
seizures, 95
sexual dysfunction, 99
use in special populations, **75–76**
elderly patients, 25
withdrawal symptoms with, 92
Ventricular premature contractions, lithium-induced, **367**
Verapamil
for bipolar disorder, 400–401, 421–422
drug interactions with
carbamazepine, 343, **373**
lithium, 343, **370**
selective serotonin reuptake inhibitors, **63**
tricyclic antidepressants, **60**
side effects of, 401
Vertigo. *See* Dizziness, drug-induced
Vesprin. *See* Triflupromazine
Violence. *See* Aggressive behavior
Visual disturbances, drug-induced
antidepressants, **37**
tricyclics, 22, 111
antipsychotics, 144, **171**
anxiolytics, **278**, **279**
mood stabilizers
carbamazepine, **363**, 426
lamotrigine, **364**
oxcarbazepine, **364**

Vitamin C, for selective serotonin reuptake inhibitor–induced bleeding, 96
Vivactil. *See* Protriptyline
Volume of distribution, 8

Warfarin interactions, 10
  with antidepressants, 103
    selective serotonin reuptake inhibitors, **61**
    tricyclics, **60**
  with benzodiazepines, 311
  with carbamazepine, 343, **373**
WCA (World Council of Anxiety) treatment guidelines, 291–292
Weakness, drug-induced
  benzodiazepines, 257, **278**, 306
  buspirone, **278**
  lithium, **367**
  valproate, 427
Weight changes, drug-induced
  antidepressants, **37**, **49–50**
    selective serotonin reuptake inhibitors, 25, 112
    tricyclics, 23
  antipsychotics, 144, **163**
    atypical agents, 205, 208, 223
    management of, **172**
  anxiolytics, **278**
  mood stabilizers
    carbamazepine, 342
    lithium, **360**, **368**, 411, 425
    topiramate, **172**, 402
    valproate, 342, **365**
Wellbutrin, Wellbutrin SR, Wellbutrin XL. *See* Bupropion
Withdrawal symptoms
  from antipsychotics, 207
  from benzodiazepines, 257, **281**, 308–309
  from beta-blockers, 307
  from lithium, 397–398, 412
  from meprobamate, **262**
  from nonbenzodiazepine hypnotics, 257
  related to drug elimination half-life, 9
  from selective serotonin reuptake inhibitors, 92
  from tricyclic antidepressants, 91–92
  from venlafaxine, 92
  from zolpidem, 309–310
World Council of Anxiety (WCA) treatment guidelines, 291–292

Xanax. *See* Alprazolam
Xerostomia in cancer patients, 111

Yohimbine
  for drug-induced sexual dysfunction, **59**, 99, **172**
  side effects of, **59**

Zaleplon, 253, **263**
  discontinuation of, 257, **263**, 309
  dosage of, **261**, **263**
  drug interactions with, **285**
  formulations of, **261**
  for insomnia, **263**, 296
  mechanism of action of, 255, **272**, 303–304
  pharmacodynamics of, **273**
  pharmacokinetics of, 256, **263**, **276**
  in pregnancy, 258, 316
  side effects of, 257, **263**
  use in elderly and/or dementia patients, **288**
Zinc supplementation, for valproate-induced hair loss, 415

Ziprasidone, 139
  cost of, **152**
  dosage of, **148, 151**
  drug interactions with, **177**, 214
    nefazodone, 24
  elimination half-life of, 142, **161**
  formulations of, **151**
  indications for
    bipolar disorder, **156,** 338
      acute mania, 140, 190–191, 389
    schizoaffective disorder, 191
    schizophrenia, 191, 198
    Tourette's syndrome, **158**
  intramuscular, 188
  pharmacokinetics of, **161**
  receptor affinities of, **159**
  side effects of, 143, **163,** 188, 208
    extrapyramidal symptoms, 202
    hypomania, 390
    sexual dysfunction, 205
  use in special populations
    elderly patients, 223
    pregnancy, **185**
Zoloft. *See* Sertraline
Zolpidem, 253, **263**
  abuse liability of, 310
  dependence on, 310
  discontinuation of, 257, **263**
  dosage of, **261**
  drug interactions with, 258, **285**
  formulations of, **261**
  for insomnia, 57, **263,** 295–296
  mechanism of action of, 255, 272, 303–304
  pharmacodynamics of, **273**
  pharmacokinetics of, 256, **263, 276**
  in pregnancy, 258, 316, 323
  side effects of, 257
  withdrawal from, 309–310
Zonegran. *See* Zonisamide
Zonisamide, for bipolar disorder, 338, 402–403
Zopiclone, 253, **264**
  dependence on, 310
  drug interactions with, 258, **285**
  mechanism of action of, 255, **264, 272**
  pharmacodynamics of, **273**
  pharmacokinetics of, 256
Zydis. *See* Olanzapine
Zyprexa. *See* Olanzapine